Road to USMLE
Step 2 CS

**Vital Checklist Communication and
Clinical Skills Workbook— Second Edition**

Road to USMLE
Copyright ©2016 Harpreet Singh

ISBN 978-1506-906-46-1 PRINT

LCCN 2016933189

December 2016

Published and Distributed by
First Edition Design Publishing, Inc.
P.O. Box 20217, Sarasota, FL 34276-3217
www.firsteditiondesignpublishing.com

ALL RIGHTS RESERVED. No part of this book publication may be reproduced, stored in a retrieval system, or transmitted in any form or by any means — electronic, mechanical, photo-copy, recording, or any other — except brief quotation in reviews, without the prior permission of the author or publisher.

Chief Medical Author
Harpreet Singh MD, FACP
Talk Medicine Radio Show—Patient Education via Airwaves
Chief Experience Officer—Michigan Primary Care Partners
CEO and Founder—Vital Checklist and (iCrush)
Board Certified Internal Medicine Physician— Michigan Primary Care Partners
Patient Experience Coach—Vital Checklist Workshop for Health Caregivers
Health, Wellness and Weight Loss Expert—(iCrush) Lifestyle Loss Institute for patients
USMLE Instructor—Vital Checklist Workshop for Step 2CS
Speaker, Inventor and Medical Author for (iCrush) Series and Patient Education Guide
Medical School—KMC, Manipal, India
Residency—MSU Grand Rapids Medical Education Partners
Residency—Mercy Health and Spectrum Health, Grand Rapids, Michigan

Associate Medical Authors

Himanshu Deshwal MD
Medical School-AFMC Pune

Ankur Sinha MD
Medical School-AFMC Pune

Avantika Singh MD
Medical School-VMMC, New Delhi

Krishna Adit Agarwal MD
Medical School-VMMC, New Delhi

John Lobo MD
Urology Surgeons—Grand Rapids
General Surgery and Residency In Urology—Mayo Clinic in Rochester MN

Assistant Medical Authors

Dilip Rajasekharan MBBS
Medical School—KMC, Mangalore

Navneet Kaur MBBS
Medical School—Gian Sagar Medical College, Punjab

Rachit Chawla MD
Medical School—Manipal College of Medical Sciences, Pokharan, Nepal

Dinesh Kumar MBBS, MS
Chief Consultant in General Surgery at Christian Medical College & Hospital, India

Medical Illustrators
Harpreet Singh MD
Himanshu Deshwal MD
Gagan Pal Singh

Contributing Medical Authors

Gurpreet Singh MBBS
KMC Manipal
GS Clinic, Ludhiana, Punjab

Shafi Rana
American University of Antigua
College of Medicine, Woods
Antigua and Barbuda

Arushi Devgan MBBS
Medical School- VMMC, New Delhi, India

Tanya Paul MD
Medical School—KMC, Mangalore

Noni Rana
American University of Antigua
College of Medicine, Woods
Antigua and Barbuda

Peer Review by

Dr.Neil Goodman
Monica Delaney PAC
Dr.Harjeet Dhillon
Dr. Purvi Patel
Dr.Vikas Ghai MD, FACP
Dr.Sonia Ghai
Dr.Sarabjeet Singh MD, FACC
Dr. Jasleen Kaur MD
Dr. Rashmi Juneja

Medical Student who have provided valuable insight

Alanrita Taneja MBBS
Tarun Bhandari MD
Harman Tiwana MD

Proof Read by

Emily Franckowiak- Medical Student
Central Michigan University, Michigan

Dedication

To The United States of America, where 54 dollars and 50 cents can take you so far.

To my patients, who gave me the opportunity to serve them.

To my parents—Anar Singh and Ajit Kaur, who taught me the concept of hard work.

To my brother—Harvinder Paul Singh and his wife-Smita Singh, who are always there for me.

To my wife—Aroma, my rock, who never questioned my long duty hours.

To my daughters—Suhani and Sanjhvi, who still have a Disneyland trip on their bucket list.

To my family and friends, who taught me to see the world with better eyes.

Foremost, to God almighty, this formless one, for blessing me with all the opportunities to speak and overcome stuttering.

This Humble Self,
Harpreet Singh

The WHY of Vital Checklist Clinical and Communication book—Road to USMLE Step 2 CS book (R2U).

USMLE Step 2 Clinical Exam tests medical students on Communication, Interpersonal Skills, Integrated Clinical Encounter, and Spoken English Proficiency.

Consumer Assessment of Health Care Providers and Systems (CAHPS Score) test US Health Caregivers on communication, discharge instructions, pain, medications, and layman language explanations. In simple words, passing USMLE Exam is equivalent to scoring good grades on CAHPS survey. Therefore, passing this exam on first attempt is critical when applying for residency. Program directors are looking for students who have passed this test on the first go.

How to use the R2U book?

R2U is a concept book and each concept is written in such a way that one can arrive at a differential diagnosis. This book will also teach you how to involve patients in their own care. Our premise in writing this book is to improve patient experience. This book will provide you with the tools, techniques, checklists, art, and other touchpoints to explain to patients in a layman language and win their trust in USMLE Step 2 CS exam and in real life.

What is in the R2U book?

This book contains numerous checklists, tables, and art to make your life easier. It is but natural that everybody learns differently. Some are visual learners, others are aural, a few prefer reading and writing, while others use kinesthetic sensory modalities. We have done due diligence to touch each and every aspect.

Who is this book for?

Medical Students, IMG's, Physician Assistant Students, Nurse Practitioner Students, and Practicing Physicians.

Enroll in Vital Checklist Workshop for USMLE Step 2 Clinical Skills.
www.vitalchecklist.com

Invite Dr. Harpreet Singh to speak at your medical school, residency, fellowship, or health care practices to improve patient experience.
www.vitalchecklist.com
www.drsinghmd.org

Check out our Patient Experience booklets, book, and tools at www.vitalchecklist.com.

Participate in our iCrush Seminars, iCrush 5k, iCrush videos, and iCrush notes at www.icrush.org. Help spread health literacy by publishing your innovative patient education concepts at www.icrush.org/notes.

www.icrush.org is a public service venture aimed at educating masses on medical knowledge.

How to Contribute

Having right people on the bus. I strongly believe in **Marcus** Anthony **Lemonis** Principles of "The Profit" who always preaches about that people should come first, process second and profit will automatically follow. In this world, we cannot live in isolation without peers, friends and coaches. Every person on this earth has a unique purpose in life and I am a big advocate of teamwork. I would not have been able to complete this project without help of smart medical students-Avantika, Krishna, Ankur, Himanshu, Dilip, Navneet, Arushi, Rachit and Tanya.

We are looking for good people-students, nurses, physician assistants, nurse practitioners and doctors to become part of Vital Checklist Family.

Please send us your contribution and for every entry that has been selected you will get an acknowledgment in the next edition. If your contribution is significant then your name will appear as a part of contributors.

Contribute at hi@vitalchecklist.com

Acknowledgement:

I also owe to all my friends, teachers, and other influential people. Without their blessings this would have not been possible.

Many teachers have helped me reach where I am today, but if I speak about each one of them, that would take up the entire book. Some of the teachers who left a permanent memory are:

- ✓ Dr. Abha Verma (Hospitalist-Spectrum Health)
- ✓ Dr. Alberta A Garbaccio (Renal Associates of West Michigan)
- ✓ Dr. Andre Gauri (Cardiology/Electrophysiologist-Spectrum Health)
- ✓ Dr. Andrew P Maternowski (Hospitalist-Spectrum Health)
- ✓ Dr. Ashutosh Chaudhari (Hospitalist-Spectrum Health)
- ✓ Dr. Asif Azeem (Gastroenterology)
- ✓ Dr. Benjamin Horn (Hospitalist-Spectrum Health)
- ✓ Dr. Benny J Kieff (Gastroenterology- Spectrum Health)
- ✓ Dr. Bernard Eisenga (Internist-Spectrum Health)
- ✓ Dr. Bohuslav Finta (Cardiology/Electrophysiologist-Spectrum Health)
- ✓ Dr. Brian Petroelje (Infectious Disease)
- ✓ Dr. Bryan Hull (Primary Care Mercy Health)
- ✓ Dr. Carlos Tavera (Internist-Spectrum Health)
- ✓ Dr. Conrad Fischer (Internal Medicine-Kaplan)
- ✓ Dr. Dale Wiersma (Hospitalist-Spectrum Health)
- ✓ Dr. Daniel Legault (Renal Associates of West Michigan)
- ✓ Dr. Daniel Osborne (Hospitalist-Spectrum Health)
- ✓ Dr. Danielle Light (Hospitalist- Spectrum Health)
- ✓ Dr. Darryl Elmouchi (Cardiology/Electrophysiologist-Spectrum Health)
- ✓ Dr. David Dobbie (Infectious Disease)
- ✓ Dr. David H Wohns(Cardiology-Spectrum Health)
- ✓ Dr. David Langholz (Cardiology-Spectrum Health)
- ✓ Dr. Doug Apple (Hospitalist-Spectrum Health)
- ✓ Dr. Elizabeth Neubig (Internist-Spectrum Health)
- ✓ Dr. Eugene Wiley (Neurology-Spectrum Health)
- ✓ Dr. Glenn VanOtteren (Pulmonology-Spectrum Health)
- ✓ Dr. Greg Golladay (Orthopedics-OA Michigan)
- ✓ Dr. Greg Marco (Pulmonology- Spectrum Health)
- ✓ Dr. Gregory Naegos(Pulmonology- Spectrum Health)
- ✓ Dr. Gregory Osborne (Gastroenterology-Spectrum Health)
- ✓ Dr. H.Paul Singh (Cardiologist-West Michigan Cardiology)
- ✓ Dr. Helayne Sherman (Cardiology-Spectrum Health)
- ✓ Dr. Imad Ahmad (Renal Associates of West Michigan)
- ✓ Dr. James A Visser (Renal Associates of West Michigan)
- ✓ Dr. James Baron (Hospitalist-Spectrum Health)
- ✓ Dr. James Hoekwater (Pulmonolgy- Spectrum Health)
- ✓ Dr. James Passinault (Primary Care Mercy Health)
- ✓ Dr. Jeeva Subramaniam (Internist-Spectrum Health)
- ✓ Dr. Jeffery Wilt (Pulmonologist-Borgess Health)
- ✓ Dr. Jennifer Krause (Hospitalist-IPCM)
- ✓ Dr. Jihad Mustapha (Cardiologist-Metro Health)
- ✓ Dr. Jody Banister (Primary Care Mercy Health)
- ✓ Dr. Joel Van De Riet (Hospitalist-Spectrum Health)
- ✓ Dr. John Cantor (Pulmonology-Spectrum Health)
- ✓ Dr. John Visser (Neurology-Spectrum Health)
- ✓ Dr. Juliana Grey (IPCM- Grand Rapids)
- ✓ Dr. Kevin Wolschleger(Cardiology-Spectrum Health)
- ✓ Dr. Kseniya V Filippova (Renal Associates of West Michigan)
- ✓ Dr. Lawrence Feenstra (Internist-Spectrum Health)
- ✓ Dr. Lynn J. Cronin (Cardiology- Spectrum Helath)
- ✓ Dr. Malar Vasanthan (Hospitalist-Spectrum Health)
- ✓ Dr. Marc McCleland (Pulmonology- Spectrum Health)
- ✓ Dr. Mark Boelkins (Renal Associates of West Michigan)
- ✓ Dr. Mark Koets (Pulmonology-Spectrum Health)
- ✓ Dr. Mathew Lee Marvin (Hospitalist-Spectrum Health)
- ✓ Dr. Michael Bergquist (Hospitalist-Spectrum Health)
- ✓ Dr. Michael Dickinson (Cardiology- Spectrum Health)
- ✓ Dr. Michael Harrison (Pulmonology-Spectrum Health)

- ✓ Dr. Michael Lozek (Cardiology-Spectrum Health)
- ✓ Dr. Michael Puff (Gastroenterology- Spectrum Health)
- ✓ Dr. Michael Vrendenberg (Cardiology-Spectrum Health)
- ✓ Dr. Mimi Emig (Infectious Disease-Spectrum Health)
- ✓ Dr. Nagib Chalfoun (Cardiology/Electrophysiologist -Spectrum Health)
- ✓ Dr. Naseer Khan (Internist & Hospitalist-Saint Mary's Hospital)
- ✓ Dr. Philip Goushaw (Renal Associates of West Michigan)
- ✓ Dr. Randal Meisner (Gastroenterology-Spectrum Health)
- ✓ Dr. Raymond Roden (Cardiology-Spectrum Health)
- ✓ Dr. Richard McNamara (Cardiology-Spectrum Health)
- ✓ Dr. Richard Switzer (Program Director-Medicine Pediatrics)
- ✓ Dr. Rima Shah (Internist-Spectrum Health)
- ✓ Dr. Robert Camp (Hospitalist-Spectrum Health)
- ✓ Dr. Russel Lampen (Infectious Disease-Spectrum Health)
- ✓ Dr. Shaukhat Khan (Gastroenterology)
- ✓ Dr. Simin Beg (Hospitalist-Spectrum Health)
- ✓ Dr. Sohail Qadir (Internist and Spectrum Health)
- ✓ Dr. Srivilliputtur G Santhana "Krishnan" (Renal Associate of West Michigan)
- ✓ Dr. Stephen Fitch (Pulmonology Spectrum Health)
- ✓ Dr. Steven Triesenberg (Infectious Disease)
- ✓ Dr. Tejinder Mander (Cardiologist-West Michigan Cardiology)
- ✓ Dr. Terrance Barnes (Pulmonology-Spectrum Health)
- ✓ Dr. Thomas Rupp (Gastroenterology- Spectrum Health)
- ✓ Dr. Timothy Daum (Pulmonologist- Spectrum Health)
- ✓ Dr. Timothy Fritz (Cardiologist-Spectrum Health)
- ✓ Dr. Timothy Thoits (Neurology-Spectrum Health)
- ✓ Dr. Vidyulatha Talla (Hospitalist-Spectrum Health)
- ✓ Dr. Wael Berjaoui (Pulmonology-Spectrum Health)

I would also like to specially thank:
Dr. A.k. Handa (my Botany teacher at Arya College, Ludhiana)
Dr. Vivek Pandey (MS-Orthopedics, my one year senior and my guide in medical school)
Both of whom deserve a special mention, as they have always kept pushing me to aim higher.

Dr. Craig Rosenburg and Dr. Derik King of ECI Healthcare Partners deserve special mention for giving me my first opportunity to lead a hospitalist program. What an amazing organization (www.ecihealthcarepartners.com) to work for! Their philosophy of "People First" is forever etched in my mind, as this is the organization that will walk the talk.

How can a doctor become successful without supportive nurses?

I am indebted to Joyce Wideman RN, who taught me how, and what to speak, and Emily Smith RN who, most importantly, taught me what not to speak.

Infinite nurses have helped me to take care of my patients. I am so grateful to all of the nurses of Spectrum Health-Blodgett, Butterworth, and Big Rapids Hospital who have helped me to achieve my goal.

How can I forget Three Rivers Health nurses, unit clerks, and chief nursing officer? What a great experience for me to learn and lead a program in a smaller setting! I appreciate all the help provided by Hope Bailey (CNO), Liz Fueling, Karen Long, and many more nurses from Three Rivers Health who supported me in each and every way during my stint at that facility. I am grateful to Mecosta County Nurses and Dena Durante RN for providing valuable feedback on communication cards.

I have been blessed to meet so many other good people at Three Rivers Health—pharmacists (Leonard Darling and crew), social workers (Chris Johnson), and physical, occupational, and speech therapists, but the one person who was extremely helpful was acute care unit clerk, Pattey Lakey. Her passion for reading books really got me started reading all of the business books.

I would like to thank my present and past CEOs, Program Director, and CNO's for providing excellent leadership from which I learned great people skills—

- Pete Coogan (*CEO-GRMEP*)
- Dr. Mark Spoolstra (Program Director-Internal Medicine Residency)
- Dr. John O'Donnell (Program Director-Internal Medicine Residency)
- Mr. Richard Breon (CEO- Spectrum Health)
- Dr. Khan Nedd (CEO-HOWM)
- Dr. Adam Singer (CEO-IPCM)
- Dr. Jeffrey Schilinger (CEO-HPPartners)
- Dr. Girsh Juneja (CEO-MPCP)
- Bill Rusell (CEO-Three Rivers Health)
- Robert M. Williams, MD, Dr.PH,FACEP; Chairman of the Board-ECI Healthcare Partners
- Dr. Craig Rosenberg (Regional Director- ECI Healthcare Partners)
- Dr. Derik King (President and CEO-ECI Healthcare Partners)
- Dr. Ken Epstein (CMO-ECI Healthcare Partners)
- Mr. Sam Daugherty, (CEO-Big Rapids Hospital-Spectrum Health)
- Netty Cove (CNO-Big Rapids Hospital-Spectrum Health)
- Hope Bailey (CNO-Three Rivers Health)

Last, but not the least, I am thankful to all from whom I learned the valuable lessons of life. These inspired leaders and their books helped me to attain my goal. Some of them are:

Simon Sinek, Atul Gawande, Charles Duhigg, Jeffery Liker, Josh Kauffmann, Anthony Robins, Steve Jobs, Bill Gates, Clayton M. Christensen, Douglas Conant, Mette Norgaard, Dave Ramsay, Perry Marshall, John Medina, Michael Gerber, Jim Collins, Oprah Winfrey, Eric Ries, Daniel Pink , Tony Hsieh, Sachin Tendulkar, Eliyahu Goldratt, Gregory Miller, Taiichi Ohno, Quint Studor, Ken Fortier.

This list of acknowledgements is probably incomplete and I apologize for that, as many more people, teachers, and coaches have influenced my life.

Dale Carnegie, Vital Smarts, Net Plus Connections Coaching and Workshops trained me to connect positively with people.

Friends are forever! Without close friends it would not have been possible. They encouraged me through the tough times. Though many people supported me, a few who were helpful in those times of stuttering—Preeti Ahuja, Bhavana Rai, Birinder Ahuja and Amit Sofat in Sacred Heart Convent School; Ashish Chandwani in Arya College; Srirang Abkari, Rishi Swarup, Veerinder Taneja, and many more in KMC, Manipal; and Harjeet S.Dhillon, Atif Rizwan, Nehal Lakhani, Chethan Rajappa, Purvi Patel, Erica Bracamontes-Woolley, Anna Willard, Raj Dasgupta, Nim Goraya, Jad Goraya, J. Chong, Khurram Abbas for their support in Residency. Many more friends like—Sarabjeet Singh, Jasleen Duggal, Vikas and Sonia Ghai have shown the right prospective of what is important and what is irrelevant.

Thank you everybody,

Dr.Harpreet Singh

Disclaimer

Medicine is an ever-changing and ever evolving science. Clinical experiences and research broaden our knowledge and understanding of a subject on a daily basis. The authors and publishers of this work have checked the information material for accuracy from multiple sources, and believe that the knowledge is generally in accord with the standards that are acceptable at the time of publication. However, in view of the possibility of human error, and changes in medical science, neither the authors nor any other party involved in the publication of this book claim that all information contained in this book is accurate in all respects or complete. They disclaim all responsibility for any errors or omissions or from any results that were obtained from use of the information contained in this material. This material is for informational purposes only. The content is not meant to be a substitute for professional medical advice, diagnosis or treatment. Always seek the advice of your physician or other qualified health provider with any questions you may have regarding a medical condition. Never disregard medical advice or delay in seeking it because of something you have read here. We do not endorse or recommend any tests, physicians, products, procedures, opinions or any other information that may be available on the website. Reliance on any information provided by the Vital Checklist website, the (iCrush) website, (iCrush) patient education booklets, the Vital Checklist employees or others appearing on the website or visitors is solely at your own risk.

Sincerely
Vital Checklist and (iCrush) Team.

Foreword

I have known Dr. Harpreet Singh when he first started his training as a 1st year intern. From day one I saw the passion in his eyes and heart to be best clinician and educator for his patients and students. I am very proud of all of his accomplishments both personal and professional. I know his book, Road to USMLE Step 2 CS truly reflects all the hard work and knowledge he has accumulated in his career so far to help students succeed and conquer the USMLE Step 2 CS. I wish him all the best in the future and hope you enjoy his book.

Raj Dasgupta MD, FACP, FCCP, FAASM
Assistant Professor of Clinical Medicine
Division of Pulmonary, Critical Care and Sleep Medicine
Keck School of Medicine of USC, Department of Medicine
University of Southern California
Assistant Program Director, Internal Medicine Residency
Associate Program Director, Sleep Medicine Fellowship
Author of Medicine Morning Report: Beyond the Pearls

Preface

Sheri Jo's voice still rings in my ears, "Dr.Singh, by being a standardized patient (a model patients who portrays clinical scenarios), I have become a better patient. I ask doctors more relevant questions regarding my illness. I am an intelligent patient, now." This was six years ago when I started Vital Checklist Workshop and trained medical students.

Sheri Jo left us at the age of 42 because of breast cancer.

Her voice still reminds me that not only medical students will benefit from this coaching, but also the standardized patients will learn the art of asking the right questions to the doctors.

If we need to save money and FLIP THE HEALTHCARE, we need to activate both fronts—medical students who are the foundation and torchbearers of medicine and the patients who have hard time understanding the medical jargon. To train medical students I had to train lay people to become standardized patients. CPR (Cardiopulmonary Resuscitation) and ACLS (Advanced Cardiovascular Life Support) training can be done on simulators and mannequins, but communication and clinical skills have to be trained by the humans on the humans.

Since 2009, I have trained communication and clinical skills to many students who have passed USMLE Step 2 Clinical Skills exam in first attempt. In this process, I have been able to activate many lay people to become smart model patients (standardized patients) and that has helped them to ask better questions in real life scenarios.

Being a standardized patient myself and training lay people as the standardized patients, I have gained insight of the problems patients face on daily basis. I have gained life-changing experiences, which I have implemented in my daily routine of examining patients. I have done no double-blind randomized control trials that are published in the most reputed journals, but have received love from my patients who have showered me thank-you cards, testimonials, and comments on social media. This has become my proof of concept and now I have started iCrush.org portal to *educate patients with love* in different languages, in different settings.

In 2009, I trained my first medical student. It was serendipity. I received a call from a student—Deepak, and he wanted to get trained in communication and clinical skills, and I agreed hesitantly as I did not know where to start. I spent three months developing my curriculum and read many clinical skills book available. However, something was missing. How can I teach customer service to the young minds? How can I show a young doctor about respecting patients and the value of talking politely with love and respect? This is when I resorted to business theories and adapted and changed customer experience principles to patient experience. I read Jim Collins book—Good to Great, and that taught me Hedgehog Concept, and during this time, an idea came to make medical student "Good to Great" Doctors. However, I have taken this a step further after I read Porter's Five Forces. As per him, being best is a self-destructive phenomenon. Don't try to be the best, try to be UNIQUE. We want to make medical students "Best-to-Unique" health caregivers and not just the "Pamphlet Doctors."

A pamphlet doctor is a doctor who hands a pamphlet to the patient and leaves the room without discussing the problem with the patient. A pamphlet doctor *assumes* that patient is educated, activated and understands their disease process by just reading a pamphlet. A pamphlet doctor checks the box in the electronic health record and feels happy about fulfilling the benchmark.

However, in real setting patient just keeps the pamphlet on the bedside table, throws it in a trash, shreds it or stores it in drawer. Do you know how many times the patient leaves the education material in the car trunk and never opens it again? Some patients may actually read it, but can they recall after 24 hours.

Trust is not equal to checking the box.

Trust develops when you Love Communicating or Hyper-Communicate with the patient.

I have not reinvented any wheel and the concepts in this book are not mine. These concepts are derived from various books, TED talks, Google Talks, You Tube Videos and various inspirational and business leaders and have taken me six years to develop. I have practiced with numerous students and standardized patients. Aroma—my better half has sacrificed family time and helped me to coach medical students. Without her help, I could not even fathom to complete this project and develop meaningful concepts.

Everything happens with the blessings of God, family members, and parents. My mother—Ajit Kaur, has always blessed and guided me to the path of righteousness. My brother—Dr.Paul Singh, a cardiologist by trait, laid the foundation of patient experience in me when I followed him in his clinic. I owe my clinical skills to him and communication skills to my sister-in-law Smita Singh. I would not have been able to accomplish this humongous project without the help of Gagan Pal Singh who has helped me to develop business model and strategy.

I am a big believer of people first, process second and then everything falls in its place. Next is the list of students who have co-authored this book with me—Dr. Himanshu Deshwal, Dr.Avantika Singh, Dr. Krishna Agarwal, and Dr. Ankur Sinha. As we were discussing the concepts and theories, we toiled day in and out. Dr. Sinha was in England, Dr. Avantika and Dr. Agarwal in India and me in the US. Holding a video meeting in three times zones was one of the difficult tasks. With my busy schedule, I had limited time. These three brilliant doctors took time out, and I taught them, and they wrote for me. Our first draft took at least 13 months. We needed an illustrator, though I could draw rough sketches, we needed a professional person, and this was when Dr. Deshwal came into the picture. He wrote many articles with me, drew pictures, and sat with me: He even changed his sleeping and exercise schedule for me. I came back from work at 7 or 8 p.m. and Dr.Deshwal sat with me for next 5 to 6 hours reading, correcting and editing the Road To USMLE Step 2 CS Book. It is a blessing to know them and I am very excited that everybody has matched in his or her dream residency programs

Many more students—Dr.Dilip Rajashekharan, Dr, Navneet Kaur, Dr, Rachit Chawla, Dr. Dinesh Kumar, Dr. Tanya Paul and Dr. Arushi Devgan have helped me to complete this initiative. I will always be indebted to them.

As I was completing the preface of this book, my spiritual teacher—Nirankari Baba Hardev Singh Ji left for heavenly abode. He taught me the lessons of empathy, love and respect, which I have used for Patient Experience.

I still remember the days when I struggled to speak a word and stuttered. Speaking my name--Harpreet was a chore for me. Everybody made fun of me in the class, on the playground and everywhere else. Even my relatives bullied me and called me a "Stutterer." When everybody was teasing me, He knew how to cure me and help me. He had planned my future. He gave me His stage to speak or give discourse. I still remember that day when I spoke for 12-13 minutes and in one setting my stuttering was gone. Since that day in the year 1993, I have not stuttered again. From the days of stuttering to now being an orator, teaching medical students Communication and Clinical Skills and now being a Co-Host of Talk Medicine radio show. He taught me the lessons of love, compassion, and empathy, which I have used in my patient care and teach my medical students. I have inculcated in my daily routine His life lessons. His congregation is a "MASTER CLASS" and I have learned so much from them.

Last year, when His mother passed, he explained to us how He used to seek blessings from His mother. Being a Guru, His mother never allowed him to touch her feet. So, in an attempt to seek blessings, He used to tell that he was doing pulse examination of her feet. One of my patients gave me a Bible, and I read this verse- Jesus Washes His Disciples' Feet (Matthew 26:14-39; Luke 22:24-

27; John 13:1-17). All noble Men have taught us lessons which we human beings imbibe. Since that day, I have included this practice in my patient care whenever I examine my patient's feet, I not only do pulse examination but also seek blessings from my patients so that I can help them. Being a pawn of God Almighty, I am just an instrument or tool. My guiding light and my GPS-God Positioning Satellite will guide me with the medical knowledge where I can help my patients.

His message of "Religion Unites, Never Divides" and "Blood should run in veins, not in drains" is what we have to strive for and unite everybody. Let's live in unity and harmony and be tolerant of each other. I often use His quotes in my patient care, "To bow in front of others is the strength, not weakness."

I have used these principles of Baba Hardev Singh Ji in my upcoming books on Patient Experience. My Guruji gave so much for the welfare of the humanity-- starting blood donation camps, opening schools and colleges for the under-privilege, cleaning campaigns and as a mark of respect for Him, I pledge to contribute in the field patient education and patient experience and walk on the path of love as shown by my Guruji.

This humble self,
Harpreet Singh

Table of Contents

Section A - Introduction 1
Making Better Doctors 8
Communication and Interpersonal Skills 8

Section B – Doorway Information 16
Basics of Communication and Clinical Skills 16
Opening Strategy: Doorway Information 16
Opening Strategy: Managing the Blue Sheet 17
Managing the Blue Sheet 19
Blue Sheet Template 21

Section C – History Physical 26
HISTORY TAKING: Case Based 26
HISTORY TAKING: General 34
Physical Examination 46

Section D - Approach to Common Cases 66
Approach to Abdominal Case 66
Approach to Chest Pain 79
Approach to Shortness of Breath 83
Approach to a Case of Syncope 88
Approach to Dizziness 94
Approach to Fatigue 101
Approach to Hearing Impairment 109
Approach to Insomnia 123
Approach to Joints and Extremities 130
Approach to Urinary Incontinence 157
Approach to Headache 167
Approach to a Pediatric Case 174
Approach to a Case of Muscle Weakness 180
Approach to a Case of Edema 183

Section E - The Art of Answering Challenging Questions 190
Practice Sheets 194

Section F - Counseling 238
Closure: General Framework - ADICA 238
VITAL CHECKLISTS 245
Counselling: Case or Disease Based 263
How to Improve Health Literacy? 273

Section G – Differential Diagnosis ... 298
Narrowing the Diagnosis ... 298
Differential Diagnosis ... 300

Section H - Approach to Investigations ... 333

Section I – Recap or Recall ... 362

Section J - Common Medications ... 414

Section K – Practice Cases ... 420

Section L – Patient Notes ... 432
How to create a good patient note? ... 432
Examples of Patient Notes ... 437
To get your patient note corrected, ... 442
please contact hi@vitalchecklist.com ... 442
Practice Material ... 443
Headache ... 446
Loss of Consciousness ... 446
Dizziness ... 446
Numbness and Tingling ... 447
Muscle Weakness ... 447
Tremors ... 447
Seizures ... 448
Confusion ... 448
Memory Loss ... 448
Loss of Vision ... 449
Hearing Loss ... 449
Chest Pain ... 449
Palpitations ... 450
Shortness of Breath ... 450
Cough ... 451
Sore throat ... 451
Snoring ... 452
Abdominal Pain ... 452
Dysphagia ... 452
Weight Loss ... 453
Vomiting ... 453
Diarrhea ... 453
Jaundice ... 453
Bloody Vomiting ... 454
Bloody Stools ... 455
Fatigue with Pallor ... 455
Polyuria ... 456
Weight gain ... 456
Neck Mass ... 456
Knee pain ... 457

Ankle Pain 457
Elbow pain 457
Shoulder pain 457
Back Pain 458
Bloody urine 458
Burning Urination 458
Incontinence 458
Lower abdominal pain 459
Pregnancy 459
Unable to conceive 459
Erectile Dysfunction 460
Vaginal Bleeding 460
Pain During Sex 460
Depressed Mood 461
Hallucinations 461
Insomnia 461
Anxiety 462
Dehydration 462
Seizures 462
Enuresis 462
Wheezing 463
Fever 463

Section M – Vital Checklist Workshop and Health Care Strategy 466
Who benefits and how do they benefit? 466
Shortage of doctors! Medical practices are being disrupted. We need more physician assistants and nurse practitioners. 467
Praise for Dr. Harpreet Singh's Vital Checklist Workshop 472
Putting yourself in your patients' shoes: Communication is about emotions 479
Theory of Constraint + Lean Principles = Vital Checklist Workshop 479
An easy to remember and hard to forget way to recall the steps: 480
(iCrush) Mission, Vision Goals and Objectives 486

Section N - Testimonials 488
Student Experience: Praise of Vital Checklist Workshop for STEP 2 CS 488
Patient Experience: Praise from Real Life Patients 491

Section O – Authors 518

Section A

Introduction

Section A - Introduction

Why USMLE Step 2 Clinical Skills Test?

Health Literacy is called The Sixth Vital Sign. Poor health literacy is the main reason of increase morbidity, mortality and poor compliance with medications. According to the report, Low Health Literacy: Implications for National Health Policy "Low health literacy is a major source of economic inefficiency in the U.S. health care system." The report estimates that the cost of low health literacy to the U.S. economy is between $106 billion and $238 billion per year.

Though technology is trying to bridge this gap, we still need conscientious, health caregivers who work with their head, heart and hands to win the patient's trust.

As per Bill Gates, "Real technological advancement would come when the system is overhauled."

Overhauling the entire process starts with the people (caregivers). As per Marcus Lamonis famous TV show on CNBC—The Profit, it all starts with the people, followed by process and then followed by the profit.

Effective Communications by health caregivers create a positive and life changing impact on the patient. However, every caregiver is different and connects in a different way with their patients, but nowadays caregivers have to meet benchmarks and therefore standardization is required. To achieve this, medical students are being graded on a standardized USMLE Step 2 Clinical Skills test and it is a mandatory for a student to pass this test in all three sub-domains together at one go — Integrative Clinical Encounter (ICE), Spoken English Proficiency (SEP), Communication Interpersonal Skills (CIS) before they start the clinical practice. If we want healthcare culture to change, we need our foundation to be strong, which means we need to start young. The "Road to USMLE, Residency and ultimately "The Match" is the bottom-up approach that will help the medical student to create a sound basis at the start of their career rather than in residency, fellowship or clinical practice. Old habits are difficult to change and this is the reason we want to tap the medical students when they are young and easy to mold and make a strong foundation. We hope that this Road to USMLE workbook will help the students to score high in the patient satisfaction surveys and thus provide Very Important Patient Experience (VIP experience).

This USMLE Step 2 CS exam helps the Program Directors to screen the candidates with excellent communication and clinical skills. Failing this exam poses a challenge to the students and thus decreases the chance of residency match. You must wonder why does this happen?

Communication and Clinical skills of the physicians are compared and scored at the national level with Press Ganey Score, Hospital Consumer Assessment of Healthcare Providers and Systems (HCAHPS) or The Clinician and Group Consumer Assessment of Healthcare Providers and Systems (CG CAHPS) survey. The reimbursements are now being based on these scores and whether we can make patients happy. Patients are rating hospitals, physicians, nurses, physician assistants', and nurse practitioners and thus failing this communication and clinical skills exam may mean you are not up to the speed with American healthcare.

Only 74% of examinees from Non-US/Canadian schools passed their exam in 2013-2014 while 95% was the passing rate of examinees from US/Canadian Schools during the same calendar year. 26% of foreign medical students and 5% of American medical graduates failed their exam or could not impress standardized patients in USMLE Step2 CS with their communication and clinical skills. Now, are these medical students ready to become full-fledged doctors? Maybe! Maybe not!

How do we coach medical students for their USMLE Step 2 Clinical Skills exam?

We have developed Vital Checklist Theory of Patient Education and Empathy (ViCTOPee). ViCTOPee is the conglomerate of many theories adopted from various visionary leaders—Jim Collins, Eliyahu Goldratt, Michael Porter, Simon Sinek, Dr. Atul Gawande, Dr. Pronovost, George Miller, Allan Paivio, Neil Fleming, Tony Robbins, Charles Duhigg, Nir Eyal, Ryan Hoover, Dr. John Medina, Douglas Conant, Mette Norgaard, Perry Marshall, Michael Hyatt, Dr. Ramachandran, Steven Covey, Dale Carnegie, Dr. Judith Hibbard, Dr. James Merlino, Dr. Toby Cosgrove, Paul Spiegelman, Charles Kenney, Dr. Adrienne Boissy and many more thought leaders.

We believe in "Catch them before they fall." USMLE Step 2 CS exam is a very tricky exam as it assesses the candidates in many domains.

Some students will rush to the exam and fail the exam. However, this rash decision of giving USMLE Step 2 CS exam quickly because of the time constraint is hard to rectify afterward when applying for residency. Failing this exam will leave a black mark on their resume for life.

There are four types of students, and we have aligned these students in four boxes which we have derived from statistics formula—the first kind of students are the students who know that they have strong communication and clinical skills and have 100% confidence of passing the exam (TRUE Positives). In the second category are students who have weak communications and clinical skills but have 100% confidence of passing the exam (False Positives). The third subset has good/okay communication and clinical skills but has no confidence in passing the exam (False Negatives). Last but not the least, a fourth category--The True Negative, is composed of students have has poor communication and clinical skills and have no confidence in passing the exams.

	Test+ Strong Communication and Clinical Skills	Test − Weak Communication and Clinical Skills
Low stress, low anxiety, high confidence or <u>overconfidence</u>	Good or Okay Communication and Clinical Skills + 100% Confidence of passing the exam (True Positive)	Weak Clinical Skills + 100% Confidence of passing the exam or may be overconfident (False Positive)
High stress, high anxious, <u>low confidence</u>	Good or okay Communication and Clinical Skills + No Confidence of passing the exam (False Negative)	Weak or poor Communication and Clinical Skills + No Confidence of passing the exam (TRUE Negative)

Most of the American graduates and many IMG's have excellent communication and clinical skills and have 100% confidence in passing the exam, and we will place them in TRUE POSITIVE category. They may benefit from our training thus improving their HCAHPS, CGCAHPS score or other patient satisfaction surveys. However, this can also wait until the residency. The other way this book can help is better documentation in the clinical encounter thus fulfilling the meaningful use criteria. Improving communication and clinical skills may impact patient safety.

Next in line are the foreign medical graduates who have a good command of English and thus may be over confident. However, they forget that this is also an integrated clinical encounter (ICE) and Communication Interpersonal Skills (CIS) exam. They will appear without preparing for the exam and fail the exam because of their overconfidence. Time and again, we have seen that some medical graduates from foreign countries, especially from good institutes, who have good score fall in this trap and don't seek help.

The third subsets of students have excellent communication and clinical skills but have little confidence. This subset usually gets stress during the exam and may fail the exam. Our standardized patients help them to restore the faith in them so they can have smooth sailing during the exams.

Last but not the least, are the students who have poor communication and clinical skills and are low confidence. These students are easy to mold into American culture and have never taken history in English. Our approach with the students is to start from the bottom. Before going to the exam, you have to realize which category you belong.

Before we immerse medical students into coaching, we look for the constraints in them and try to pinpoint these and overcome these bottlenecks one by one. We have adapted this theory from Eliyahu Goldratt's "Theory of Constraint". Our customized workshops are unique and focus on one student at one time. Medical students ask this question frequently—How much time should I give for USMLE Step 2 CS preparation? Usually, I have to interview a student to answer this question, and it depends on whether the student is well versed with English grammar or not. Though USMLE Step 2 CS exam is not an American accent-testing exam, sometimes it is nice to know the basic culture etiquettes. This workbook complements our Vital Checklist Workshop for Step 2 CS and is designed in a way to save preparation time for a medical student.

What is our purpose?

Make "Best-to-Unique" health caregivers who can promote patient experience. At Vital Checklist, we believe that Patient Experience starts with Patient Education. Not only this, we need empathetic caregivers with the excellent learning environment, which will encourage the patients to ask questions proactively rather than react to their diseases. By-Asking-Doctors questions, patients are activated and hopefully stay healthy and stay fit. Smart patients are happy patients and thus less stressed out. In the era of Dr.Google or Dr.Bing, patients are going to ask questions as they have information available to them at the touch of a button. Our modus operandi is rather than being reactive, let's be proactive in our approach. Let's educate, activate and engage with the patient when they are with you. BE PRESENT at the moment and win the trust of patients. This provides phenomenal job satisfaction for doctors in the era of meaningful use.

Patient Experience= Patient Education X Patient Activation X Patient Engagement X Empathy X Environment.

Patient Experience is the product of all these elements, and they work in all-or-none fashion. The patient experience starts with the health literacy.

Health literacy is not just checking the box in electronic health record, handing a pamphlet, giving that 79-page heart failure booklet, making an app or a flashy website. The real health literacy is easy to understand and hard to forget medical information. Is the patient at fault of not remembering medical knowledge? We as caregivers have spent decades in training, and we expect patients to learn every bit of information in last 15-20 minutes of hospital stay and adhere those instructions. The real health literacy is providing patient education in which they can act to take control of their health and are empowered to make their decisions.

Though Vital Checklist started as a USMLE Step 2 Clinical Skills coaching program but on seeing the success of my students in their exam with standardized patients (patients who portray clinical scenarios or model patents), I used these same concepts, business theories for my real-life patients in my clinic and wanted to make my patients my raving fans. My vision in this book is teaching medical students' how to provide real health literacy and an ultimate patient experience or VIP experience. We have done no ground-breaking research or any randomized control trials, but these are my observations in my clinical practice followed by thank you letters, testimonials and patient experience videos which provide proof of concept. I am not teaching any rocket science in this book but have taken many business theories and fused them to make one Vital Checklist Theory of Patient Education and Empathy (ViCTOPee)

In one line, The Purpose of this Book is:

Don't Make Pamphlet Doctors! Make Real Doctors.

Introduction: How to prepare for USMLE Step 2 Clinical Skills?

The number one mistake a student makes in USMLE Step 2 CS exam is taking this exam for granted. Every student thinks that this exam is a cakewalk, and they will nail this exam in one or two weeks. However, failing this exam means your Road to USMLE will be tough as the competition is stiff.

Do's

1) Have a study partner.
2) Make sure to study for a **minimum** of one month for this exam.
3) Practice cases with the study partner
4) Try to give this exam after USMLE Step 1.
5) If you have not taken history in the English Language, make sure to give an extra time for your preparation.
6) Learn American culture by immersing yourself in externship and observerships.

Don't

1) Follow blindly what other medical students are doing. Use your neurons and if somebody says that they nailed the exam after studying for 7 days, this does not mean the same rules applies to you. It all depends on the cases and the day you will give the Step 2 CS Test. Everybody is different and learn differently.

Why one month for Step 2 CS?

Road to USMLE Step 2 CS is a very exhaustive book, and you need to practice the concepts before you sit for the exam. A few students will think that they don't need to learn differential diagnosis and associated symptoms, but they are wrong as this is the key to generate the differential diagnosis.

How to prepare for Step 2 CS?

We call this funnel approach. When you see a clinical scenario, make sure that you pay attention to the vital signs as you can gauge the patient sickness from the abnormal vital signs. Draw a picture of the body part so that remembering the differential diagnosis is easier. If you cannot remember the anatomy, physiology and cannot draw a diagram, make sure you write differential diagnosis. You can write differential diagnosis with an acronym or checklist V.I.T.A.L S.I.G.N.S

Vital Signs: An easy way to remember differential diagnosis	
V	❏ Vascular
I	❏ Infections
T	❏ Trauma
A	❏ Autoimmune
L	❏ Labs and Blood work
S	❏ Surgery
I	❏ Inflammation
G	❏ Genetics
N	❏ Neoplasia
S	❏ Sexually transmitted disease

© 2016 Harpreet Singh MD, FACP | Vital Checklist | (iCrush)

After making a mental note of the differential, proceed to history and ask all the possible questions. We have designed Road to USMLE book in a way so that reaching to the diagnosis becomes easiest. It is important to ask associated symptoms, as this will help you to narrow the diagnosis. The funnel keeps on narrowing as you proceed and then you ask the general history questions followed by the physical exam.

After that comes the counseling and explanation in layman language of the disease process.

Lastly, typing the patient note. If you are not well versed with the typing, please make sure you practice note writing.

Making Better Doctors

Communication and Interpersonal Skills

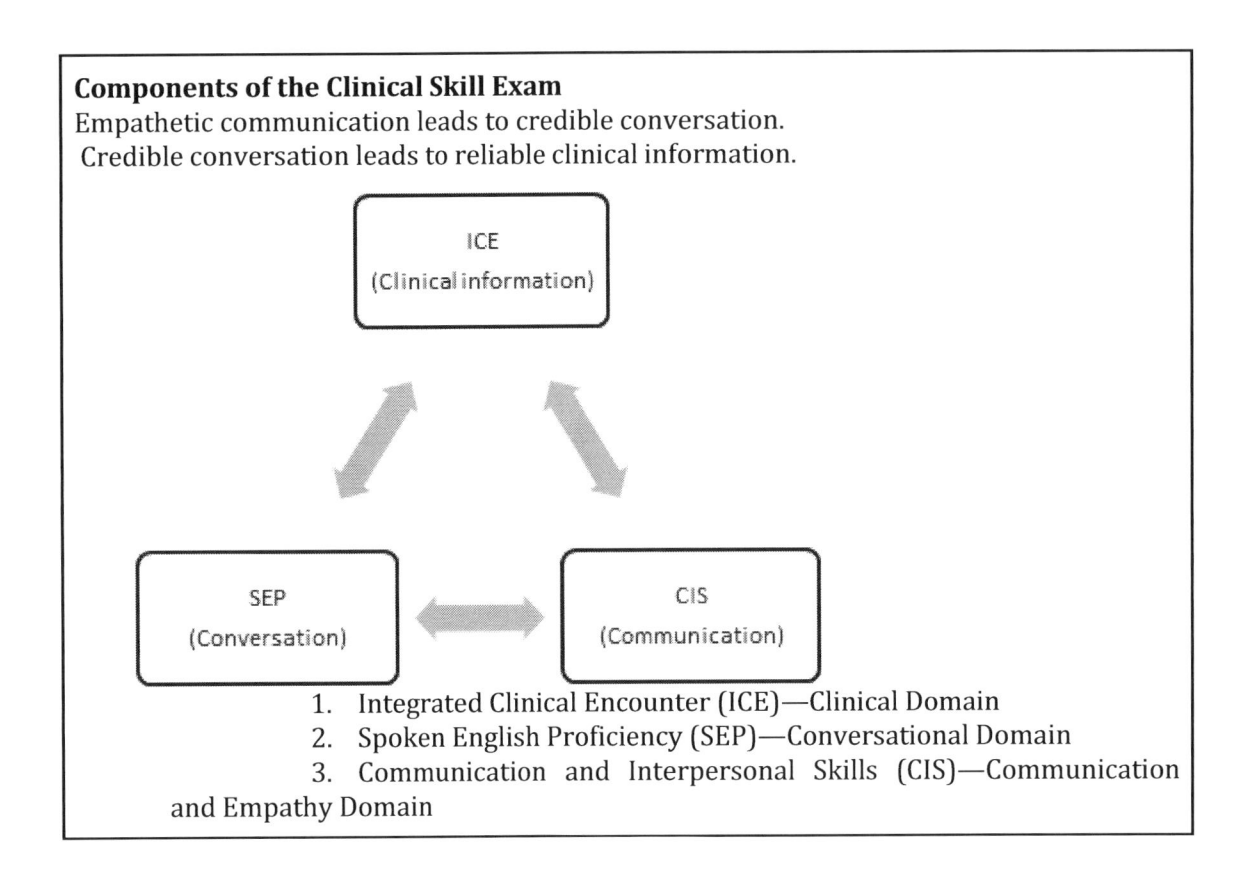

Components of the Clinical Skill Exam
Empathetic communication leads to credible conversation.
Credible conversation leads to reliable clinical information.

```
           ICE
    (Clinical information)
         ↙     ↘
   SEP    ⟷    CIS
(Conversation)  (Communication)
```

1. Integrated Clinical Encounter (ICE)—Clinical Domain
2. Spoken English Proficiency (SEP)—Conversational Domain
3. Communication and Interpersonal Skills (CIS)—Communication and Empathy Domain

The examination scenario is a high intensity situation where the stress levels are bound to be very high. With millions of thoughts, one will naturally think about questions to ask, differentials to keep in mind, and procedures and examinations to follow. In the process, we get so involved in our thoughts that we forget to focus on the patient's grievance and worries, and we lose marks on communication and interpersonal skills. This creates a negative impact and we will lose points, as we have failed to connect with the patients. We at Vital Checklist recommend making a plan of action at doorway.

Once in front of the patient, it is recommended to live the moment and listen to the patient, giving them adequate opportunity to express their complaints. One should also motivate the patient to speak more about the concern.

By doing so, you not only reveal a lot of crucial information, but also develop a clear approach to the case scenario as well as a connection with the patient.

Our methodology is designed in such a way that we focus on developing new synaptic connections via immersion coaching (neuroplasticity). This will not only help you to pass USMLE Step 2 CS exam in your first attempt, but also enable you to score high on HCAHPS and CG CAHPS Survey in real life practice.

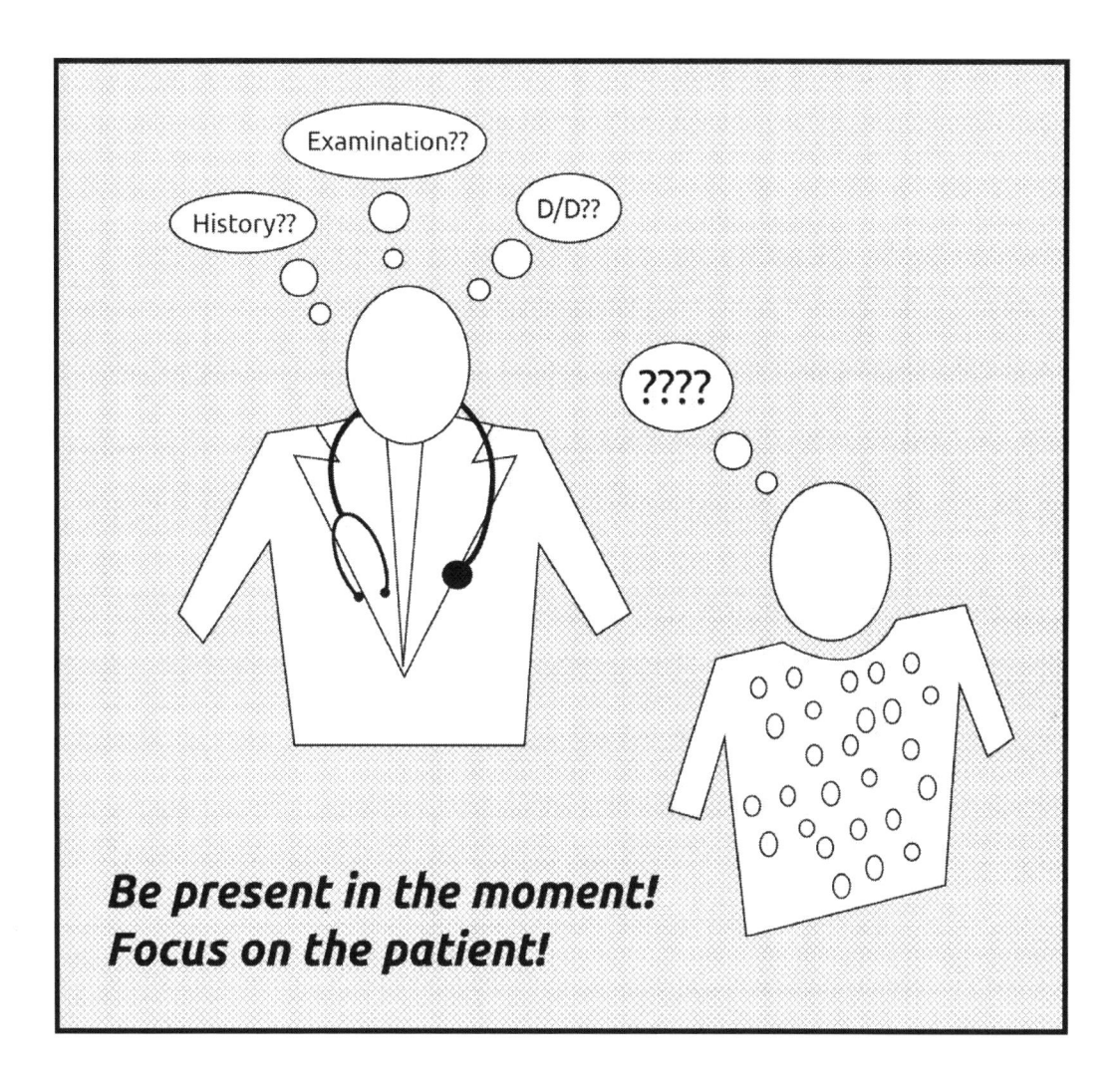

**Be present in the moment!
Focus on the patient!**

Here is an overview of what is expected from the student during the exam.

Knock

- ✓ The first thing to do after reviewing the doorway information, and before entering the room, is to KNOCK on the door! Do not enter without knocking and without the patient's permission. It is one of the most basic etiquettes a physician needs to take note of.

Introduce and Handshake

- ✓ After entering the room, greet the patient, introduce yourself, and shake the patient's hand. This ensures basic contact with the patient. Don't forget to make eye contact with him/her during the introduction. For example, "Good morning Mr. Joseph, I am Dr. Kurtis and I am going to be your physician today."

Drape

- ✓ Many times, the patient will already have the cloth, or paper, draped over their lap. If they are not draped before starting with the examination, ensure they have been draped prior to the examination. This will make them comfortable and ensure a proper interaction.

Draw out the foot end of the bed when the patient is required to lie down

- ✓ Whenever a patient has to lie down for examination, gently pull out the foot support of the examination table so that their legs do not hang off the edge. Make sure to get accustomed to the examination table and the instruments (otoscope, ophthalmoscope, etc.) during the initial 15 minutes before the real exam starts.

Empathy

- ✓ The importance of empathy cannot be stressed enough. It is one of the major pillars of understanding the patient's problem and also of ensuring a good patient experience. When this is achieved, offer support to them. Gently pat the patient's back, shoulder, or touch the elbow to convey empathy more effectively.

Paraphrase

- ✓ If the patient did not grasp the meaning of a particular sentence, make sure to rephrase it in easier words. There should be mutual understanding between doctor and patient for there to be a successful and meaningful office visit. Don't use medical jargon, instead, use simple layman words to ensure that they understand everything being said.

Open-ended questions

- ✓ Q: "How can I help you?" Let the patient speak.

If you want to start with the doorway information, for example, a case scenario of chest pain, always ask, "Can you describe the problem in your own words?"

An open ended question gives us an insight into the patient's problem in much more detail, as the reply is never a one word answer, but a detailed expression of their concerns and feelings. Also, open ended questions give the patient full control of what information they share. They build trust with the physician since they allow the patient to control the scenario. Open ended questions usually begin with 'Why,' 'How,' or 'Tell me more.'

Closed ended questions often end in a 'Yes' or 'No' reply and may deviate the patient and physician from the real problem.

- ✓ Q: "Is the pain sharp in nature?" One should use these closed ended questions to help the patient express their concern only if the patient is unable to express clearly.

It is crucial to ask open ended questions, because if we lead the patient in a particular direction using closed ended questions, it limits the amount of information we can extract from the patient.

Transition

- ✓ When going from one question to another, make the transition smooth. Don't jump from one topic to the other. Nonverbal gestures are as important as verbal gestures. Therefore, you must use your eyes and hands while transitioning to further topics.

Interruptions should be avoided

- ✓ Try to achieve a flow and minimize interruptions in the history and examination. Follow the checklists provided in this book to have a plan in mind before entering the room. It will help to avoid wasting time, as well as to avoid looking blank in front of the standardized patient.

Sanitation

This is really important! Ensure proper sanitation while examining the patient. Ideally, washing the hands before examining every patient is the best. However, due to time constraints, washing hands during every patient encounter is not possible, so gloves are recommended. Wearing fresh gloves before examining every patient is equivalent to washing the hands.

> Action Box:
>
> We have been asked this question time and again. Should we use gloves or wash hands?
>
> Let us say that you enter the examination room and plan to wash your hands during this clinical encounter. You successfully fulfil your objective and take a stunning history, writing down everything in your notes. Now you leave your clipboard aside, wash your hands, and examine the patient.
>
> What if, something falls down? You have to pick up that stuff and then invest your time in washing your hands again.
>
> What if you need to pick up the clipboard again? The clipboard is a fomite and carries a lot of germs. Since you touched the clipboard, you are supposed to wash your hands again before re-starting the examination. After finishing the exam, you are supposed to counsel, explain, and answer all the challenging questions. As in the USMLE Step 2 CS exam, we have a time constraint, it might not be feasible to wash your hands again, and you may have to leave the room when the bell rings. If you do not wash your hands again, you might be carrying germs to the computer to write your patient

note. The whole purpose is defeated. In an ideal setting, you must wash in and wash out.

However, if you use gloves to examine the patient, you do not have to wash your hands again and again, thus saving a lot of time.

Additionally, the patient will not complain that your hands are cold if you are wearing gloves.

Obtain consent for examination

- ✓ Before embarking on the physical exam, always ask the patient for their permission. Ask, "Will it be okay if I examine you now?"

Explain all the tests

- ✓ After receiving verbal consent to examine the patient, start the physical exam while explaining every test that will be performed on them. Explain the "why" of the test, as well as the "what." Keep talking to the patient, and keep them engaged during the physical exam.

Summarize

- ✓ After completing the history and physical exam, summarize them for the patient. Tell the patient what has been gathered through the history and physical exams, then ask if there is anything that might have been missed, or anything that they would like to add. Sometimes important information is revealed by the patient on reinforcement, which would have been missed on regular history.

Answering questions

- ✓ Usually, after summarizing, the patient will ask one or more questions about the condition. These are called "Challenging Questions," because they are aimed at challenging the doctor's knowledge and ability to answer them in an appropriate way. It often will determine the score on the CIS component. **Please refer to The Art of Answering Challenging Questions chapter for more details.**

Listen with the intent to understand the patient

- ✓ As mentioned earlier, listening to the patient is very important. The patient will share their complete history if they are asked open ended questions and listened to carefully. Listen with the intent to understand the patient's situation, and not merely to make notes. Seek to understand patients first.

Eye contact

- ✓ Establishing eye contact with the patient is an essential part of the clinical encounter. Start making eye contact with the patient right from the beginning of the encounter. This will help form a relationship with the patient and gain their confidence.

Now, let's summarize these points and make a checklist!

Remember, ***KID DEPOT IS ON SALE!*** ™

☐	K	Knock
☐	I	Introduce and Handshake
☐	D	Drape
☐	D	Draw out the foot end of the table during examination
☐	E	Empathy
☐	P	Paraphrase
☐	O	Open Ended Questions
☐	T	Transition
☐	I	Interruption should be avoided
☐	S	Sanitation- Wear gloves or wash your
☐	O	Obtain consent for examination
☐	N	Now, explain all the tests
☐	S	Summarize
☐	A	Answer all the questions and doubts
☐	L	Listen with the intent to understand the patient
☐	E	Eye contact

The above Vital Checklist can be a good scoring guide when you are practicing with your study partners and preparing for your exams. However, when you are doing observerships or externships, you need a crisp and concise approach for the hospitals which can help you to score high on all the possible domains in HCAHPS Survey. We call this a HISWEPT™ Approach.

HISWEPT	
H	Hand wash, Hand shake, Hello ✓ Did you wash or sanitize your hands? Did you shake hands and say hello to the patient? ✓ Trust develops when you shake hands.
I	Introduce ✓ Did you introduce yourself and your hospital?
S	Summarize and Survey the subjective Symptoms ✓ Summarize the previous day story/previous visit story; ✓ Ask any subjective symptoms! ✓ Most importantly, sit, don't rush.
W	Worries (Concerns) ✓ Any worries-depression/anxiety or anything else? ✓ Worry about the discharge needs?
E	Evaluate, Examine, and Explain ✓ Patient's objective examination and trying to explain why you are doing this particular examination.
P	Plan it! Picture it! ✓ Plan the assessment and draw a picture to explain the patient.
T	Treatment plan and Thank You ✓ Treat the patient, tell the disposition, and thank the patient.

We know that remembering each and every Vital Checklist is difficult, but when you practice these with standardized patient this will start making sense. *It is not the practice that makes perfect but the **perfect** **practice** that makes perfect.*

Section B

Doorway Information

Section B – Doorway Information

Basics of Communication and Clinical Skills

Opening Strategy: Doorway Information

At the beginning of each patient encounter, the first step is to scrutinize the doorway information. We recommend spending at least 40-45 seconds at the doorway reading and analyzing the information, followed by quickly writing a checklist. The following elements MUST be noted:

Name of the patient:

Make sure to read the:

- ✓ Salutation: Carefully note the salutation (Mr./ Ms./ Mrs./ Dr.) and address the patient appropriately. Don't confuse or ignore Ms. (pronounced as mizz) and Mrs.
- ✓ **Second name/Family name**: The patient should be addressed by this name throughout the encounter.
- ✓ In pediatric cases, always confirm the legal guardian of the child for medico-legal and consent purposes.

Age:

- ✓ Age is an important factor not only to build an appropriate differential diagnoses, but also to counsel about preventive measures, E.g. If the patient is above 50 years of age, always recommend colonoscopy.
- ✓ If the patient is a **minor**: always seek consent before physical examination. It may be mentioned as: "His mother has given oral consent on phone for physical examination and is on her way to the hospital."
- ✓ If you have a female patient aged between 12-50 years, never forget to do a urine pregnancy test after counseling the patient about the need for the test.

Gender:

- ✓ A myriad of differential diagnoses may come to mind based on gender. Remember, some questions are specific to female patients (menstrual, obstetric history, etc.), and some to male patients (prostate symptoms in elderly, etc.).

Chief complaint:

- ✓ Write down the chief complaint and quickly formulate a plan, including provisional diagnoses, history, and physical examination. Always keep in mind if any special tests will be needed or not (e.g Kernig's/ Brudzinski sign for headache with fever patient.)

Vital Signs:

Carefully note any abnormal vital signs. There are various ways to mention vital signs in the patient note:

- ✓ Vital signs: Within normal limits
- ✓ Tachycardia to 140/minute with other vital signs within normal limits
- ✓ Vital Signs: BP: 130/70 mmHg, Temp: 98.4°F, RR: 15/minute, HR: 78/minute, regular

Examining Tasks:

- ✓ Taking history
- ✓ Performing appropriate and focused physical examination
- ✓ Explaining your assessment and further plan of care to the patient.
- ✓ Writing a patient note

Opening Strategy: Managing the Blue Sheet

Front Side

A blue sheet is provided during the examination for convenience. Appropriately managing the blue sheet will help elicit a good history and write a good patient note.

We have developed various easy ways to remember mnemonics for history taking, examination, and counseling of the patient, which will help you to manage the blue sheet effectively and also save time. At first, you will feel overwhelmed with the number of mnemonics, but after practice, you will feel confident.

Back Side

The backside of the rough sheet should be used as a patient education and counseling sheet.

- ✓ Spend 2-3 minutes on closure and counseling.
- ✓ Make sure you address the patient's concerns/challenging questions.
- ✓ Draw 2-D diagrams and explain the disease / organ system involved / pathogenesis / progression / planned imaging studies / etc. to the patient.

VITAL CHECKLIST TRIVIA:

As per Neil Flemming, there are four types of learning methods—Visual, Aural, Reading, and Kinesthetic. We should use all possible avenues for better understanding and recall of complex medical concepts. This is why 2D diagrams must be drawn when explaining the disease process to the patient.

Remember: **"A picture speaks a thousand words."**

Patients appreciate the effort put into explanations and drawing 2D diagrams. These skills will help you ace the USMLE Step 2 CS examination and become a better physician in the future. A great doctor is one who is able to effectively communicate and connect with his patients in layman language.

Managing the Blue Sheet

You are standing outside the exam room door and reading the clinical scenario for your next encounter. This is your first encounter of USMLE Step 2 Clinical Skills. Your heart is pounding and you are about to enter the room. What is going on in your mind? Will the standardized patient cooperate or not.

Bell rings. There comes a voice from the overhead intercom, "Examinees you may begin the clinical scenario."

You flip the paper on the door and start reading the clinical scenario—

George Smith, a 56-year-old man comes in with a headache.

Vital Signs:
Blood pressure- 160/80 mm of Hg
Heart Rate-92 beats per minute
Pulse Ox-92%;
Respiratory Rate -18 breaths per minute

Instructions

> - Obtain a history pertinent to this patient's problem.
> - Perform a relevant physical examination (Do not perform a breast, pelvic/genital, corneal reflex, or rectal examination).
> - Discuss your impressions and any initial plans with the patient.
> - After leaving the room, complete your patient notes on the given form or computer.

After reading the clinical scenario, you rush into the room, however, lights are dimmed and patient is lying in the bed with his hips and knees flexed. Patient is anxious and when you switch on the lights, patient starts shouting at you because lights hurt him and you as a naïve medical student get scared and freeze and forget all the pertinent questions. You get into the **_Cognitive Tunneling_**. Charles Duhigg in his book— Smarter Faster Better: The Secrets of Being Productive in Life and Business has defined it has _Cognitive tunneling can cause people to become overly focused on whatever is directly in front of their eyes or become preoccupied with immediate tasks._ Because of this mishap, you cannot think straight and spoil your entire clinical scenario. Not only this, you start thinking of your first clinical encounter when you are doing eleven other cases.

> - Has this happened to your peers? Yes.
> - Can a patient get mad at you in real life? Yes.

What can you do to overcome this block of cognitive tunnel?

Making a checklist or to-do list will help you to overcome from this tunnel vision and allow you to proceed. This is called **_Reactive Thinking_** and helps you to proceed automatically. This will help in habit formation but sometimes they can become so automatic and you will forget to empathize with the patient.

Cognitive tunneling and reactive thinking happens in split seconds and our brain focuses from dim to bright spotlight.

However, we don't want this spotlight to fade away. This is the reason why we make mental pictures and tell stories. At Vital Checklist Workshop, we believe in teaching and coaching how to overcome these bottlenecks.

If you use blue sheet judiciously for writing the Vital Checklist and making 2-dimensional diagrams for differential diagnosis, you will never lose track of the real problem at hand.

Blue Sheet Template

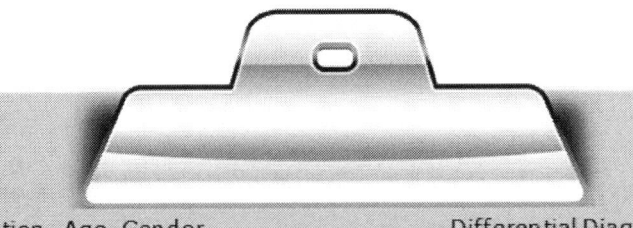

Name with salutation, Age, Gender   Differential Diagnosis:

Vitals

Chief Complaint

Symptom

	Location
	Grade
D	Duration (Including frequency)
O	Onset
C	Characteristic
T	Time of the Day
O	Occasion
R	Radiation
A	Associated Symptoms
I	Increasing factors
D @	Decreasing factors
P	Past Medical History for this symptom
M	Medications

General History Taking

What	Worries
I	Insomnia
F	Fever, Fatigue
P	Past medical history (Blood pressure, Sugar)
A	Allergies and manifestations
M	Medications
S	Surgeries
Family	Family history (Blood pressure, Sugar, Heart disease)
S	Social history (Tobacco, Alcohol, Recreational drugs)
H	Hospitalization
O	Obstetric and gynecological history (LPGA)
U	Urogenital and bowel problems
T	Travel
S	Sick contacts and sexual history
Vaccinateem	Vaccination history Empathy to be shown

Counseling:

Dr	Doctor Follow-up
S	Symptoms, Smoking
A	Activity, alcohol
W	Weight, Wine
M	Medications
D	Diet and driving

Examination:

		Skin
G: General	G: Glands
H: Heart	H: HEENT
A: Abdomen	U: Urogenital
L: Lungs	L: Lymph Node
E: Extremities	A: Buttocks/Prostate
N: Neurological	M: Musculoskeletal
	Psychiatric

Name with salutation, Age, Gender   Differential Diagnosis:

Vitals

Chief Complaint

Symptom   **General History Taking**
L   What
G   I
D   F
O   P
C   A
T   M
O   S
R   Family
A   S
I   H
D @   O
P   U
M   T
                                     S
                                     Vaccinate
                                     em

Counseling: **Examination:**
Dr   Skin
S   G: General   G: Glands
A   H: Heart   H: HEENT
W   A: Abdomen   U: Urogenital
M   L: Lungs   L: Lymph Node
D   E: Extremities   A: Buttocks/Prostate
                                     N: Neurological M: Musculoskeletal
                                                  Psychiatric

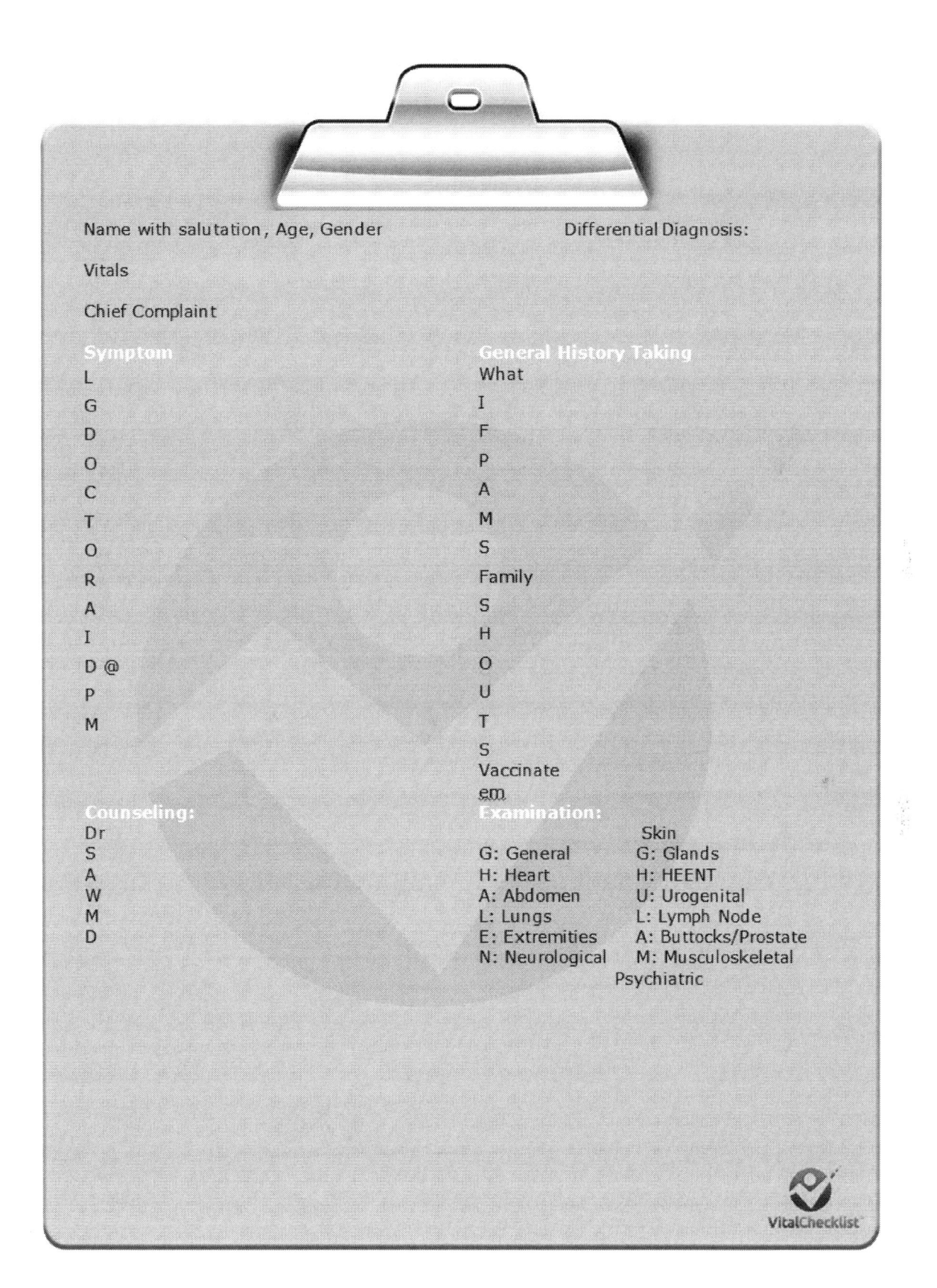

NOTES -

Section C

History Physical

Section C – History Physical

HISTORY TAKING: Case Based

The art of eliciting a good history in a limited amount of time under stressful exam conditions takes practice. The history should be relevant and thorough. Everyone has a personalized technique for history taking, honed over years of medical school training; however, such a technique should be flexible enough so that the examinee is not taken aback upon hearing a symptom they haven't previously encountered or practiced.

Once the patient describes a symptom, a methodical and comprehensive history can be elucidated using a simple mnemonic:

If the symptom is pain, use the mnemonic: **Life isn't Good, DOCTOR AID @ PM©**. If it is a non-pain symptom, use only the second part of the mnemonic: **DOCTOR AID @ PM©**. Repeat the mnemonic for each symptom, one by one.

Symptom: PAIN Life isn't Good, DOCTOR AID @ PM©		Practice the mnemonic here:
Life isn't	Location	
Good	Grade	
D	Duration (including frequency)	
O	Onset	
C	Characteristic	
T	Time of day	
O	Occasion	
R	Radiation	
A	Associated symptoms	
I	Increasing factors	
D @	Decreasing factors	
P	Previous medical history of similar symptom	
M	Medications used to relieve this symptom	

Symptom: PAIN
Life isn't Good, DOCTOR AID @ PM

Now, let's delve into the details of how to take the history for a patient with PAIN as a symptom (e.g. a patient complaining of chest pain):

Location: Ask the patient to point out the location of the pain with a finger.

- ✓ Q: "Where do you feel the pain?"
- ✓ Q: "Can you show me exactly where you are feeling the pain?"
- ✓ Q: "Can you point with your finger where exactly are you feeling maximum pain?"

The patient may use their finger to point out epigastric pain. They may hold their clenched fist over their chest to describe ischemic chest pain/pressure (Levine's sign)

Grade: Ask the patient to grade the severity of the pain.

- ✓ Q: "On a scale of 0 to 10, 10 being the worst pain you've ever had, how do you rate this pain?"

Challenging Question: The patient might say, "I'm sorry, I do not understand." You should then rephrase your question: "Can you tell me where you would rate this pain on a scale of 0 to 10, where 0 refers to no pain and 10 describes the worst pain you've ever had?" This is a must ask question.

Duration: Ask the patient about the duration of the pain.

- ✓ Q: "When did the pain start?"
- ✓ Q: "Since when have you had this pain?"
- ✓ Q: "How long have you had this pain?"

The patient may have had this pain for a few hours, a few days, or even a few years. If it's a chronic pain, it is important to ask:

- ✓ Q: "Is this pain the same as before, or is it different?"
- ✓ Q: "Do you think this is a new pain?"

The importance of differentiating the current pain from the underlying chronic pain can be gauged from the following examples:

A 46-year-old male patient is complaining of having a backache for four years that is particularly painful while sitting in a chair. The patient is asking for a disability note. One question that should be asked is: "Is this pain different from your old pain?" The patient answers, "Yes doc! Actually, my pain became worse after I sneezed."

This is a case of facet arthritis, four years in duration, presenting with a possible disc herniation.

A 45-year-old male patient with a chronic backache, which becomes better on bending and worse on extension of the back, is suffering from lumbar stenosis. He complains of the backache getting worse after having a bout of coughing. He needs to be evaluated for a probable disc herniation.

After the patient describes the duration of the pain, ask him if it is continuous or intermittent.

- ✓ Q: "How long does the pain last?"
- ✓ Q: "Does the pain come and go?"
- ✓ Q: "How often does it come?"

Onset: Ask the patient about the onset of the pain.

- ✓ Q: "Does the pain begin suddenly or gradually?"

Pain due to ischemic heart disease is usually sudden, but it may be gradual in onset if the plaque ruptures slowly. (Very important to discuss about non STEMI and STEMI)

Characteristic: Ask the patient open ended questions that help describe the pain.

- ✓ Q: "Can you describe the pain in your own words?"
- ✓ Q: "What is the pain like?"
- ✓ Q: "Can you explain the nature of the pain you are experiencing?"

If the patient is unable to answer open ended questions, help him or her by asking close ended questions:

- ✓ Q: "Is the pain sharp or dull? Is it throbbing?"
- ✓ Q: "Does it feel like an elephant is sitting on your chest?"
- ✓ Q: "Is it a constricting pain?"
- ✓ Q: "Do you feel a burning pain"

Time of day: Ask the specific time of the day when the patient experiences the pain.

- ✓ Q: "Can you tell me what time of day you feel this pain?"

Occasion: Always ask the patient what they were doing when the pain started.

- ✓ Q: "Can you describe what you were doing when the pain began?"

Radiation: Ask about the radiation of the pain.

- ✓ Q: "Is the pain travelling anywhere else?"
- ✓ Q: "Has there been any change in the location of the pain since it started?"
- ✓ Q: "Do you think your pain is radiating anywhere else?"
- ✓ Q: "Does your pain go anywhere?"
- ✓ Q: "Does your pain spread anywhere?"

Associated symptoms: Ask about associated symptoms one by one. Do not ask two questions or two symptoms at once. Give the patient time to respond to one symptom, then quickly move on to the next. Use expressions and body language to help save time.

- ✓ Q: "Is the pain associated with fever?" *pause...* "Chills?"
- ✓ Q: "Any abdominal pain?" *pause...* "Any flank pain?" *pause...* "Back pain?"
- ✓ Q: "Do you experience any shortness of breath with the pain?"
- ✓ Q: "Are you struggling to take deep breaths?"

If the patient has described chest pain, ask all of the above associated features. Also, ask about feeling any chest pressure, **since patients often describe it as a separate entity to chest pain.**

- ✓ Q: "Do you have any palpitations?" The patient might say: "Sorry doc, I don't understand you!" Rephrase: "Do you have episodes of your heart racing?"

You can demonstrate by tapping your palm on the clipboard to differentiate between regular and irregular types of palpitation.

> *Action Box:*
>
> *An easier way to approach the associated symptoms is to do a mini systems review (from head to toe).*
>
> *Mini systems review is explained in great depth in a later part of the book.*

Increasing factors: Ask about aggravating factors.

- ✓ Q: "What makes your pain worse?"
- ✓ Q: "Does anything make your pain worse?"
- ✓ Q: "Is there anything that you do that makes your pain worse?"
- ✓ Q: "Is there anything you eat that makes the pain worse?"
- ✓ Q: "Is there any posture in which the pain worsens?"

Decreasing factors: Ask about relieving factors.

- ✓ Q: "What makes your pain better?"
- ✓ Q: "What do you do to make your pain go away?"

Previous history of similar symptom: This is referring only to the history of **similar** pain episodes.

- ✓ Q: "Have you had previous episodes of this pain?"
- ✓ Q: "Did you experience such a pain in the past?"

Medications: Ask about medications taken for the pain.

- ✓ Q: "Do you take any pills for this pain?"
- ✓ Q: "Do they help?"

Now, let's practice questions that will be asked when a patient complains of pain. Phrase and write questions in each row below:

Symptom: PAIN		Write the questions here:
Life isn't	Location	
Good	Grade	
D	Duration (including frequency)	
O	Onset	
C	Characteristic	
T	Time of day	
O	Occasion	
R	Radiation	
A	Associated symptoms	
I	Increasing factors	
D @	Decreasing factors	
P	Past medical history for this symptom	
M	Medications	

Symptom: Non-Pain
DOCTOR AID @ PM

For any symptom other than pain, questions about location and grade need not be asked. Strike out the first part of the pain mnemonic and use the remainder.

For Pain: **Life isn't Good, DOCTOR AID @ PM**
For Non-pain: **DOCTOR AID @ PM**
The 'R' here stands for rate of progression (radiation in the pain mnemonic).

Symptom: Non-Pain (e.g. Dizziness) DOCTOR AID @ PM©		Practice the mnemonic here:
D	Duration (including frequency)	
O	Onset	
C	Characteristic	
T	Time of day	
O	Occasion	
R	Rate of progression	
A	Associated symptoms	
I	Increasing factors	
D @	Decreasing factors	
P	Previous history of similar symptoms	
M	Medications	

Now, let's learn how to take the history for a patient with a non-pain symptom (e.g. a patient complaining of dizziness):

Duration: Ask the patient about the duration of the symptom.

- ✓ Q: "When did the dizziness start?"
- ✓ Q: "Since when have you had this dizziness?"
- ✓ Q: "For how long have you had this dizziness?"

After the patient has described the duration of the symptom, ask whether it is continuous or intermittent.

- ✓ Q: "How long does an episode of dizziness last?"
- ✓ Q: "Do you constantly feel dizzy?"
- ✓ Q: *For a patient with cough*, ask: "How often do you cough?"

Onset: Ask the patient if the symptom began suddenly or gradually.

- ✓ Q: "Did the cough develop suddenly or over time?"

Characteristic: Ask the patient open ended questions that help describe the symptom.

- ✓ Q: "Can you explain the dizziness in your own words?"

If the patient is unable to describe his or her symptom, help by asking close ended questions:

- ✓ Q: "Do you feel that you are spinning, or that the room is spinning around you?"
- ✓ Q: "Did you feel as if you were going to pass out?"

For a patient with cough, ask: "Tell me more about your cough."

- ✓ Q: "Do you bring up any sputum/phlegm with your cough?"
- ✓ Q: "Is it a dry cough?

Time of day: Ask the specific time of day when the patient experiences the symptom.

- ✓ Q: "Can you tell me at what time of day do you usually feel dizzy?"
- ✓ Q: "Is there a particular time of day when you feel dizzy?"

Occasion: Always ask the patient what they were doing when the symptom started.

- ✓ Q: "Can you describe what you were doing when the dizziness began?"
- ✓ Q: "What causes this dizziness to happen?"

Rate of progression: Ask about the progression of the symptom.

- ✓ Q: "Has this dizziness worsened over time?"
- ✓ Q: "Do you think your dizziness has progressed over time?"
- ✓ Q: "Has there been any change in the severity of the cough since it started?" (If the clinical scenario is pertaining to cough)

Associated symptoms: Ask about associated symptoms one by one. Do not ask two questions, or two symptoms, at once. Give the patient time to respond to one symptom, then quickly move on to the next. Use expressions and body language to help save time.

- ✓ Q: "Is the dizziness associated with nausea?" *Pause...* "Or vomiting?" *Pause...*
- ✓ Q: "Any headache?"
- ✓ Q: "Did you lose consciousness?"
- ✓ Q: "Have you noticed any change in your hearing?"
- ✓ Q: "Do you hear any ringing or buzzing sound?"

> **Action Box:**
> As time is a limiting factor in the exam, asking detailed associated symptoms can be counterproductive. The rule of thumb is to pause for three seconds between each question.

Increasing factors: Ask about aggravating factors.

- ✓ Q: "What makes your dizziness worse?"

Decreasing factors: Ask about relieving factors.

- ✓ Q: "What makes you feel better?"

Previous history of similar symptoms: Only the history of episodes of this symptom.

- ✓ Q: "Have you had previous episodes of dizziness?"
- ✓ Q: "Did you experience such dizziness in the past?"

Medications: Ask about medications taken for the symptom.

- ✓ Q: "Do you take any pills for this?"
- ✓ Q: "Do they help?"

Now, let's practice questions that will be asked when a patient complains of dizziness. Phrase and write questions in each row below:

Symptom: Dizziness		Write the questions here:
D	Duration (including frequency)	
O	Onset	
C	Characteristic	
T	Time of the day	
O	Occasion	
R	Rate of progression	
A	Associated symptoms	
I	Increasing factors	
D @	Decreasing factors	
P	Previous medical history of similar symptoms	
M	Medications	

HISTORY TAKING: General

The importance of a proper and complete history was stressed at the beginning of this chapter. This section lays out a format for taking past medical history, family history, social history, etc.

You can remember it with the mnemonic: "**What IF PAM'S Family SHOUTS? Vaccinate 'em!**" ™
It might sound overwhelming with the number of mnemonics used for history taking; however, by the time you reach the end of this book, you will realize that there are only four key mnemonics to be used. This book is designed in such a way that you will memorize them subconsciously, through constant use and repetition in conjunction with practice.

What IF PAM'S FAMILY SHOUTS? Vaccinate 'em!™	
What	Worries
I	Insomnia
F	Fever, with or without chills and rigors; Fatigue
P	Past medical history (Blood pressure, Blood Sugar, Cancer, Heart Disease, and Stroke)
A	Allergies and type of reactions
M	Medications
S	Surgeries
Family	Family history (Blood pressure, Blood Sugar, Cancer, Heart Disease, and stroke)
S	Social history (Occupation, Cohabitation, Tobacco, Alcohol, Recreational drugs)
H	Hospitalization
O	Obstetric and gynecological history (L-PGA)
U	Urogenital and bowel problems
T	Travel history
S	Sick contacts and sexual history
Vaccinate	Vaccination history
em	Empathy

These salient points have been further described below for better understanding.

Worries: Ask the patient about the effect the disease has on his/her life.
What are the main concerns?

- ✓ Q: "Can you please tell me if you are worried about this?"
- ✓ Q: "Can you please describe your worries for me? What troubles you the most?"

Insomnia: Ask the patient if he/she is experiencing any sleep problems because of his/her current complaints or otherwise.

- ✓ Q: "Mr. Doe, tell me about your sleep"
- ✓ Q: "How is your sleep these days?"

Please see the detailed questionnaire in the latter part of this book.

Fever: Ask the patient if he/she noticed and documented any fever during this episode.

- ✓ Q: "Did you feel warm during this period?" *Pause…* "Did you measure your temperature?"

Fatigue: Ask the patient if he/she felt tired during this episode of illness.

- ✓ Q: "How do you feel about your energy levels since this illness started?"
- ✓ Q: "Do you think you get tired easily these days?"

Please see the detailed questionnaire in the latter part of this book.

Past medical history: Important medical histories to be asked in every patient encounter are high blood pressure, blood sugar, heart disease, stroke, and cancer. DO NOT use the terms hypertension or diabetes. Instead, refer to **'blood pressure'** and **'blood sugar.'**

- ✓ Q: "Mr. Doe, can you tell me if you have any blood pressure problems?"
- ✓ Q: "Can you please tell me if you have any blood sugar problems?"
- ✓ Q: "Mr. Doe, have you ever been diagnosed with a blood pressure problem?"
- ✓ Q: "Mr. Doe, have you ever been diagnosed with a sugar problem?"
- ✓ Q: "How long ago was that diagnosis?"
- ✓ Q: "Are you taking any medications for it?"
- ✓ Q: "When was your last blood pressure measurement?"
- ✓ Q: "When was the last time your sugar was measured?"
- ✓ Q: "Do you measure your blood pressure/sugar regularly at home?"

Allergies: It is important to ask the patient about any drug, food, or environmental allergy and a description of the allergic reaction.

- ✓ Q: "Can you please tell me about your allergies, if any?"
- ✓ Q: "Can you please tell me if you are allergic to any medication?" "Any particular food?" "Anything in the environment?"
- ✓ Q: "Can you please describe the allergic reaction for me?"
- ✓ Q: "What happens when you are exposed to this agent?"
- ✓ Q: "Do you use any medications to prevent the allergic reaction?"

- ✓ Q: "Do you carry an Epi-pen (epinephrine) with you?"

It is important to ask this question, as it gives you an additional point for counseling.

For example, "Mr. Doe, I would advise you to always carry your Epi-pen with you to prevent serious allergic reactions like anaphylaxis. If you do not have one, I will prescribe you one and you can collect it from the pharmacy."

Medications: A detailed history of the patient's current medications should be elicited.

- ✓ Q: "Are you currently taking any medications?"

Some patients might hand you a card with a list of their medications. Note the drugs on the blue sheet and **give the card back to the patient!**

- ✓ Q: "Do you remember the dose of the Alprazolam (example) tablet you are taking?"
- ✓ Q: "Are you taking any over-the-counter medicines?"
- ✓ Q: "Are you taking any over-the-counter supplements?"
- ✓ Q: "Any other medication that you would like to tell me about?"

Surgeries: Ask the patient if he/she has had any surgeries in the past. If yes, take a detailed history of the procedure, its indication, and the postoperative period.

- ✓ Q: "Mr. Doe, have you had any surgeries in the past?"
- ✓ Q: "Which surgery was it?"
- ✓ Q: "Why were you advised the surgery?"
- ✓ Q: "How was your post-operative period?"
- ✓ Q: "Have you undergone any other procedures in the past?"

Family history: There are some important points about the family history that have to be elicited from all patients. Ask about any family history of 'blood pressure,' 'blood sugar,' and any death related to heart disease before the age of 60 years. Make sure to ask about stroke and cancer as well. It is also important to ask about other diseases in immediate family members.

- ✓ Q: "Mr. Doe, do you have a family member suffering from a similar condition?"
- ✓ Q: "Does anyone in your family have a blood pressure problem?"
- ✓ Q: "Does anyone in your family have a blood sugar problem?"
- ✓ Q: "Any premature deaths in your family due to events related to the heart?"
- ✓ Q: "Mr. Doe, tell me about your family. Any significant diagnosis that I should be aware of?"

Social history: Social history consists of a wide variety of questions related to the patient's life. It includes questions on their occupation, who they are living with, and questions regarding their habits. Be very polite and non-judgmental when asking questions regarding tobacco, alcohol, or any recreational drug use. Never use the term 'illicit drugs' with the patient, as some of these drugs can be used for medicinal purposes. Also, certain states of the US have made marijuana consumption legal.

- ✓ Q: "Mr. Doe, what do you do for a living?"
- ✓ Q: "Who do you live with?"
- ✓ Q: "Mr. Doe, do you consume tobacco in any form?"
- ✓ Q: "Mr. Doe, do you consume alcohol in any form?"

If the patient gives a history of alcohol consumption, it is recommended to ask the CAGE questionnaire to evaluate for alcohol addiction.

- ✓ Q: "Mr. Doe, do you ever feel the need to **cut down** on your alcohol consumption?"
- ✓ Q: "Do you ever feel **annoyed** if someone suggests that you quit drinking?"
- ✓ Q: "Do you feel **guilty** after drinking?"
- ✓ Q: "Do you need alcohol first thing in the morning, or as an **eye opener**?"
- ✓ Q: "Mr. Doe, I assure you these questions are purely confidential and will stay between us, but I need to know a few things to have an overall view about your health. Is that okay?" *pause...* "Are you using any recreational drugs?"

> **Action Box:**
> Note the CAGE evaluation as 0/4 to 4/4 depending on the number of questions they answer as 'yes'.
> A CAGE questionnaire more than or equal to 2/4 has a specificity of 77% and a sensitivity of 91% for considering alcoholism.

Certain patients might object to these questions and tell you, for example, "Do I look like a person doing drugs to you doc!" Politely tell them that asking these specific questions is part of protocol, and that every patient gets asked these questions. "I am sorry Mr. Doe, but this is just a part of our protocol. We ask every patient these questions."

Hospitalization: This segment will help cover any previous medical episodes (ER visits), and surgeries that might have been missed in the past medical and surgical history segment.

- ✓ Q: "Have you ever been hospitalized?"
- ✓ Q: "Did you ever visit an emergency room before?"
- ✓ Q: "Can you please tell me the reason for the visit?"
- ✓ Q: "Were you admitted overnight for that episode?"

Obstetrics and gynecological history: It is important to ask every female patient about her gynecological history. As a RULE, all female patients between the ages of twelve and fifty should be advised to get a pregnancy test. Politely tell them that asking these specifics are part of the protocol. Any obstetric history should be discussed under four headings – LMP, Parity, Gravida, and Abortions/Miscarriages (This can be remembered as **LPGA – LMP, Parity, Gravida, Abortions/Miscarriages).**

One must always keep in mind that obstetric and gynecological history is very personal to the patient, and her privacy must be respected at all times.

- ✓ Q: "Ms. Doe, if you do not mind, can I ask you a few questions regarding your reproductive system/ menses?"

A.) **Gynecological history**: It should cover the last menstrual period, amount of flow, duration of flow, and if any symptoms like pain, breast tenderness, and/or mood changes are present during the menstrual flow.

- ✓ Q: "Ms. Doe, when was the last time you had a period?" – **LMP**
- ✓ Q: "How many pads/tampons do you need to change per day?"
- ✓ Q: "How long does the flow last?"
- ✓ Q: "Do you have any symptoms like abdominal pain, mood swings, or breast tenderness, etc. during your menstrual flow?"

B.) **Obstetric history**: This section covers the number of pregnancies, mode of delivery, number of abortions or miscarriages, and if any ectopic pregnancy was detected.

- ✓ Q: "Ms. Doe, can you please tell me about your previous pregnancies, if any?"
- ✓ Q: "Can you please tell me how many times you have conceived so far?" – **Gravida**
- ✓ Q: "Have you had any abortions or miscarriages?"
- ✓ Q: "Ms. Doe, how many children do you have?" – **Parity** (assuming that all her fetuses that crossed the age of viability were delivered and are alive)
- ✓ Q: "How was the child born?" *pause...* "Was it a normal vaginal delivery, or a Cesarean section?"
- ✓ Q: "I know conceiving a child is a life changing event, how is motherhood treating you, Ms. Doe?"
- ✓ Q: "What is the name of the child?" Patient replies, "We named him Charlie." "Oh! That is a beautiful name." "Is Charlie's growth according to his age?"

> **Action Box:**
> This phase of your history taking can be vital in building a rapport with the patient. You must show concern towards her worries and feelings about conception and also inquire about the baby. You can ask if the child cried during birth, or developed well according to age. One sympathy touch point can be to ask how motherhood has been treating her.

Urinary problems: It is important to ask the patient about his/her urinary and bowel habits, any variations, and/or any disturbances recently. A simple mnemonic to help remember the urinary history is "**Painful Bloody Frequent U.R.I.I.N.E.™**"

Painful, or Dysuria- This refers to painful micturition. It is an important symptom of urinary tract infections or stones.

- ✓ Q: "Mr. Doe, is there any pain on urination?"
- ✓ Q: "Could you elaborate on the pain?"

Bloody- "Is there any blood in your urine?" *pause...* "Are there any clots?"

Frequency- Another lower urinary tract symptom useful to evaluate for prostatic enlargement.

- ✓ Q: "Mr. Doe, how often do you need to use the bathroom?"
- ✓ Q: "Do you feel that you need to use it more often than before?
- ✓ Q: "Has it increased from before?"

U – Urgency- Another lower urinary tract symptom useful to evaluate for prostatic enlargement.

- ✓ Q: "Mr. Doe, do you feel that you need to hurry up to the bathroom every time you want to urinate?"
- ✓ Q: "Can you control the urge to pass urine until you get to a bathroom?"

R – Retention leads to Hesitancy- This is an important question in an elderly male as he could be suffering from benign prostatic hypertrophy.

- ✓ Q: "Mr. Doe, can you please tell me about your urine?"
- ✓ Q: "Have you noticed any difficulty in urination lately?"

Urinary retention in a young male should raise suspicion for a chlamydial or gonococcal infection forming a stricture in the urethral tract.

I – Intermittency- Another lower urinary tract symptom useful to evaluate for prostatic enlargement.

- ✓ Q: "Mr. Doe, do you feel that your urinary stream is intermittent? Does it stop and come back again and again?

Some patients may complain of *Dribbling*. This is again a lower urinary tract symptom to evaluate for prostatic enlargement.

- ✓ Q: "Mr. Doe, how is your urinary stream? Is there any dribbling of urine?"

I – Incontinence- An important condition that should be evaluated in a female with urogenital problems. Always differentiate between stress, urge, and mixed Incontinence. Urine leakage is the primary symptom of incontinence. This is a feature of urinary incontinence due to sphincter dysfunction in old age. A detailed description on clinical approach to urinary incontinence is mentioned later in this book.

- ✓ Q: "Mr. Doe, do you ever lose control over your bladder?"
- ✓ Q: "Do you experience any urinary leakage on coughing or sneezing?"
- ✓ Q: "Do you have to go the bathroom emergently?"

N – Nocturia- The frequent need to get up and go to the bathroom at night is called nocturia. One event per night is a normal event; however, if you have 2 or more events per night, this is abnormal. This may make the patient groggy and tired the following day.

- ✓ Q: "How many times do you need to get up at night to go to the bathroom?"

Nocturia is different from the Enuresis. In nocturia, you will wake up and go to the bathroom.

E – Enuresis- In enuresis, or bedwetting, you don't arouse, instead, you empty the bladder while still asleep.

Bowel problems: After taking the urinary history, move on to the bowel. Find out about the patient's normal habits and any recent changes.

- ✓ Q: "Mr. Doe, please, tell me about your bowel habits."
- ✓ Q: "Have you experienced any change in your habit recently?"

Travel history: A history of recent travel is important for diseases endemic to certain areas, as well as for diseases related to clotting and embolism.

- ✓ Q: "Mr. Doe, have you traveled recently?"

A female taking oral contraceptives and giving a history of recent long distance travel can be a typical case of deep venous clots or pulmonary embolism.

- ✓ Q: "Mr. Doe, did you travel to a third world country in the last few months?"– Tuberculosis and other infectious diseases

Sexual history: This topic should be approached carefully. NEVER judge the patient. Assure the patient that whatever he/she tells you will be strictly confidential (will remain between the patient and doctor).

- ✓ Q: "Ms. Doe, I would now like to ask you about your sexual history. This will be strictly confidential and will stay between you and me only."
- ✓ Q: "Are you **S**exually active Ms. Doe?"
- ✓ Q: "So tell me about your **P**artner." – This will help you know whether they have one or more partners and whether they are married or have a girlfriend/boyfriend.

NEVER ask the patient how many partners he/she has. It amounts to judging and will result in a lower score!

- ✓ Q: "Tell me about your **O**rientation Ms. Doe. Are you sexually active with only men, women, or both?" – This is a tricky question and might feel uncomfortable at first, but practice will build confidence and a result in the acquisition of a good sexual history.
- ✓ Q: "Do you use any method of contraception?" – This will help you determine whether or not the patient is participating in **U**nprotected sex.
- ✓ Q: "Have you ever been diagnosed with a sexually **T**ransmitted disease?"

This is the perfect time to coach the patient about Safe sex practices!
You can remember the sexual history with SPOUTS, as highlighted above.

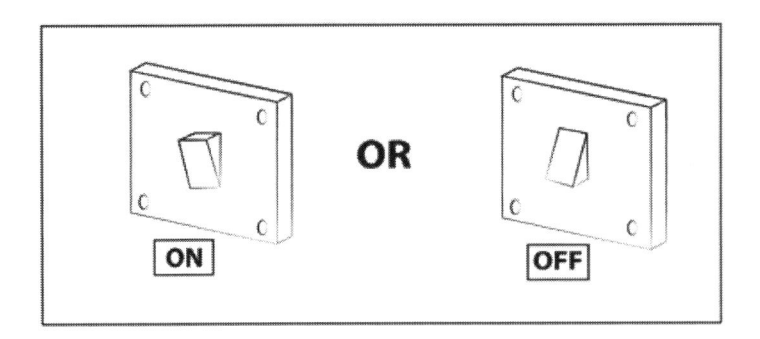

Picture-1
Are you sexually active or not?
Remember this metaphor. Don't say in the exam.
This metaphor of switch on or off is for an easy memorization of questions you will be asking SP.

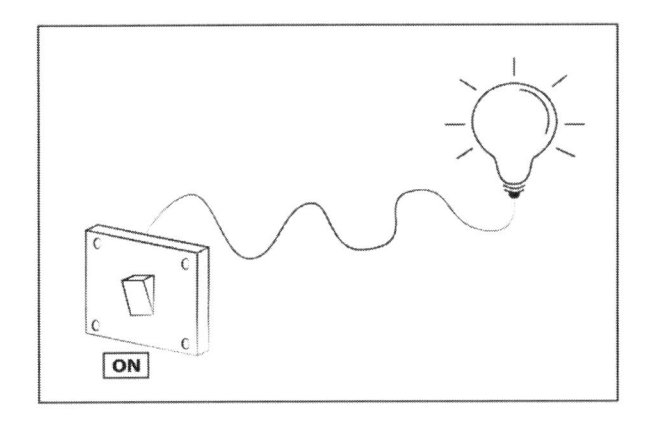

Picture -2
How many partners do you have?
Think of this metaphor of one switch is lighting up one bulb.

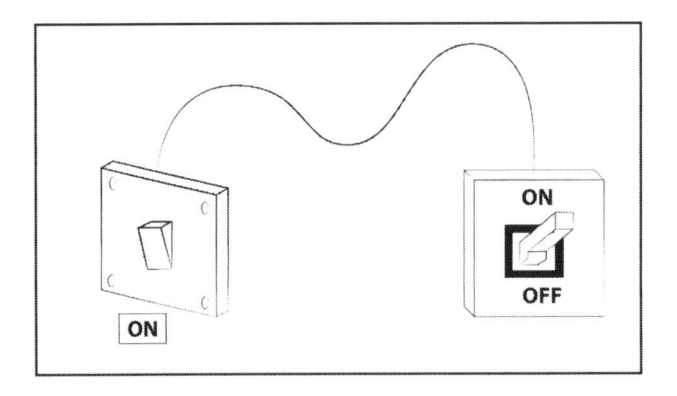

Picture -3
Do you have the same sex partners?
Remember this metaphor each switch activating each other.

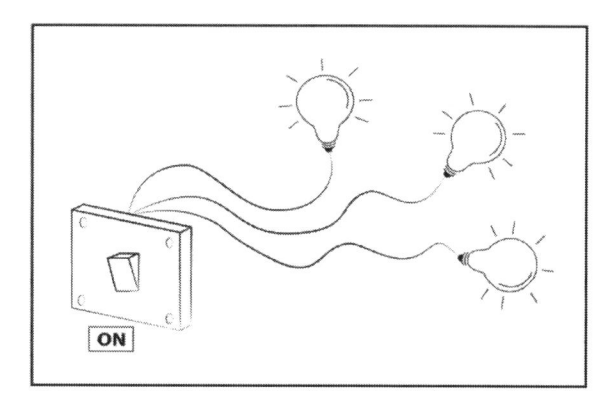

Picture-4
Do you have multiple sexual partners?
Remember this metaphor of one switch activating multiple bulbs.

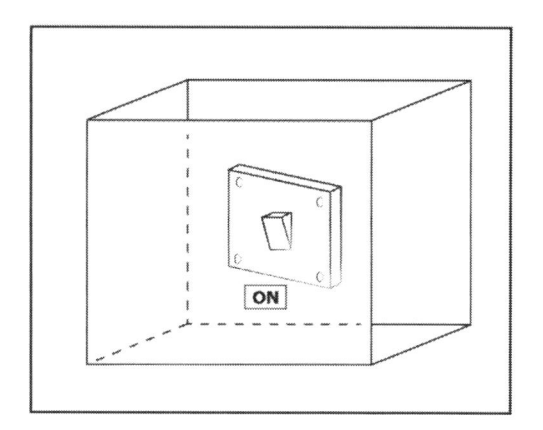

Picture -5
Do you use any protection? Remember the metaphor of weather proof outside switch box.
This question will help you to counsel the SP for using protection and prevent sexually transmitted diseases.

Sick contacts: A history of exposure to any sick contacts at home or an office has to be elicited in cases of infectious diseases.

- ✓ Q: "Does anyone else at home have a similar illness?"
- ✓ Q: "Did they have it before you?"
- ✓ Q: "Do any of your neighbors have a similar illness like this?"
- ✓ Q: "Can you think of anyone at your workplace who had a similar illness before you?"

Vaccination history: It is very important to take a complete vaccination history, specifically in a child. There won't be a child standardized patient, but there can be a parent coming to your office to consult about a child, or there can be a phone call of a child's parent! Sometimes a child's immunization card may be brought with a myriad of questions.

- ✓ Q: "Can you please tell me about their immunizations?"
- ✓ Q: "When did the child receive the last vaccine?"
- ✓ Q: "Which vaccine was it?"
- ✓ Q: "Was there any reaction to the vaccine?"
- ✓ Q: "Can I please see his immunization record?"
- ✓ Q: "Did you receive any flu vaccine?"
- ✓ Q: "Did you have any pneumonia vaccine in the last 5 years?"

Empathy: This is possibly the most important, and the most easily forgotten part of your history taking. Expressing empathy towards the patient is vital! It is not only important for scores, but it shows true understanding of the patient's feelings and that we are here to support them. Something as simple as gently patting the patient on the arm can show support. But be mindful of the safe area as depicted in the diagram below. The safe area extends from the elbow to the shoulder to ensure patting the arm is the most effective. Use body language, your eyes, and your hands to convey your feelings. Even the smallest gestures can improve the patient's experience!

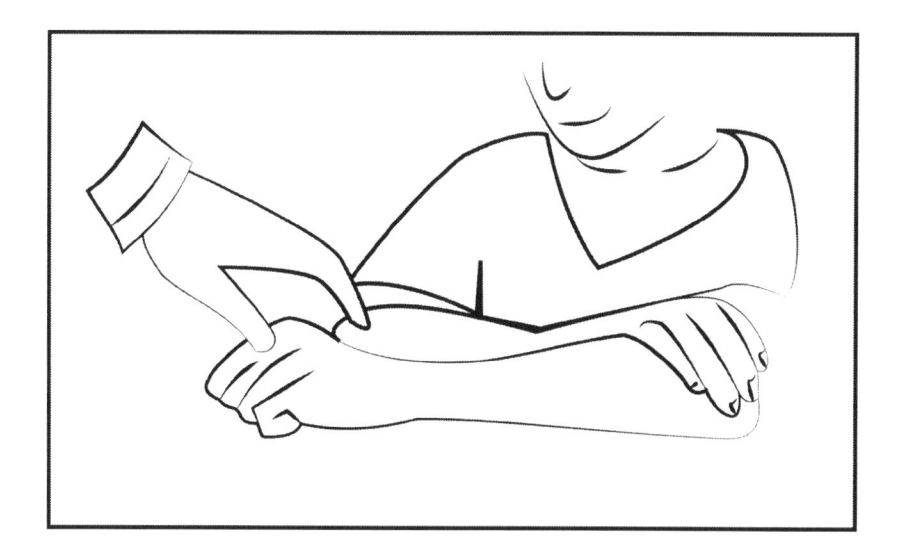

Physical Examination

Performing a **focused,** yet **comprehensive,** physical examination in a limited amount of time is a challenge. We have devised an easy to remember, and hard to forget, mnemonic to perform a thorough physical examination: **'GHALEN-GHULAM.'** **Skin** and **psychiatric** examinations can also be added to make sure the examination is truly all-inclusive.

Skin			
G	General examination	G	Glands
H	Heart (cardiovascular)	H	HEENT
A	Abdomen	U	Urogenital
L	Lungs	L	Lymph node/lumbosacral
E	Extremities	A	Anal bleeding-buttocks/prostate
N	Neurological	M	Musculoskeletal-muscles and joints
Psychiatric			

Always remember that the key here is to do a **FOCUSED** physical examination, as Step 2 CS is a **timed** exam. You are not only tested on your clinical skills, but you also have the additional burden of proving yourself in a limited time. Hence, this checklist will come in handy to help you remember the core-areas you must touch upon.

It is only your clinical judgment which will help you decide the **primary system** that you will like to thoroughly examine for a particular case. Information gathered from the doorway information as well as the history-taking will be enough for you to make a clear decision on this.

Before performing the physical examination:

1. CONSENT: Always take the patient's permission before performing any maneuver, or even before touching the patient.

2. WEARING GLOVES or WASHING HANDS?
Always remember: the first rule is 'DO NO HARM,' so wash hands with soap and water, dry them, and warm them up before touching the patient; or you could wear gloves. It is recommended that you wear gloves because:

a. It helps save crucial time during a timed patient encounter
b. It protects not only the PATIENT, but also the DOCTOR from unwanted infections, especially if you have paper cuts or open sores on hands

While performing the physical examination:

- ✓ Don't stop engaging the patient. Continue talking to the patient and explaining to them the why-how-what of the tests you are performing. Appreciate their patience.

"Now let us take a good look at the rest of your belly... *(pause)*... I see no abnormal veins... *(pause)*... no swellings... *(pause)*... no stretch marks... (pause)... no scars or discolorations..."

"Now I am going to listen to your bowel sounds... *(pause and listen)*... I hear good bowel sounds... *(pause)*... Now I am listening for any squish or bruit in your major arteries..."

- ✓ Be gentle. Don't perform unnecessary examinations. Don't repeat painful maneuvers.

After performing a physical examination:

NEVER LIE ON THE PATIENT NOTE. Never mention tests you did not perform or findings you did not obtain. Falsification of records may mean failure in the exam.

Physical examination explained:

Let's explore each of the above mentioned sub-headings:

General Examination:

- ✓ Assess the general state of the patient.
- ✓ Pick up the patient's most apparent emotion and mention it in the patient note (e.g. in acute distress/ cheerful/ anxious/ angry/ sad/ flat faced).
- ✓ Assess the patient's level of consciousness and orientation to time, place, person, and situation. (Remember it is no more AO X 3, instead it is AO X 4; Alert & Oriented X 4)
- ✓ Assess the patient's level of comfort in the surroundings and general appearance (tidy/unkempt).
- ✓ Notice the posture of the patient (decubitus).
- ✓ Pick up gross abnormalities, swellings, or malnutrition (under nutrition/obesity) in the patient. Malnutrition can be assessed not only from the build of the patient but also from hair. Nails can reveal a number of abnormalities as well, as mentioned elsewhere in this book.
- ✓ Assess for presence of anemia/ cyanosis/ jaundice/ edema in the patient.

How to report in a patient note:

"Cheerful, alert, and oriented to time, place, person, and situation, obese."
"Sad, AO X 4, of average build, with poor personal hygiene."
"Patient is in no acute distress, looks sad, AO X 4."
"Patient is in no acute distress, but looks tired. Has a flat affect, speaks and moves slowly."

Heart: Cardiovascular Examination:

- ✓ Since the vital signs are already provided in the doorway information, it is pertinent to assume they are correct.
- ✓ However, if you believe that this case requires a thorough cardiovascular examination, make sure you take the pulse, as well as the blood pressure yourself. Mention all qualities of the pulse in the patient note if you have taken it. Take blood pressure in both lying down and standing position.
- ✓ If you believe that time is not on your side when you begin your physical examination, but feel that a more detailed analysis of pulse and blood pressure is required, then you can mention this in the patient note (**postural vital signs/orthostatics**).
- ✓ At all times (including for the patient note) assume that the vital signs mentioned in the doorway information are correct (even if you find different values when you check the vital signs during the patient encounter yourself).

Pulse:

Notice the rate, rhythm, volume, condition of the artery wall, and any special character of the pulse. Compare the bilateral pulses. If you suspect, look for the presence of radio-femoral delay. (Remember: the key here is to do a focused examination in a limited amount of time; hence, be specific about these details only if you have ample time and are aiming for a high level of performance). Look for the presence of all peripheral pulses and compare them bilaterally. Check the radial, carotid, femoral, popliteal, posterior tibial, and dorsalis pedis artery.

Blood Pressure/Postural Vital Signs/Orthostatics

Neck Veins:
Assess whether neck veins are engorged or not. Asses for the hepato-jugular reflex and JVD.

Heart:

Look: Look at the precordium and back; shape of precordium (any deformity/bulging), apical impulse, superficial engorged veins, any abnormal pulsations, and/or scar marks of previous surgery or trauma.

Listen: Cardiac rate, rhythm; listen for heart sounds and adventitious sounds (murmurs/rubs/gallops). Listen in the mitral area, tricuspid area, aortic area, and pulmonary area.

Feel/Touch/Palpate: Feel for an apex beat or any thrill.

Carotid Artery: Auscultate for bruit after asking the patient to hold their breath. Never obstruct both the carotid arteries at once.

Renal Artery: Auscultate for bruit.

Pedal Edema: Check bilaterally for pitting or non-pitting pedal edema.

How to report your findings in a patient note:

Pulse and BP are reported with the vital signs.
If you want to elaborate on the characteristics of the pulse (regular, low volume, no radio-radial delay, no special character, no abnormality in arterial wall, all peripheral pulses palpable) then you can add it with the pulse rate in vital signs, or mention it separately under the cardiovascular system on the patient note.

"S1, S2 heard. No murmurs, rubs, or gallops. JVP not raised. No carotid or renal bruit. No pedal edema."
"S1 S2 +, No murmurs/rubs/gallops."
"Apical impulse not displaced. RRR. Normal S1/S2. No murmurs, rubs, or gallops."

Abdomen

Remember to:

- ✓ **Look** (Inspection)- Examine for scars, sinuses, bruises and/or rashes (Grey Turner's sign in pancreatitis), abnormal distension or masses, distended veins, etc.
- ✓ **Listen** (Auscultation)- Listen for bruits and bowel sounds.
- ✓ **Feel/Touch** (Palpation)- Light touch followed by deep palpation to look for abnormal masses and hepatosplenomegaly.
- ✓ **Tap** (Percussion)- Tap to differentiate gaseous distension from solid masses and fluid in the peritoneal cavity (ascites).
- ✓ **Special Tests**- In certain clinical scenarios, some special tests may be required. One must always remember to inform the patient about these tests, their procedures, and the reason for performing them. For example: Murphy's sign for right upper quadrant pain, CVA tenderness in case of flank pain, rebound tenderness, Rovsing's sign and psoas sign for right lower quadrant pain.

Never do any test aggressively in order to get a result, as you may compromise the patient's comfort and may worsen his/her pain.

How to report your findings in a patient note:

"Soft and non-tender. BS +. No hepatosplenomegaly. No evidence of ascites."

"Soft, non-distended, C-section scar present. Mild RUQ tenderness. No rebound tenderness or guarding. Murphy's –ve, BS +ve, no organomegaly or masses. No ascites."

"Soft, non-distended, non-tender abdomen, BS are heard, No hepatosplenomegaly. Mild right CVA tenderness present."

> Action Box:
> Why is auscultation done before palpation of the abdomen?
>
> Gaseous distension of various parts of the bowel remains relatively static in the supine position.
> If palpation is done before the auscultation, this could stimulate peristalsis and lead to fallacious results on the exam.
>
> When you are examining the abdomen, have a systematic approach. Though it does not depend where you stand, it is always advisable to pick one side of the patient. This will enable you to develop your approach and never miss anything. For example, if you stand on the right, start with palpation of the right upper quadrant, then move up to the epigastrium followed by left upper quadrant. Next, move to left lower quadrant, followed by the right lower quadrant, ending at the umbilicus. Make sure you also perform bimanual palpation of the kidneys to check for ballotability and renal angle tenderness.
>
> During this process, it is of paramount importance that you keep informing the patient about the region/organ you are currently palpating, so that he is aware of the anatomy and also feels a sense of satisfaction that the whole of his abdomen was examined by the physician in detail.
>
> If the patient has a pain in the right lower quadrant, always start examination in the opposite quadrant, considering the patient's discomfort.

Lungs (Respiratory System)

Make sure you do the respiratory examination in sitting position.

Upper Respiratory Tract:

- ✓ Assess the nose (congestion, discharge, hypertrophied turbinate, polyps, nasal septum deviation).

- ✓ Assess the sinuses (examine for presence of frontal or maxillary sinus tenderness). Pharynx can either be assessed here or along with HEENT examination.

Lower Respiratory Tract (Chest)

Inspection- Assess the respiration (Assume the rate given in the doorway information is correct.

- Assess the rhythm, type, depth, and breathing pattern of the respiration).
- Observe for abnormal respiration, bilateral chest movements, scars, sinuses, and rashes.
- Look for tracheal deviation, supraclavicular hollowing, intercostal retraction, crowding of ribs, or change in the shape of chest wall (barrel shaped chest in COPD, vertebral anomalies leading to restrictive pattern disease).
- Assess the use of the accessory muscles of respiration.

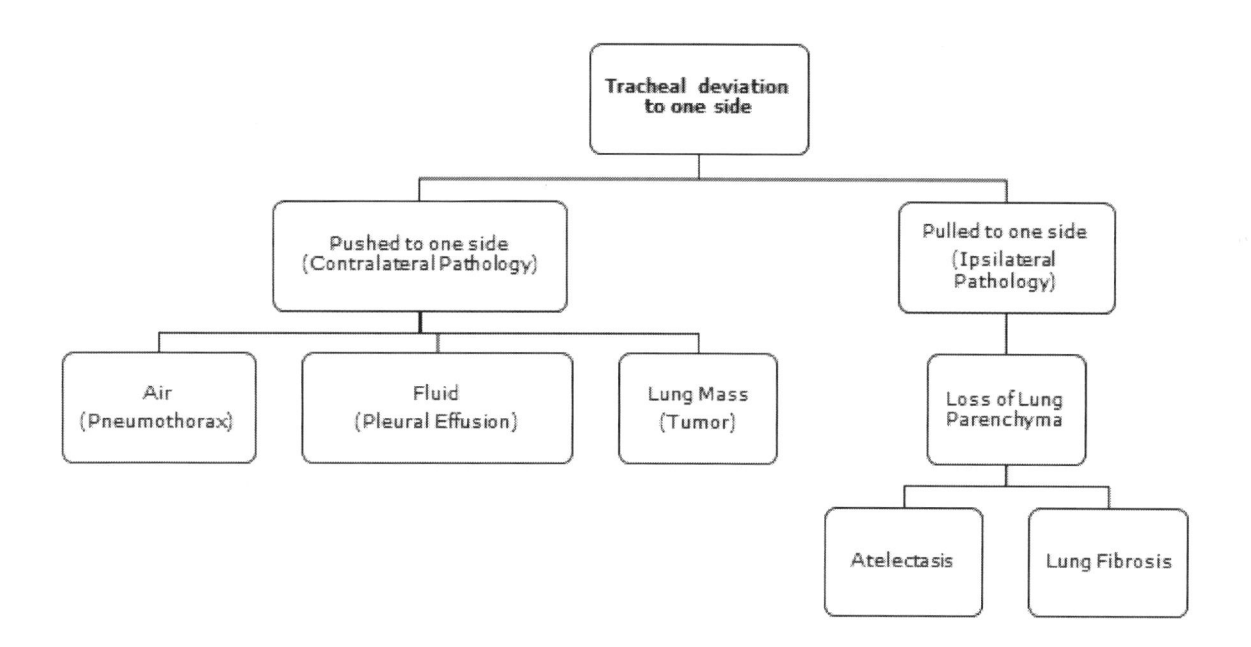

```
                    Tracheal deviation
                       to one side
                            |
            ┌───────────────┴───────────────┐
   Pushed to one side              Pulled to one side
   (Contralateral Pathology)       (Ipsilateral Pathology)
            |                               |
   ┌────────┼────────┐                Loss of Lung
   Air    Fluid    Lung Mass          Parenchyma
(Pneumothorax) (Pleural Effusion) (Tumor)    |
                                    ┌────────┴────────┐
                                 Atelectasis      Lung Fibrosis
```

Auscultation:

- Auscultate bilaterally for breath sounds and identify any adventitious sounds (rhonchi, crepitation, pleural rub and wheeze).
- Assess for vocal resonance, whether it is increased or decreased.
- Listen for whispered pectoriloquy and egophony.

> **Action Box:**
> Mechanism of whispered pectoriloquy- Ask the patient to whisper a few words while you auscultate various parts of his lungs. In case of consolidation, the sound will appear magnified as sound travels faster through fluids and solids as compared to air.

Mechanism of Egophony :

On auscultation:

- ✓ <u>Clear lung field:</u> You will hear an unchanged sound (i.e. the articulated sound is heard clearly).
- ✓ <u>Consolidation:</u> The patient's spoken 'E' is heard like an 'A'. This is because the solid mass will disproportionately dampen the higher acoustic overtones more than the others. This is referred to as **"E to A transition."**

"When E becomes A, its pneumonia."

Which words should you ask the patient to articulate?

Using the phrase **'blue balloons'** has been found to be more effective than asking the patient to articulate 'ninety-nine'

Palpation:

- ✓ Palpate for surface temperature, tenderness, and position of trachea.
- ✓ Measure chest expansion and assess chest movement bilaterally.

Percussion:

- ✓ Percuss bilaterally.
- ✓ Assess hepatic and cardiac dullness.

Why is percussion important? It tells us the consistency of the tissues by the quality of reflected sound and palpable vibrations.

How is this done?

- ✓ Place the volar aspect of the middle finger firmly on the chest and tap with the other hand's middle finger.
- ✓ Listen and feel the vibrations.

What does it indicate? A loud resonating sound (hyperresonant) indicates air between the pleura (pneumothorax) and tympanic in case of hyperinflation of lungs in COPD.

A dull non resonating sound suggests consolidation of the lung parenchyma (pneumonia) or a solid mass lesion.

A stony dull sound usually suggests fluid between the pleura (pleural effusion/empyema). The tapping sound is not reflected back as it is dispersed by the multiple solid-liquid interfaces that it travels through on percussion; therefore, it lacks the resonating quality.

Where should the percussion be done?

- ✓ Anteriorly- Midclavicular line; from top to bottom.
- ✓ Posteriorly- Interscapular region bilaterally.
- ✓ Never do this on the scapula.
- ✓ Axillary region.

Vocal and Tactile Fremitus:

Vocal fremitus gives us an idea of any abnormality in the chest. It works on the same principle as an ultrasound, except that we feel and listen to the sound generated by the patient.

When we palpate or listen to various regions of the chest, we ask the patient to speak diphthong words. Diphthongs are words formed by combining two vowels, specifically when they start as one vowel sound and go to another, creating a resonating high frequency sound (e.g. blue moon, ninety nine, etc.).

'Ninety nine' is very commonly used while testing for vocal fremitus, however, it is a low frequency diphthong and is not as sensitive as other high frequency diphthongs (blue balloons, blue moons, Scooby-doo). It is, therefore, suggested to use high frequency diphthongs for a better examination experience and result.

> **Action Box:**
> Sound travels faster in :
> Solids >> Liquids >> Gas
> In Pneumonia - Tactile Fremitus (TF)/Vocal Fremitus (VF) *increases* due to consolidation of lung parenchyma.
> In Pleural Effusion - Tactile Fremitus (TF)/Vocal Fremitus (VF) *decreases* due to an additional liquid interface.

How to report your findings in a patient note:

"B/L CTA, no wheezing, no rales." (B/L = bilateral, CTA= clear to auscultation)

"Clear breath sounds bilaterally."

"B/L CTA, no adventitious sounds."

"Two large bruises on right chest, right sided tenderness over the ribs, decreased breath sounds over all of right lung field, left lung fields clear with no adventitious sounds."

Extremities:

This must involve a thorough examination of all peripheral pulses, along with the extremity examination. However, in a clinical skills exam, avoid palpating femoral pulses in order to respect the patient's privacy by exposing minimum body surface.

Always document edema and varicose veins. Pay close attention to any hair loss, as this could indicate peripheral vascular disease. Also document any scars, sinuses, or rashes. Make sure to note any changes on the skin of a diabetic patient. You can consecutively perform a quick neurological examination of the extremities to evaluate for neuropathy.

How to report your findings in a patient note:

"Tremor seen on outstretched fingertips."

"No edema, peripheral pulses 2+ and symmetric."

"No asterixis, no edema."

"Inspection: Right calf red, swollen as compared to left; muscle contours normal; no ulcers, sinuses, bruises, or pigmentation. Palpation: Right leg is warmer compared to left; pitting pedal edema present on the right side; dorsalis pedis pulse felt and equal on both sides; range of motion WNL at ankle joint, knee, and hip joint; Homans' sign positive on right side. Sensations intact to pin prick and soft touch."

"Extremities- Pulses: posterior tibialis and dorsalis pedis 2+ bilaterally. Position: bilateral feet held in pronation. Mobility: normal at hip, knee, ankle, and foot joints. Tender to palpation over medial calcaneal tuberosity and plantar fascia. On passive extension of toes, plantar heel and arch pain +. Sensations intact to pin prick and soft touch. DTR: intact."

"No clubbing, cyanosis, or edema."

"On palpation, diffuse tenderness over middle and upper right arm and right shoulder; pain and restricted ROM on flexion, extension, abduction, and external rotation of right shoulder. ROM at right elbow and wrist normal.

"Pulses: 2+ & symmetric in brachial and radial arteries. Unable to assess muscle strength due to pain. DTRs intact and symmetric. Sensation intact to pinprick and soft touch."

Neurological Examination:

Higher Function: Conscious, Cooperative

Alert and oriented to time, place, person, and situation (AO X 4)

- ✓ Q: "Mr. Doe, Can you please tell me where you are now? What is the time? What is the date? Can you tell me who am I? What is the purpose of your visit?"

Emotional state:

- ✓ Sad, anxious, angry, euphoric, hostile
- ✓ Observe the emotional state, as this will be helpful to empathize.

Memory:

Always be very observant of the patient's activities. Is this patient coming with a family member (which might reflect dementia)? Always ask one question that will differentiate the short term memory loss from the long term memory loss.

"Mr. Joe, can you repeat these three words after me, '**A pen, a table, and a chair.**' I want you to remember these words, as I will ask you to repeat these words at the end of the examination as well."

- ✓ Q: What did you eat this morning?
- ✓ Q: What is your date of birth?

If the patient is forgetful and has short term memory loss, always question him/her about activities of daily living (who cooks food, buys groceries, does laundry, etc.), as this could shed light on the patient's functionality. These patients may have Alzheimer's dementia, so paying close attention to who is handling the financial aspect is also a key consideration.

Cognition:

"Can you spell "WORLD" backwards for me?" or "Can you subtract 7 from 100 backwards (100-7=93, 86, 79, etc.)" Keep going until the patient reaches 65. Document it as "Serial 7's," intact or not intact.

- ✓ Speech
- ✓ Handedness

> **Action Box:**
> Sometimes it becomes imperative to differentiate between true dementia and pseudo-dementia, which is often seen in depressed patients. In true dementia, patients are unaware of their memory loss and can be combative when someone tells them that something is wrong (anosognosia). They are often brought to the hospital by their loved ones/family.
>
> In pseudo-dementia, patients are usually aware that they are forgetting things, and will come themselves to the hospital complaining of memory loss.

Cranium and Spine

Neck: Rigidity, Kernig's sign, Brudzinski's sign, straight leg raising test.

Cranial Nerves:

Olfactory Nerve examination is usually skipped

A. **Optic:** Visual acuity, field of vision (confrontation perimetry)

B. **Oculomotor, Trochlear, and Abducens**: Assess the extraocular muscles and their movement. Look for nystagmus and ptosis. Compare bilateral pupils (size, shape). **Do the light reflex, consensual light reflex, and accommodation reflex.**

C. **Trigeminal**: For motor function, check the muscles of mastication (masseter, pterygoids, and temporalis). For sensory function, check the sensations over the face. We usually avoid the corneal reflex. **Jaw jerk** can be performed.

D. **Facial**: Showing the teeth, blowing, whistling, eye closure, comparison of angle of mouth on both sides, comparison of nasolabial folds, drooling of saliva from angle of mouth. Check the taste sensation on anterior 2/3rd of tongue (can be skipped during step 2 CS exam). Make sure you assess whether the upper half of the face is escaped or not. This will help differentiate between UMN and LMN facial nerve palsy. **(Remember the upper face escapes in upper motor neuron palsy)**

E. **Vestibulocochlear**: Assess the patient's hearing. Do Weber's test and Rinne's test.

F. **Glossopharyngeal and Vagus Nerve**: Look at movements of soft palate on saying 'aah.' Avoid gag reflex with standardized patients.

G. **Spinal Accessory**: Shrugging of the shoulder against resistance to check the power of trapezius. Turning the chin to the opposite side against resistance to check for the power of individual sternomastoid muscle. The muscle on the opposite side of the chin movement becomes prominent.

H. **Hypoglossal**: Deviation of the tongue on protrusion (deviates towards the paralyzed side as the healthy genioglossus pushes the tongue to the paralyzed side). Any atrophy or fasciculations.

Motor Examination:

Compare bilaterally for nutrition, tone, power, coordination, and involuntary movements.

Sensory Examination:

A. **Superficial sensations:** Pain and touch (temperature can be avoided in Step 2 CS examination). Pins and cotton are provided during the examination.

B. **Deep or proprioceptive:** Vibration sense can be assessed by using tuning forks provided during the step 2 CS exam in the patient encounter room. Position sense can also be performed.

C. **Cortical:** Stereognosis and graphesthesia can be assessed. For sterenognosis, ask the patient to close his eyes and hand him a pen, pencil, toothpick, or a knee hammer and ask him to recognize the object. Ideally a key or a coin is used in a physical examination, but they are not allowed in the Step 2 CS exam. You can utilize whatever is present in the room.

For graphesthesia, you can draw using the blunt side of a pen on the palm of the patient and ask them if they can recognize the design.

Reflexes:

A. **Superficial: Abdominal reflex and plantar reflex.** Don't perform cremasteric reflex in Step 2 CS exam.

B. **DTRs:** Biceps, triceps, knee, ankle.

C. **Cerebellar functions:** Intention tremor, finger-nose test, dysdiadochokinesia.

D. **Autonomic system examination:** Abnormal sweating, postural hypotension.

E. **Gait** examination and **Romberg's** test

How to report your findings in a patient note:

"Mental status: AO × 4, spells backward but can't recall 3 objects. No neck rigidity. Cranial nerves: 2-12 intact. Motor: Strength 5/5 in all muscle groups except 3/5 in left arm. Sensation: Intact to pinprick and soft touch. DTRs: 3+ in left upper and lower extremities, 1+ in the right, Babinski –ve bilaterally. Cerebellar: no abnormalities. Gait: normal. Romberg: -ve."

"AO X 4, memory intact. Motor: Strength 5/5 in bilateral lower extremities. Sensation: Decreased pinprick; soft touch, vibratory, and position sense in bilateral lower extremities. DTRs: Symmetric 2+ knee jerks, absent ankle jerks. Babinski –ve bilaterally."

*(Notice that in the above patient note excerpt, the examinee has deliberately not mentioned the cranial nerve examination or upper extremity examination. The examinee may not have had time to perform a thorough examination, but nevertheless performed a focused and essential examination. This examinee will not lose out on the score because: **the examinee did not skip the essential exam**. Also the examinee did not lie in the patient note!)*

Glands

- ✓ Check the thyroid gland for any swelling. Do other tests for thyroid abnormalities:
- ✓ Palpation of thyroid gland in the beginning should always be done from behind by using both hands. Ask the patient to slightly flex the neck. Place your thumbs at the nape of the neck. Note the size, shape, surface, and mobility (Ask the patient to swallow by offering a glass of water).
- ✓ This can be followed by palpation from the front using the Lahey's method.
- ✓ Check for signs of hyperthyroidism, including the ophthalmopathy and cardiovascular signs. Assess for presence of Pemberton's sign (Retrosternal goitre can obstruct the venous

outflow of the head causing congestion of the face when the patient is asked to raise their hands above their head).
- ✓ Auscultate for a thyroid bruit.
- ✓ Look for tonsillar hypertrophy.
- ✓ Check other glands (parotid, submandibular, etc.)

> **Action Box:**
> **Thyroid Bruit:** more prominent in the upper part of the neck (superior thyroid artery arises from external carotid artery)
> **Carotid Bruit:** more prominent over the lower part of the neck (over common carotid artery)
> **Venous Hum:** disappears on pressing with the bell of a stethoscope

HEENT Examination:

Head: Look and palpate for signs of trauma, hydrocephalus, etc. Palpate the sinuses and temporomandibular joints. Transillumination of sinuses may be done if they are tender (dim the light of the room first).

Eye: Assess for color of conjunctiva and sclera, look for nystagmus, and perform a fundoscopic exam. Assess the extraocular muscles. Do light reflex and accommodation reflex and compare the pupils of both eyes.

Ear: Perform external examination by inspection and palpation, then follow with an otoscopy. Assess hearing. Do Rinne's test and Weber's Test. Use a different disposable specula at the end of the otoscope for each ear.

Nose: Inspect the nose. Look at the color of the mucosa, determine the presence of any discharge (color of discharge if present), examine the middle and inferior turbinates, and look for the presence of polyps.

Throat/Neck: Inspect the mouth, teeth, and throat. Assess the soft palate, hard palate, tonsils, and uvula. Look for any pharyngeal erythema, pooling of discharges, inflammation, etc. Look and palpate for cervical lymphadenopathy. Look for thyroid enlargement or any other swellings (midline neck swellings/lateral neck swellings). Assess the carotid and thyroid bruit. Make sure to press on only one carotid artery at a time.

How to report your findings in a patient note:

"Sclera, conjunctiva normal. PERRLA. Nasal turbinates erythematous but not hypertrophied. Oral cavity examination unremarkable. Mucosa moist. Oropharynx examination shows 3+ tonsillar hypertrophy bilaterally. No pooling of secretions in the posterior oropharynx and no post-nasal drip. Left ear examination shows normal external auditory meatus, TM with positive Light Reflex, landmarks clearly visible. No discharge was noted. Right ear examination shows normal external auditory meatus, TM with positive Light Reflex, landmarks clearly visible. No discharge."

"PERRLA, no funduscopic abnormalities."

"NC/AT, non-tender to palpation, PERRLA, EOMI, no papilledema, no nasal congestion, no pharyngeal erythema or exudates, dentition good.
(Here NC/AT: Normocephalic, atraumatic.
PERRLA: Pupils equal, round, reactive to light and accommodation.
EOMI: Extraocular movements intact/extraocular muscles intact)

"NC/AT, PERRLA, EOMI, no nystagmus, no papilledema, no cerumen bilaterally, TMs normal, mouth and oropharynx normal."

"No conjunctival pallor, mouth and pharynx WNL."

"NC/AT, PERRLA, EOMI, no nystagmus, no papilledema, cerumen not seen. TMs with light reflex, no stigmata of infection, no erythema or tenderness of auricle, preauricular, or external auditory meatus. No lymphadenopathy, oropharynx normal. Weber test revealed no lateralization; Rinne test is positive (revealed air conduction > bone conduction)."

Urogenital Examination:

- ✓ Urogenital examination is **NOT** to be done in the Step 2 CS examination on standardized patients.
- ✓ However, you must mention the need to perform a urogenital examination in case the chief complaint or history warrants a need to do so. You must mention this to the patient during the closure, as well as in the patient note under the work up plan (along with further examinations and investigations).

How to report your findings in a patient note:

REPORT UNDER DIAGNOSTIC WORK-UP HEADING:
"Urogenital Examination"
"Pelvic Examination"

Lymph Nodes

Palpate the lymph node groups and assess:

✓ Size: Determine whether lymphadenopathy is significant or not:

Insignificant if < 2cm enlargement
In axilla and inguinal area, insignificant if < 3cm
For cervical lymphadenopathy and in the supraclavicular fossa > 1cm is significant

✓ Consistency: It may be soft/rubber/hard/etc. A rubbery lymph node suggests lymphoma. A hard lymph node suggests malignancy.

Tenderness: Suggests inflammation.
Matting

Lymphadenopathy can be termed as generalized when there is enlargement of more than two non-contiguous lymph node groups.

How to report in a patient note:
You can mention the state of lymph nodes either with HEENT or neck or in the general physical examination:

"Neck: No lymphadenopathy, thyroid gland is normal."

"HEENT: No lymphadenopathy."

Rectal Examination

✓ Prostate/rectal examination is **NOT** to be done in the Step 2 CS examination on standardized patients.
✓ However, you must mention the need to perform prostate examination in case the chief complaint or history warrants a need to do so. You must mention this to the patient during the closure, as well as in the patient note under the work up plan (along with further examinations and investigations).

How to report your findings in a patient note:

REPORT UNDER DIAGNOSTIC WORK-UP HEADING:

"Prostate Examination"
"Digital Rectal Examination"
"Proctoscopy/Sigmoidoscopy"

Musculoskeletal Examination

The musculoskeletal or the locomotor system examination comprises of examination of the muscles, bones, joints, and soft tissue structures (e.g. ligaments and tendons).

Inspection:

- ✓ Joint or joints involved (monoarticular/pauciarticular/polyarticular)
- ✓ Attitude of the limb
- ✓ Presence of any swelling
- ✓ Presence of any deformities and whether these are reducible
- ✓ Signs of inflammation (rubor, calor, dolor, tumor, functio lesia)
- ✓ Compare muscles bilaterally
- ✓ Presence of any skin changes (pigmentation/ulcers/sinuses/scars)

Palpation:

- ✓ Surface temperature
- ✓ Tenderness
- ✓ Palpation of swelling for consistency, fluctuation
- ✓ Crepitus

Special tests have been explained in detail in the chapter on approach to joints and extremities.

Muscle power and movements:

Restriction of movements or excessive mobility; any pain on movement, any muscular spasms

Grade the muscle power on a scale of 0 to 5 for each limb.

Grade 0: Complete paralysis
Grade 1: Only a flicker of contraction is present
Grade 2: Active movement with gravity eliminated
Grade 3: Active movement against gravity present
Grade 4: Active movement against gravity and against some resistance
Grade 5: Normal power

Measurements:

Compare the length, as well as circumference, of the limbs. Since time is a major constraint in the clinical skill examination, it is advisable to measure the dimensions of the limbs only if gross difference is visible.

How to report your findings in a patient note:

"Inspection: Right calf red, swollen as compared to left; muscle contours normal; no ulcers, sinuses, bruises, or pigmentation. Palpation: Right leg is warmer compared to left; pitting pedal edema present on right side; dorsalis pedis pulse felt and equal on both sides; Range of motion WNL at ankle joint, knee, and hip joint; Homans' sign positive on right side. Sensations intact to pin prick and soft touch."

Skin Examination

- ✓ Finally, examine the skin of the patient. Look for any scar marks (previous trauma/surgeries), discoloration, pigmentation disorders, keloids, or peculiar findings (café au lait spots, melisma, linea nigra). Always measure the scar.
- ✓ Examination of hair and nails can be performed and mentioned under this heading as well.
- ✓ In psychiatric examination, timing of the onset of the patients symptoms is the key. Be vigilant about the time of onset and duration of symptoms.

Psychiatric history taking and examination:

- ✓ Ensure that you evaluate for the presence of any psychiatric disorders. Comment about the presence of any particular facies, anxiety, stigmata of depression (D.I.G.E.S.T P C.A.Psule), schizophrenia, or OCD. Ask the patient about any recent stressor in life that might be troubling them.
- ✓ Psychiatric history has been re-emphasized here in the examination section so that you do not miss out on this integral component.

Action Box:

If you suspect that the patient might be suffering from depression, always ask them about their mood, "Are you sad?" "Have you been sad for most of the days in the last 14 days/2weeks?"

If the patient says 'Yes,' follow it up with a questionnaire covering all components of

D.I.G.E.S.T P. C.A.Psule.

D-Depression
I-Insomnia
G-Guilt
E-Energy loss
S-Suicide ideation
T-Time period more than 2 weeks
P-Pleasure loss/Anhedonia
C-Concentration
A-Appetite
P-Psychomotor retardation (Flat affect)

NOTES -

Section D

Approach to Common Cases

Section D - Approach to Common Cases

Approach to Abdominal Case

In this chapter, we are going to learn how to approach a case of a patient with abdominal complaints and how to reach a quick differential diagnosis.

It is crucial for physicians to ask all the relevant questions regarding the patients' clinical scenario. This starts right before entering the examination room and goes up to the time the physician leaves the room.

Based on doorway information

The doorway information will mention the chief concern that brought the patient to the hospital, along with the patient's vital signs. Make a note of the vital signs in your patient note. If they are abnormal, you should not take it for granted.

As you scroll through the information, you will realize it is probably a gastrointestinal case.
It can be made easy by imagining the following.

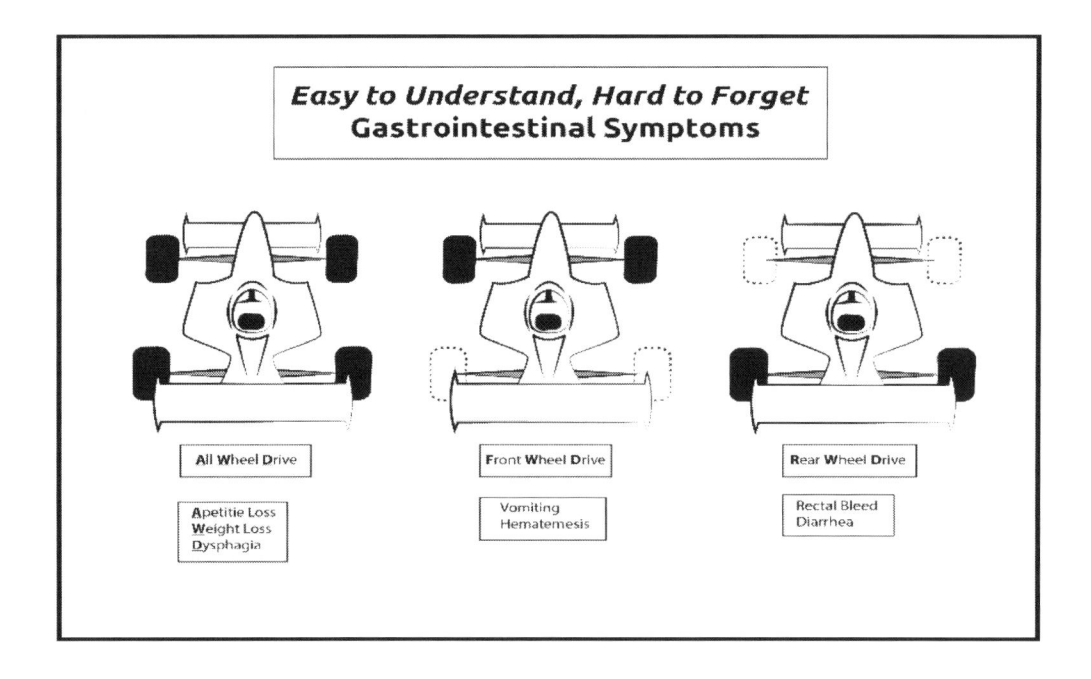

Easy to Understand, Hard to Forget Gastrointestinal Symptoms

All Wheel Drive	Front Wheel Drive	Rear Wheel Drive
Apetitie Loss, Weight Loss, Dysphagia	Vomiting, Hematemesis	Rectal Bleed, Diarrhea

All-<u>W</u>heel <u>D</u>rive	Front-Wheel Drive	Rear-Wheel Drive	Other Symptoms
A-Abdominal pain A-Appetite gain or loss A-Anorexia	Reflux and Halitosis	Diarrhea	Itching (Cholestasis)
W- Weight loss	Vomiting	Bleeding PR	Jaundice
D- Dysphagia	Hematemesis	Constipation	Abdominal Mass

Figure: Here we have used an analogy of all-wheel drive, front-wheel drive, and rear-wheel drive cars. This will help you to memorize what to ask from the patient when you have limited time.

Based on history and examination

A step-by-step approach is prudent for organizing all of the symptoms and generating a good list for the differential diagnosis.

Let us begin with the most common symptom.

Abdominal Pain

Take a generic history with 'Life isn't Good, Doctor Aid @ PM;' however, pay close attention to these aspects--quadrant, quality, and the associated factors.

- ✓ **Quadrant (Location)** - First, determine the location of the abdominal pain. This also helps to narrow down the list of suspected organs involved based on anatomic location.
- ✓ **Quality** – Assess the quality and nature of the pain (dull, sharp, or colicky?)
- ✓ **Other characteristics of the pain** – Radiation, duration, and aggravating and relieving factors.
- ✓ **Associated symptoms-** Is the pain associated with other symptoms like diarrhea, vomiting, abdominal mass, jaundice, bleeding, etc.?
- ✓ **Arriving at the differential diagnosis-** The information collected determines how we arrive at a differential.

Funnel Approach

(Start with all the information and narrow down to a specific differential diagnosis)

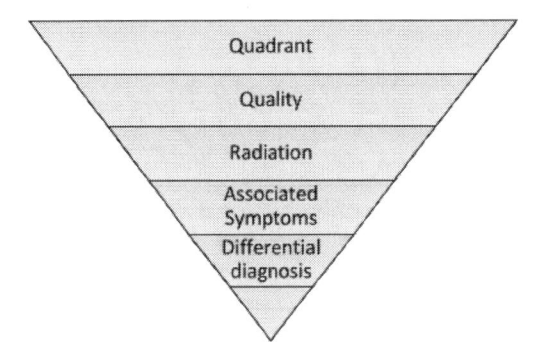

```
         Quadrant
         Quality
         Radiation
         Associated
         Symptoms
         Differential
         diagnosis
```

STEP 1: Find out: Quadrant/Location of the pain:

Ask the patient:

- ✓ Q. "Can you point with your finger to the exact location of the pain?"
- ✓ Q. "Can you tell me where the pain is the worst?"

The patient may not use one finger to point out the location of the pain. He/she might use his/her hand to describe this pain. Why is this important? It indicates diffuse pain that might reflect peritoneal irritation.

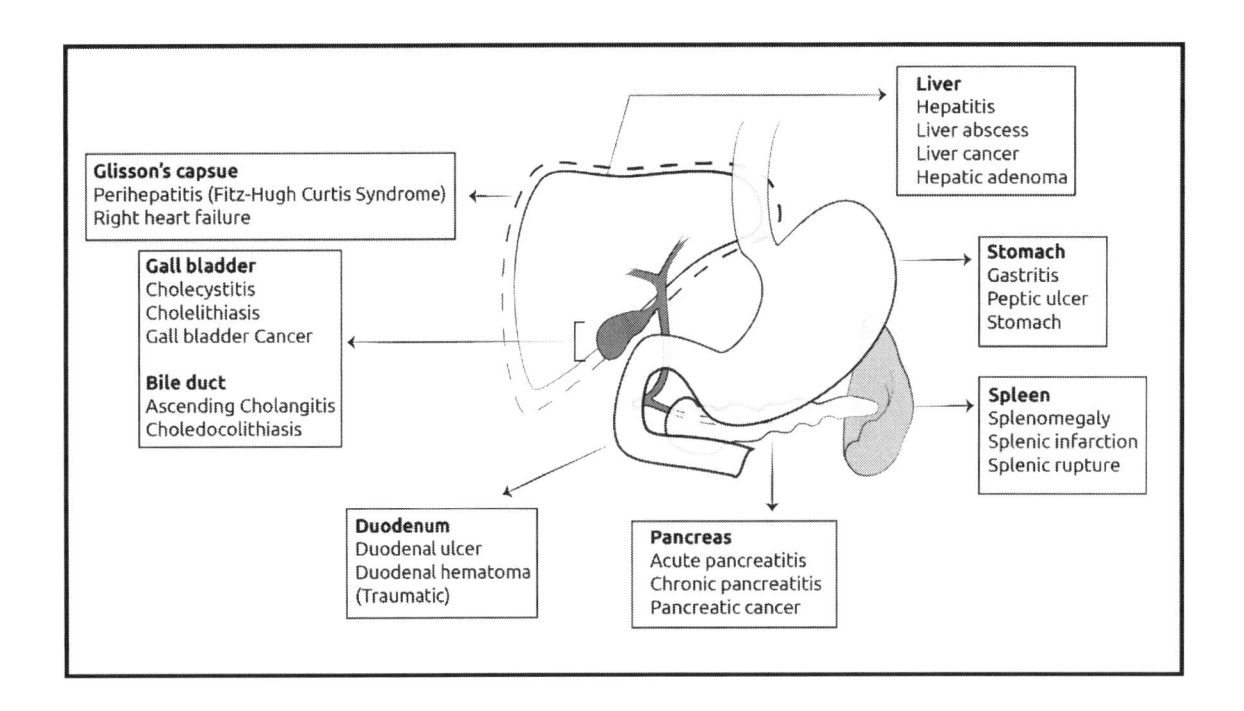

Glisson's capsue
Perihepatitis (Fitz-Hugh Curtis Syndrome)
Right heart failure

Gall bladder
Cholecystitis
Cholelithiasis
Gall bladder Cancer

Bile duct
Ascending Cholangitis
Choledocolithiasis

Duodenum
Duodenal ulcer
Duodenal hematoma
(Traumatic)

Pancreas
Acute pancreatitis
Chronic pancreatitis
Pancreatic cancer

Liver
Hepatitis
Liver abscess
Liver cancer
Hepatic adenoma

Stomach
Gastritis
Peptic ulcer
Stomach

Spleen
Splenomegaly
Splenic infarction
Splenic rupture

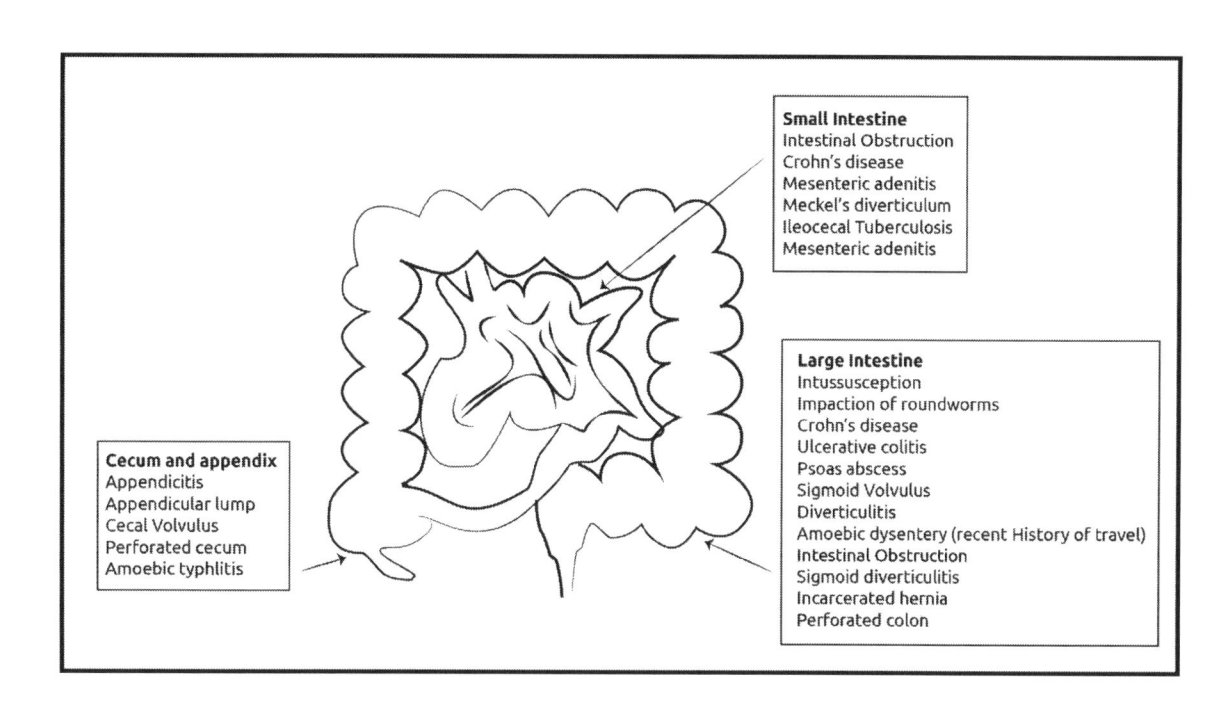

Small Intestine
Intestinal Obstruction
Crohn's disease
Mesenteric adenitis
Meckel's diverticulum
Ileocecal Tuberculosis
Mesenteric adenitis

Large Intestine
Intussusception
Impaction of roundworms
Crohn's disease
Ulcerative colitis
Psoas abscess
Sigmoid Volvulus
Diverticulitis
Amoebic dysentery (recent History of travel)
Intestinal Obstruction
Sigmoid diverticulitis
Incarcerated hernia
Perforated colon

Cecum and appendix
Appendicitis
Appendicular lump
Cecal Volvulus
Perforated cecum
Amoebic typhlitis

Organs Located In Various Quadrants

Right Upper Quadrant (RUQ):
- ✓ Liver
- ✓ Gall bladder
- ✓ Duodenum and other parts of small intestine
- ✓ Pylorus of stomach
- ✓ Right kidney
- ✓ Hepatic flexure of the colon
- ✓ Part of ascending colon
- ✓ Part of the transverse colon
- ✓ Head of the pancreas
- ✓ Right adrenal gland

Left Upper Quadrant (LUQ):
- ✓ Liver: tip of the medial lobe
- ✓ Spleen
- ✓ Stomach
- ✓ Left kidney
- ✓ Pancreas (Body)
- ✓ Splenic flexure of the colon
- ✓ Part of transverse colon
- ✓ Part of descending colon
- ✓ Small Intestine
- ✓ Left adrenal gland

Right Lower Quadrant (RLQ):
- ✓ Small Intestine
- ✓ Appendix
- ✓ Cecum
- ✓ Ascending colon
- ✓ Bladder
- ✓ Right ovary
- ✓ Uterus if enlarged
- ✓ Right spermatic cord
- ✓ Right ureter

Left Lower Quadrant (LLQ):
- ✓ Small Intestine
- ✓ Sigmoid colon
- ✓ Descending colon
- ✓ Bladder
- ✓ Left ovary
- ✓ Uterus
- ✓ Left spermatic cord
- ✓ Left ureter

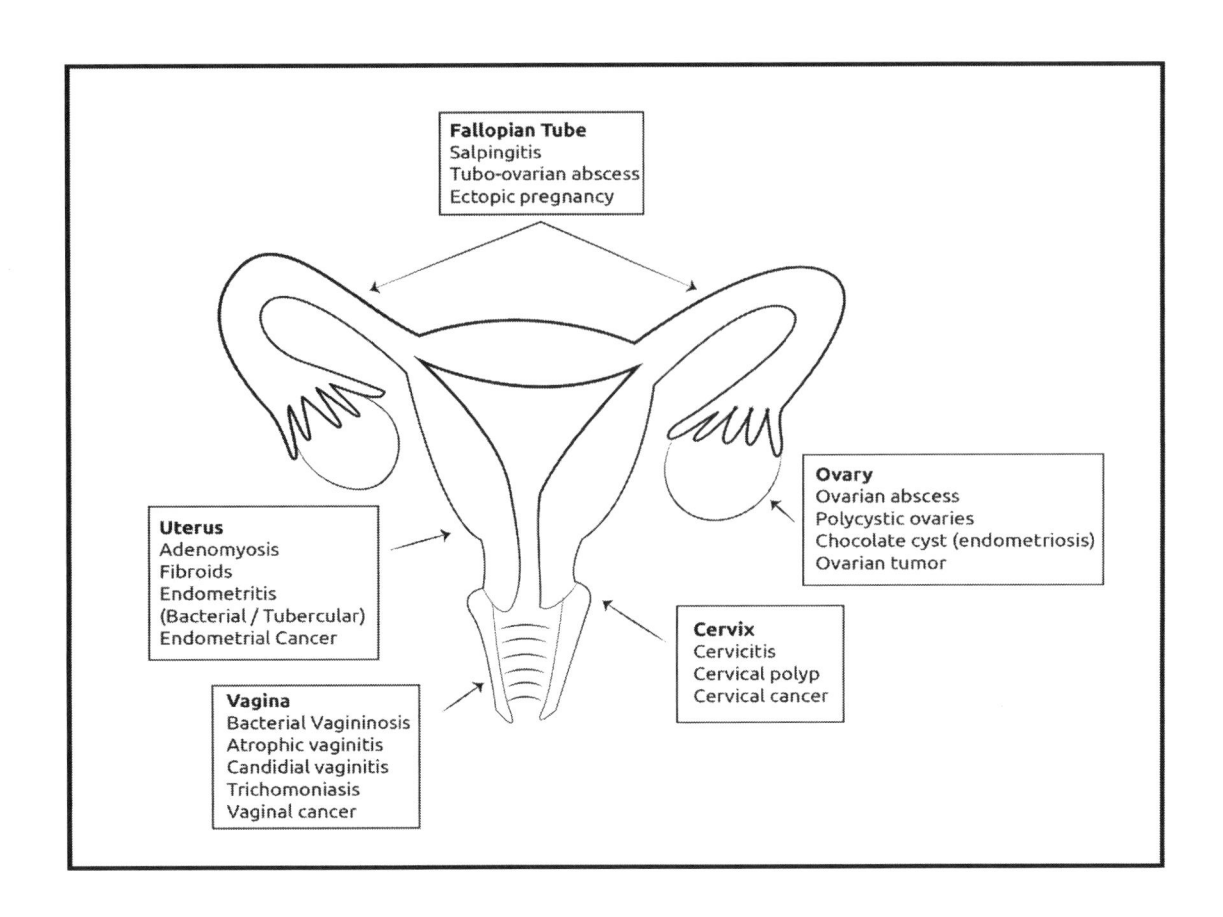

Fallopian Tube
Salpingitis
Tubo-ovarian abscess
Ectopic pregnancy

Ovary
Ovarian abscess
Polycystic ovaries
Chocolate cyst (endometriosis)
Ovarian tumor

Uterus
Adenomyosis
Fibroids
Endometritis
(Bacterial / Tubercular)
Endometrial Cancer

Cervix
Cervicitis
Cervical polyp
Cervical cancer

Vagina
Bacterial Vagininosis
Atrophic vaginitis
Candidial vaginitis
Trichomoniasis
Vaginal cancer

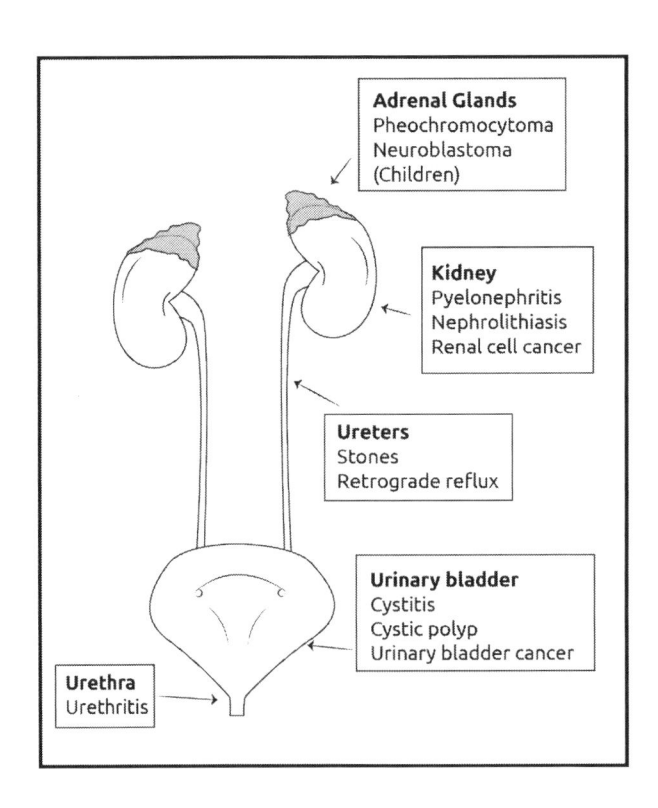

Adrenal Glands
Pheochromocytoma
Neuroblastoma
(Children)

Kidney
Pyelonephritis
Nephrolithiasis
Renal cell cancer

Ureters
Stones
Retrograde reflux

Urinary bladder
Cystitis
Cystic polyp
Urinary bladder cancer

Urethra
Urethritis

STEP 2: Narrow down: Quality of the pain

Ask the patient:
- "Does the pain come and go?"
- "Is the pain cramping?"
- "Is the pain intermittent?"
- "Is the pain constant?
- "Is the pain sharp or stabbing?"

Colicky pain:
Colicky pain is a sharp, intermittent pain that comes and goes. It indicates pain related to a hollow organ. This pain is usually experienced when there is some resistance to the outflow of these organs or if the walls of these organs are irritated. The initial pain is colicky, but if an obstruction exists, the pain gradually changes to visceral pain due to dilation.

Intestinal colic:

- Bowel obstruction, Gastroenteritis, Crohn's Disease, Irritable Bowel Syndrome.
- Jejunum/Proximal Ileum: Colic appears in waves, at intervals of 3-5 minutes, and the pain lasts for 30 seconds.

Terminal ileum: the interval is longer, at approximately 8-10 minutes. Site of colicky pain can give hints about the site of obstruction:

- Small intestinal cramps are referred to the epigastric or umbilical region.
- Colonic cramps are referred to the lower abdomen (hypogastrium)

Biliary colic:

- Biliary colic is the RUQ pain that may radiate to the back or the tip of the right scapula. It usually occurs after fatty meals. Biliary Colic is a misnomer, as it is constant in nature, despite being of a hollow organ origin.
- When there is an obstruction in the CBD, the gallbladder wall contracts to overcome the obstruction, however, the gallbladder wall is a thin layer of smooth muscles, resulting in a weak contraction. This leads to a constant type of pain as compared to a colicky pain.

Q : Why biliary colic radiates to the shoulder?

A: Any diaphragmatic irritation can cause referred pain to the shoulder or acromion tip. Diaphragm is supplied by the phrenic nerve (c3,c4,c5). Phrenic nerve has motor fibres and sensory fibres. These sensory fibres also enter the cord at c3, c4,c5 levels. This segment of the cord also supplies the supraclavicular nerve via cervical plexus. The lateral supraclavicular nerve supplies the skin, directly over the acromion process thus causing the referred pain.

Renal colic:

- ✓ Obstruction of the renal pelvis with a stone (Staghorn Calculi).

Ureteric Colic:

- ✓ Ureteric colic occurs due to obstruction of the ureter with a stone. Here, pain starts in the loin and radiates down to the testis, groin, or inner thigh. (**Loin** to **Groin** pain)
- ✓ Remember to ask about the change in the character of the pain.
- ✓ The colicky pain of acute intestinal obstruction may change into the constant burning type of pain if strangulation has taken place.
- ✓ Pain in appendicitis may initially be cramping and later become constant when pus fills the organ.

Action Box:

Initially, pain starts as a Visceral pain, due to irritation of viscera or visceral peritoneum. It is

Vague, diffuse in nature, and can be colicky if a hollow organ is involved, e.g., diffuse abdominal pain or colicky pain in initial stages of acute appendicitis.

Vi- Visceral, Vague

SC- Sympathetic Chain

erAL- ALimentary Canal (esophagus to anal)

Visceral pain is followed by Somatic pain, which occurs when the parietal peritoneum is irritated. It is localized in nature, e.g., radiation of pain to RLQ in acute appendicitis.

S- Skin, Sensory

S- Six (T6-L1)

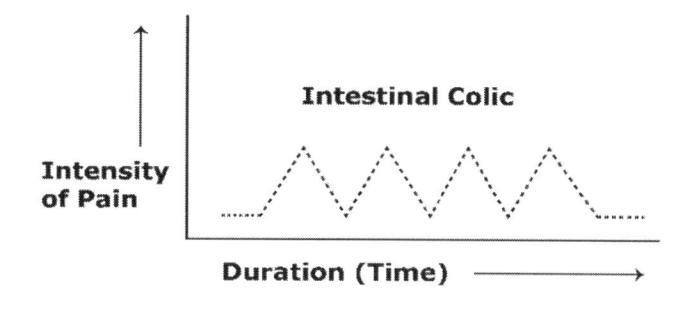

Intestinal Colic

Intensity of Pain vs Duration (Time)

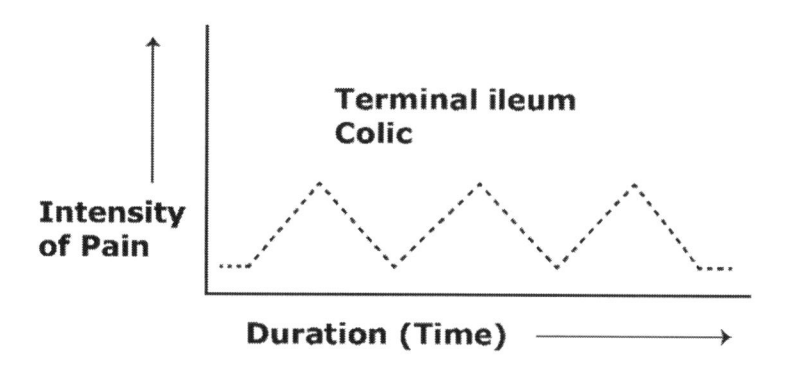

Terminal ileum Colic

Intensity of Pain vs Duration (Time)

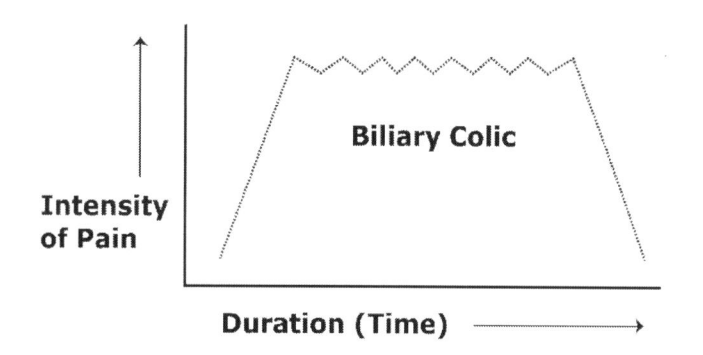

Biliary Colic

Intensity of Pain vs Duration (Time)

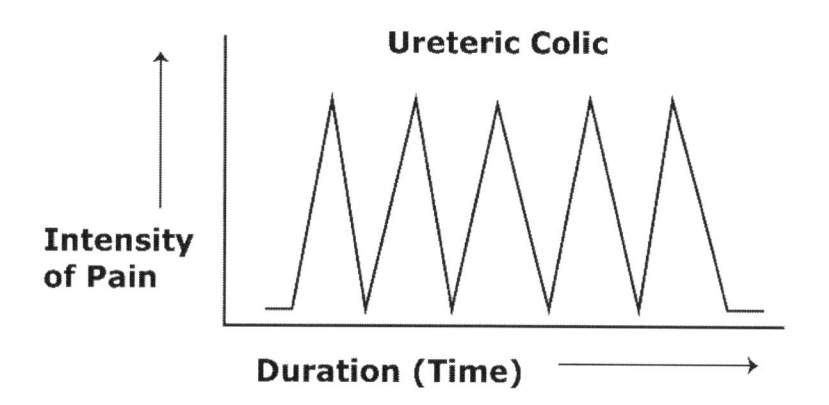

Ureteric Colic

Intensity of Pain vs Duration (Time)

Other types of abdominal pain

Dull/boring pain

Acute pancreatitis presents with a deep, boring pain that tends to become more severe when the patient lies down. The patient has a tendency of sitting on the bed and leaning forward.

It is important to note that the pain will not be colicky if the gallbladder is inflamed: there is no peristalsis in an inflamed gallbladder. Hence, this patient presents with a dull pain.

A dull pain in RUQ should point towards GB pathology (e.g. cholecystitis), before considering liver pathologies (e.g. hepatitis). This is because the pain is due to the stretching of Glisson's capsule. This stretching takes place later in the pathology, so the pain of hepatitis is a late feature.

Aching pain

- ✓ The Pain of pelvic inflammatory disease (PID) can be of an aching nature.
- ✓ Fitz-Hugh Curtis Syndrome (peri-hepatitis) can present as an RUQ pain due to the spread of infection to the liver capsule and formation of adhesions.

Tearing pain

- ✓ Acute dissection of the aorta presents with a severe tearing pain, usually radiating to the back (retroperitoneal).

Pleuritic Pain

- ✓ Sharp, catching pain that increases with respiration is called pleuritic pain. It may occur in a case of pleurisy or pleural effusion.
- ✓ Sometimes, an amoebic liver abscess can extend into the lungs above, causing a pleuritic pain.

STEP 3: Other characteristics of the pain

After locating the quadrant and understanding the nature of the pain, we have an idea as to whether the pain is originating from a luminal organ or a solid organ and whether the pain is benign or a surgical emergency. To further locate the involved organ or pathology, we have to look for other important clues like:

- ✓ Radiation of the pain- This depends on the common sensory origins of the particular organ and dermatome where the pain is referred to, e.g. cholecystitis pain is referred to the tip of the right scapular blade.

Retroperitoneal organs	
Duodenum (2nd, 3rd, and 4th part)	An **ulcer** in the 2nd part of the **duodenum** can erode the gastroduodenal artery, leading to massive bleeding.
Pancreas (except the tail, which is in the splenorenal ligament)	Acute pancreatitis
Kidneys and Ureters	Renal stone, Ureteric stone, Pyelonephritis
Ascending and Descending colon	Diverticulitis
Aorta and IVC	AAA, Mesenteric
Adjoining lymph nodes	Lymphadenopathy
Esophagus (lower 2/3rd)	Esophagitis, Barrett's Esophagus
Rectum (lower 2/3rd)	Proctalgia Fugax, Proctitis

Peritoneal organs: Rebound tenderness is a hallmark of peritoneal inflammation
Stomach
Transverse colon
Bile duct
Liver
Duodenum (1st part)
Sigmoid colon
Appendix

Duration of the pain- Pain from a duodenal ulcer, chronic pancreatitis, and gallstones can be chronic in nature due to the slowly evolving underlying pathology.

Time of day- Duodenal ulcer pain can occur more at night as compared to the day.

Aggravating factors-

- ✓ Pain in gallstone disease (Cholelithiasis) occurs after eating a fatty meal.
- ✓ A patient with a history of pancreatitis can have a recurrence on intake of alcohol, leading to acute abdomen pain.
- ✓ Pain may worsen with food in a case of bowel ischemia.

Relieving factors-

- ✓ Although nonspecific, pain due to a duodenal ulcer may get relieved on having food.
- ✓ Pain from acute pancreatitis may decrease on bending forward.

STEP 4: Associated symptoms

Using the funnel approach, we narrowed down the list of suspected organs to a few organs located in one particular **quadrant** (e.g. RUQ pains cuts down the suspicion to only organs present in the RUQ).

To further narrow the approach, we asked about the **quality** of pain, thereby ruling in or out either a luminal organ or a solid organ in that quadrant.

Other characteristics of the pain add more accuracy to our approach to the diseased organ, thereby further shortening the differential list.

In addition to this, the associated symptoms can help a person localize the symptoms to one or two organs. Some of the examples are as follows:

- ✓ Jaundice- Suggestive of a liver pathology or an obstruction to the bile duct outlet.
- ✓ Fever and shock – May suggest an infectious or septic pathology.
- ✓ E.g. Acute Cholangitis, Acute Hepatitis, Acute peritonitis, etc.
- ✓ Anorexia and weight loss in an elderly women may suggest an underlying GI malignancy, especially if paraneoplastic syndromes such as migratory thrombophlebitis, left supraclavicular lymphadenopathy are also present.
- ✓ Bleeding PR- May suggest a malignancy, intussusception, or a mesenteric infarct.
- ✓ Diarrhea- May suggest an infectious, inflammatory, or toxin mediated.

Non-Pain Abdominal Symptoms
Gastrointestinal Bleed

Ask the patient:

- ✓ Is there blood in your stools?
- ✓ Is it mixed/streaked onto the stool? Is there blood on your toilet paper?
- ✓ Is there blood in the vomitus?
- ✓ Is there blood in your urine?

Bleeding from the proximal gut (proximal to the ligament of Treitz):

- ✓ Hematemesis and Melena - Blood must remain for at least 8 hours within the gut lumen to produce melena
- ✓ <u>Melena</u> refers to <u>altered blood</u> in the stool, leading to black, tarry stools (due to the production of acid hematin). Such stools are semi-solid and offensive (acid hematin is altered by bacteria).

Bleeding from the distal gut (distal to the ligament of Treitz):

- ✓ Hematochezia
- ✓ Passage of bright red frank blood per rectum

- ✓ It may be mixed with stool or passed without stool
- ✓ Common causes are hemorrhoids, angiodysplasia, anal fissure, anal fistula, trauma, proctitis, ischemic colitis, pseudomembranous colitis, and carcinoma of colon.

> **Action Box:**
> Blood streaks on the stool + Pain = Most likely an anal fissure
> Blood on the stool, toilet paper, or in the toilet = Hemorrhoids, pruritus ani/ pinworm
> If painless- internal hemorrhoids, and if painful, then it could be due thrombosed hemorrhoids.

Malnutrition

It is very important to assess the patient for symptoms and signs of malnutrition, because the nutritional status of a person has a bearing on their other organ systems as well. Some common causes of malnutrition are:

- ✓ Inadequate intake
- ✓ Problems with digestion
- ✓ Problems with absorption
- ✓ Increased metabolic demands

Causes and examples of malnutrition	
Category	**Example**
Inadequate intake	Anorexia nervosa, bulimia nervosa, poverty
Problems with digestion	GERD, bariatric procedures, pancreatic insufficiency (chronic pancreatitis)
Problems with absorption (malabsorption)	Inflammatory bowel diseases, coeliac disease
Increased metabolic demands	Growing children, pregnant and lactating women

History findings

- ✓ Weight loss or poor weight gain in childhood
- ✓ Slowing of linear growth in childhood
- ✓ Irritability, anxiety, fatigue, weakness, etc.

Specific nutrient deficiencies:

- Iron – Microcytic anemia, fatigue, weakness, cheilosis, glossitis, nail changes
- Vitamin A – Decreased dim light vision, dry eyes, skin and hair changes
- Vitamin D – Poor bone growth, rickets in children, osteomalacia in adults
- Iodine – Goiter
- Vitamin B12 – Megaloblastic anemia, peripheral neuropathy (tingling, paresthesias etc.)
- Folic acid – Megaloblastic anemia without peripheral neuropathy, history of a baby with neural tube defects in women
- Zinc – Poor wound healing, poor growth, alopecia, acrodermatitis, features of anemia, etc.

Examination findings

- Anthropometry – A child with growth retardation, delayed growth curve
- Skin changes – Dry skin, peeling-off, patches of hypopigmentation and hyperpigmentation
- Nail changes – Spoon-shaped nails (koilonychia), etc.
- Hair changes – Thin, brittle, and sparse hair. Easily pluckable. Alternating hypo- and hyperpigmented patches (Flag sign).
- Decreased subcutaneous fat (especially on the arms and buttocks)
- Dependent edema or anasarca (hypoproteinemia)
- Abdominal distension – Hypoalbuminemia ascites and fatty liver
- Oral cavity – Angular stomatitis, cheilosis, glossitis and nonspecific mouth ulcers

Approach to Chest Pain

A patient presenting with chest pain should be evaluated for a life threatening cause. In this chapter, we discuss how to approach a patient presenting with chest pain or tightness. As mentioned earlier in the chapter on 'Approach to an abdominal case,' we will be using our 'Funnel Approach' here as well.

Like any other pain in the body, we start our approach to chest pain in a similar fashion, by asking the following:

Life isn't Good **DOCTOR, AID @PM.**

We have to pay special attention to the key findings that differentiate life threatening conditions from non-emergent ones; therefore, with the combination of symptoms and key findings, it becomes easier to channel down to one particular organ pathology and base your differential diagnosis on it in a quick and life-saving manner.

There are many reasons for the presentation of chest pain. The diagram shown below covers almost all of the organs that may cause chest pain.

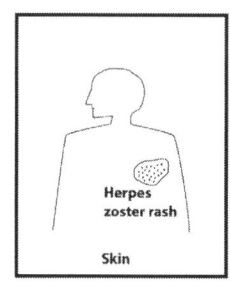

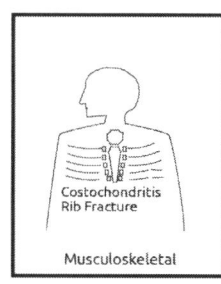

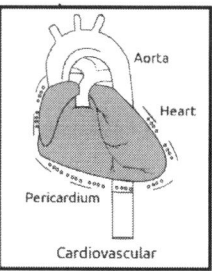

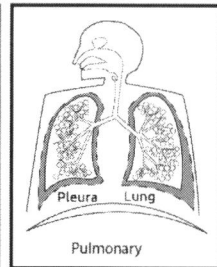

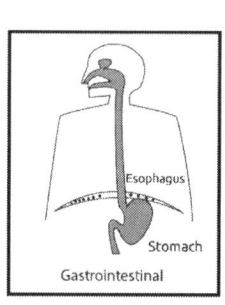

Location
The location of the pain can help rule out various diseases from the differential.

Central-

- ✓ **CVS-** MI, angina, aortic stenosis, pericarditis, cardiac tamponade, aortic dissection. Cardiac pain can be diffusely spread over the central chest.
- ✓ **Musculoskeletal-** Costochondritis can be parasternal in nature.
- ✓ **Gastrointestinal-** GERD, esophagitis. esophageal rupture can be substernal.

Peripheral-

- ✓ **Skin-** Herpes zoster is almost always unilateral/**dermatomal** as it involves a particular nerve distribution.
- ✓ **Musculoskeletal-** Costochondritis, rib fracture, sickle cell crisis. Musculoskeletal pain usually presents with chest tenderness and difficulty breathing due to pain while breathing (important to differentiate from pleurisy).
- ✓ **Respiratory-** Pleurisy, pleural effusion, pulmonary embolism, pneumonia, lung tumor.

Grade

Ask for the intensity of the pain on a scale of 0 to 10, with ten being the worst pain ever experienced.

- ✓ Herpes zoster rash may be very painful, therefore, a close inspection of the chest is mandatory. Esophageal rupture, aortic dissection, and acute myocardial infarction can all present with severe chest pain.
- ✓ On the other hand, pain due to pneumonia, GERD, and inferior wall MI may all be low in intensity.

Duration

- ✓ Q: "How long has this pain been going on?"

This describes the chronicity of the pain. Conditions like angina, costochondritis, fibromyalgia, and herpes zoster may last for weeks.

- ✓ Q: "For how long does the pain last?"

This is important to tell us the duration of the particular episode that brought the patient to the doctor. Acute thromboembolism and myocardial infarction can be of short duration and need immediate medical attention.

Onset

Differentiate between a gradual or sudden onset of pain. Sudden, severe chest pain can be an aortic dissection, pulmonary thromboembolism, or a myocardial infarction.

Characteristic

Characteristic of the pain is the most important part of the pain history. It can help you understand the nature of the disease.

- ✓ Constricting type- Acute MI, constrictive pericarditis

- ✓ Patient may complain of a sensation of squeezing, pressure, or heaviness in the chest in a case of an acute MI
- ✓ Tearing type- Aortic dissection. The patient may be diaphoretic, unstable, and complain of severe chest pain.
- ✓ Sharp pain- Pleuritic pain may be sharp in character, which may lead us to think of pleurisy, pleural effusion, pulmonary embolism, or esophageal rupture.

Time of the day

Diurnal variations may indicate towards the etiology. Post dinner chest pain can be due to GERD, as the patient is more likely to lie supine. Symptoms in asthmatic patients are worse in the early morning and night.

Occasion

Ask for the first instance when the pain was experienced.

- ✓ Q: "What were you doing when this pain happened?"

Exertional chest pain suggests a cardiovascular pathology.

Radiation

Cardiac ischemic pain may radiate to the jaw or the left arm depending on the site of ischemia. Pain from aortic dissection can radiate to the back.

- ✓ Q: "Is this pain going anywhere?"

Associated symptoms

Associated symptoms will help you pinpoint a system. The most important associated symptoms with cardiac chest pain are as follows:

- ✓ Dyspnea (Shortness of breath)
- ✓ Diaphoresis (Sweating)
- ✓ Dizziness or syncope
- ✓ Nausea or vomiting
- ✓ Palpitations

Post-palpitations diuresis (due to the release of natriuretic peptide from the heart during an episode of arrhythmia)

Increasing Factors

These are factors exacerbating the problem. Exertion exacerbates cardiac pains, food worsens GERD, and inspiration worsens pleuritic or pericarditis pain.

Decreasing factors

These are factors that improve the pain. Resting may improve anginal pain.

Previous history of similar symptoms

This is used to differentiate between an acute and a chronic problem.

Medications

A list of all medications that the patient is taking is important and can give you a clue about what you might have missed in the history.

Now analyze this information quickly to differentiate the chest pain into an emergency or a non-emergency condition. Unstable vitals are an important indicator, but elaborative history is a must. The most common life-threatening conditions that can present with chest pain are:

- ✓ Acute myocardial infarction
- ✓ Unstable angina
- ✓ Thoracic aortic aneurysm with dissection
- ✓ Esophageal rupture
- ✓ Tension pneumothorax

Once these conditions are ruled out, we can take a detailed history to make our differentials in the non-emergent conditions.

Bibliography

1. Marcus GM, Cohen J, Varosy PD, et al. The utility of gestures in patients with chest discomfort. *Am J Med*. 2007;120(1):83-89. doi:10.1016/j.amjmed.2006.05.045.
2. Launbjerg J, Fruergaard P, Hesse B, Jorgensen F, Elsborg L, Petri A. Long-term risk of death, cardiac events and recurrent chest pain in patients with acute chest pain of different origin. *Cardiology*. 1996;87(1):60-66.
3. Lindsell CJ, Anantharaman V, Diercks D, et al. The internet tracking registry of acute coronary syndromes (i*trACS): a multicenter registry of patients with suspicion of acute coronary syndromes reported using the standardized reporting guidelines for emergency department chest pain studies. *Ann Emerg Med*. 2006;48(6):666-677.e1-e9. doi:10.1016/j.annemergmed.2006.08.005.

Approach to Shortness of Breath

Introduction

Shortness of breath, also known as 'Dyspnea,' is defined by the **American Thoracic Society** as 'a subjective experience of breathing discomfort that is comprised of qualitatively distinct sensations that vary in intensity. The experience derives from interactions among multiple physiological, psychological, social, and environmental factors, and may induce secondary physiological and behavioral responses.'[1]

The most common causes of shortness of breath are as follows:

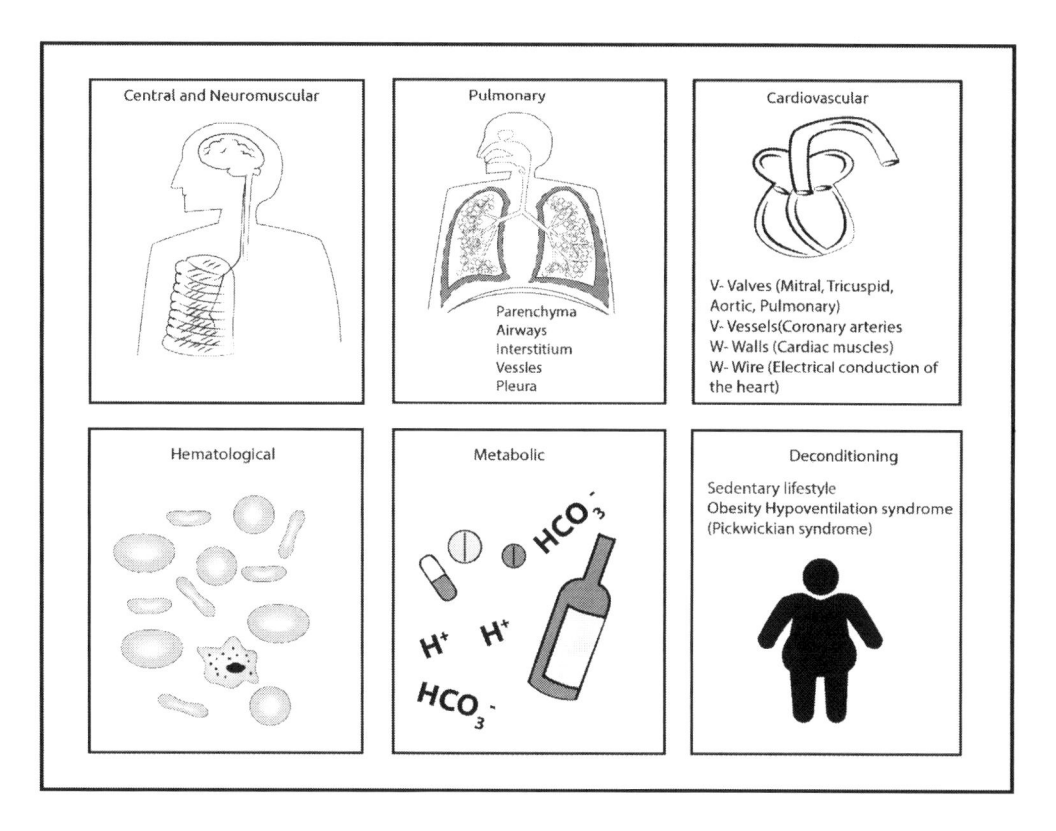

Central and Neuromuscular	Pulmonary	Cardiovascular
	Parenchyma Airways Interstitium Vessles Pleura	V- Valves (Mitral, Tricuspid, Aortic, Pulmonary) V- Vessels(Coronary arteries W- Walls (Cardiac muscles) W- Wire (Electrical conduction of the heart)
Hematological	Metabolic	Deconditioning Sedentary lifestyle Obesity Hypoventilation syndrome (Pickwickian syndrome)

Causes

Respiratory

1. **Central**- Stimulation of medullary respiratory centers, neurological insult or drugs like **salicylates** can cause an increase in the respiratory drive, leading to tachypnea and dyspnea. Other causes of central dyspnea can be hypoxia and hypercapnia due to various diseases.[3]

2. **Neuromuscular-** A defect in the respiratory muscles and their nerve supply can lead to hypoxia and hypercapnia. It may classically present as **'air hunger'** or **'urge to breathe,'**[4] e.g. Guillain-Barre Syndrome and myasthenia gravis.

3. **Pulmonary-** Pulmonary causes are either due to problems in the airway tubes, the pulmonary parenchyma, the blood vessels, or the interstitium.

    - **Parenchyma-** Acute respiratory distress syndrome (ARDS), pneumonia, direct pulmonary injury (contusion), tuberculosis, lung tumor.
    - **Airway-** Asthma, COPD, bronchiectasis, bronchogenic carcinoma.
    - **Interstitium-** Interstitial lung disease, occupational lung disease (asbestosis, silicosis), sarcoidosis.
    - **Vessels-** Pulmonary embolism, pulmonary hypertension.

4. **Pleural-** Pleural effusion, pneumothorax, hemothorax.

Cardiovascular

Cardiovascular causes are mainly due to increased congestion of the lungs due to overloading of the heart. It can be easily remembered as V_2, W_2, and its **covering**.

- **Valve-** Mitral Regurgitation, Mitral Stenosis, Aortic Stenosis
- **Vessels-** Acute coronary syndrome
- **Wall-** Cardiomyopathy, Decompensating left heart failure
- **Wire-** Arrhythmias
- **Covering-** Pericarditis, Pericardial tamponade

Metabolic

1. **Acidosis-** Metabolic acidosis can be compensated by respiratory alkalosis. It is possible only if the patient breathes quickly to wash out CO_2.

    - **DKA-** Accumulation of ketones causes ketoacidosis
    - **Ethylene glycol and methanol poisoning-** It can cause metabolic acidosis
    - **Sepsis-** Processes like pneumonia may progress to respiratory fatigue, overt sepsis and lactic acid accumulation causing end-organ hypoperfusion, acidosis, and tachypnea.[5]

2. **Toxic**

- **Salicylate-** Stimulates respiratory centers leading to hyperventilation.
- **Carbon Monoxide-** Blocks oxygen metabolism at the cellular level (oxidative phosphorylation), causing anaerobic respiration and a hypoxia-like state. Also, it binds more strongly to hemoglobin as compared to oxygen, thus interfering with end-organ tissue perfusion.[6]
- **OP poisoning-** Causes bronchoconstriction and increased secretions in the airway that may cause dyspnea.

Hematological

- **Anemia-** Decreased oxygen carrying capacity of blood due to anemia may cause fatigue, shortness of breath, and tachypnea.
- **Sickle Cell Disease/Acute chest syndrome-** Vaso-occlusion, embolization, and ischemia can precipitate severe chest pain and shortness of breath.[7]

Psychiatric

Hyperventilation- Certain psychiatric diseases can present with hyperventilation and subjective dyspnea. It becomes imperative in such scenarios to rule out serious systemic pathologies before establishing a psychiatric diagnosis.

- **Panic attack**
- **Anxiety**

Approach to a history of dyspnea

In patients presenting with shortness of breath, a quick way to align your history in the right direction is first to differentiate the source of shortness of breath.

We use the mnemonic DOCTOR AID @ PM, but we focus more on the important aspects of the symptom that help us understand the source better.

The first question that comes to mind in a case of shortness of breath, is to know whether it is coming from a cardiovascular disease or a respiratory disease.

The key distinguishing features on history suggestive of a cardiovascular disease (heart failure) are:

- **orthopnea** (breathless on lying supine) and
- **paroxysmal nocturnal dyspnea** (sudden episodes of breathlessness that wake a person up in the middle of the night).[8]

> **Action Box:**
>
> When the left heart starts to fail, the blood backs up and starts congesting the pulmonary veins coming from the lungs.
>
> As a result of the back pressure, fluid starts to diffuse out of the blood vessels and into the alveoli, causing pulmonary edema

Once you know the probable cause of breathlessness, you can grade it using the **NYHA** (New York Heart Association) classification for cardiovascular cause and the **MMRC** (Modified Medical Research Council) dyspnea scale for respiratory cause.

Scale	Modified Medical Research Council Dyspnea Scale
0	Breathless during strenuous exercise
1	Breathless on hurrying on the level or walking uphill
2	Walks slower than people of the same age group or has to stop for breath when walking at their own pace
3	Short of breath when walking 100 meters
4	Too breathless to leave the house

Scale	New York Heart Association Classification
I	Patient with cardiac disease, but no symptoms on normal activity
II	Comfortable at rest, normal activities cause symptoms (mild limitation)
III	Comfortable at rest, less than normal activities cause symptoms (marked limitation)
IV	Symptoms at rest (severe limitation)

SPECIAL CoWS™: An easy-to-remember and hard-to-forget *Vital Checklist for heart failure*		
S	**Shortness of breath**	**Do you have shortness of breath?** **S. W. E. A. T - Sleeping, Walking, Eating, ADL, Talking**
P	Pillows	Do you use pillows for sleeping? How many pillows do you use?
E	Exhaustion	Are you tired? Do you feel exhausted?
C	**Chest pain** **Confusion**	**Do you have chest pain?** **Do you have any episodes of confusion?**
I	Irregular heart beat	Do you feel your heart racing and beating faster?
A	Appetite loss	How is your appetite?
L	Lightheadedness	Do you feel lightheaded?
Co	Cough	Do you have any cough?
	Cough with pinkish phlegm	**Is there any pink phlegm with your cough?**
W	Weight gain	Have you experiences any weight gain?
S	Swelling in the legs	What about any swelling in your legs?

Bibliography

1. Parshall MB, Schwartzstein RM, Adams L, et al. An official american thoracic society statement: Update on the mechanisms, assessment, and management of dyspnea. *Am J Respir Crit Care Med.* 2012; 185:435-52.
2. Simon, P. M.; Schwartzstein, R. M.; Weiss, J. W.; Fencl, V.; Teghtsoonian, M.; Weinberger, S. E., Distinguishable types of dyspnea in patients with shortness of breath. *Am Rev Respir Dis* **1990,** *142* (5), 1009-14.
3. Simon, P. M.; Schwartzstein, R. M.; Weiss, J. W.; Lahive, K.; Fencl, V.; Teghtsoonian, M.; Weinberger, S. E., Distinguishable sensations of breathlessness induced in normal volunteers. *Am Rev Respir Dis* **1989,** *140* (4), 1021-7.
4. Banzett, R. B.; Lansing, R. W.; Brown, R.; Topulos, G. P.; Yager, D.; Steele, S. M.; Londono, B.; Loring, S. H.; Reid, M. B.; Adams, L.; et al., 'Air hunger' from increased PCO2 persists after complete neuromuscular block in humans. *Respir Physiol* **1990,** *81* (1), 1-17.
5. Casserly, B.; Phillips, G. S.; Schorr, C.; Dellinger, R. P.; Townsend, S. R.; Osborn, T. M.; Reinhart, K.; Selvakumar, N.; Levy, M. M., Lactate measurements in sepsis-induced tissue hypoperfusion: results from the Surviving Sepsis Campaign database. *Crit Care Med* **2015,** *43* (3), 567-73.
6. Hardy, K. R.; Thom, S. R., Pathophysiology and treatment of carbon monoxide poisoning. *J Toxicol Clin Toxicol* **1994,** *32* (6), 613-29.
7. Siddiqui, A. K.; Ahmed, S., Pulmonary manifestations of sickle cell disease. *Postgrad Med J* **2003,** *79* (933), 384-90.
8. Ekundayo, O. J.; Howard, V. J.; Safford, M. M.; McClure, L. A.; Arnett, D.; Allman, R. M.; Howard, G.; Ahmed, A., Value of Orthopnea, Paroxysmal Nocturnal Dyspnea, and Medications in Prospective Population Studies of Incident Heart Failure. *Am J Cardiol* **2009,** *104* (2), 259-64.

Approach to a Case of Syncope

Syncope is the sudden and transient loss of consciousness and postural tone with complete recovery of the neurological function without the need of medical intervention.

Loss of consciousness with residual deficits, inability to regain normal mental function, and/or seizure activity is not included in syncope—e.g. stroke, head injury, seizure, encephalitis metabolic (hypoxia, hypoglycemia), toxic insult (alcohol), and vertebro-basilar defects. This is known as a non-syncopal attack, or Transient Loss of Consciousness (TLOC).[1]

The primary cause of syncope is cerebral hypo-perfusion, therefore, the etiologies of presyncope and light headedness overlap with loss of consciousness.

Transient changes in cerebral blood flow can occur due to the following reasons:

- ✓ **Neural**- Reflex mediated/neural control of vascular structures, hypersensitive vascular baroreceptors, and situation based activation of reflexes leading to syncope.

- ✓ **Causes**- Neuro-cardiogenic/vasovagal syncope, situational syncope (micturition, defecation syncope etc.), and carotid sinus hyperactivity. **Orthostatic hypotension**- Failure of autonomic nervous system or significant loss of blood volume may cause the failure of the compensatory mechanism that maintains blood pressure. This may lead to decreased cerebral perfusion, causing light headedness and syncope (decrease in systolic blood pressure of more than 20 mm of Hg, diastolic pressure of more than 10 mm of Hg, or rise in heart rate of more than 20 beats per minute within 3 minutes of standing[2]).

Causes-
- ✓ *Primary autonomic failure*- Parkinson's disease, Lewy body dementia, multiple system atrophy (Shy-Drager syndrome).
- ✓ *Secondary autonomic failure*- Diabetes mellitus, hereditary autonomic neuropathy, HIV neuropathy, drug-induced.

```
Vasovagal Syncope
      ↓
Intense emotions, pain or stress
      ↓
Stimulation of vagal nerve
      ↓
Reflex bradycardia and vasodilation
      ↓
Decreased cerebral perfusion
      ↓
Syncope
```

```
Situational Syncope
      ↓
Afferent triggers in pulmonary, gastrointestinal, urogenital, heart and carotid artery
```

Disease	Key features
Parkinson's disease	Pill-rolling, slowness of movement (bradykinesia), increased resistance to passive movement, postural instability
Lewy body dementia	Dementia + episodes of black out, also known as cognitive fluctuations; visual hallucinations (classic of LBD) and Parkinsonism
Multiple system atrophy (Shy-Drager syndrome)	Autonomic failure including urogenital dysfunction, cerebellar ataxia, and pyramidal signs
Diabetes mellitus	Polyuria, polydipsia, polyphagia
Hereditary sensory autonomic neuropathy (HSAN- 5 types)	h/o congenital insensitivity to pain, distal muscle weakness, hearing loss, spontaneous distal amputation or bone necrosis, decreased sweating or tearing, abnormal swallow reflex, etc.
HIV neuropathy	h/o prior HIV diagnosis, unprotected sexual intercourse
Drug-induced	h/o drug intake, e.g. diuretic, antihypertensive drugs, antipsychotic medications

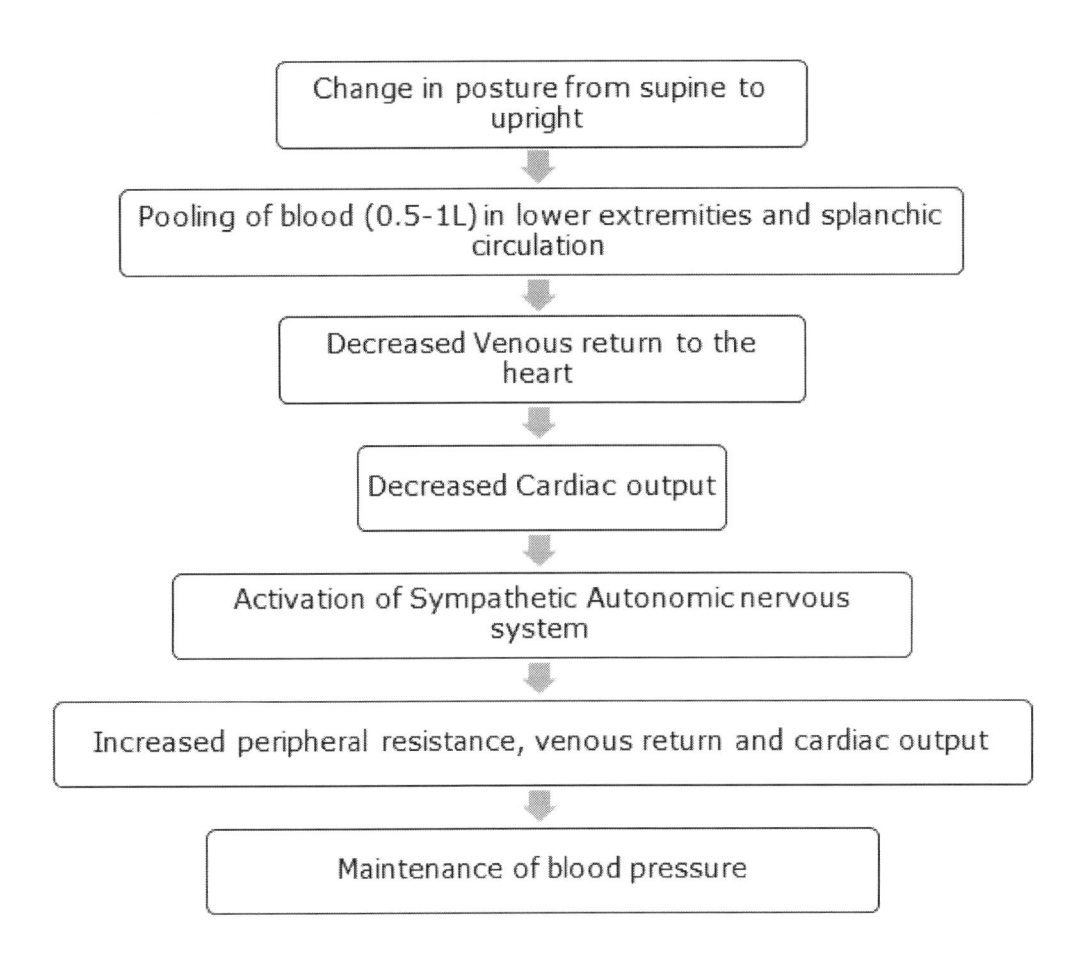

```
Change in posture from supine to upright
            ↓
Pooling of blood (0.5-1L) in lower extremities and splanchic circulation
            ↓
Decreased Venous return to the heart
            ↓
Decreased Cardiac output
            ↓
Activation of Sympathetic Autonomic nervous system
            ↓
Increased peripheral resistance, venous return and cardiac output
            ↓
Maintenance of blood pressure
```

Cardiovascular- Disease affecting the heart leads to decreased cardiac output and may cause syncope. As mentioned in the chapter on dizziness, the problem may lie in any of the following components of the heart: V2, W2-vessels, valves, walls, and/or wiring.

V- Valves	Aortic stenosis, severe pulmonic stenosis
V-Vessels	Myocardial ischemia, vasculitis, pulmonary artery hypertension, pulmonary embolism
W- Wiring	Arrhythmias, heart blocks, Brugada syndrome, long QTc syndrome
W- Walls	Hypertrophic cardiomyopathy, atrial myxoma

Psychogenic- Panic attacks and anxiety can present with syncopal attacks. It is imperative to first evaluate for life threatening etiology like cardiac arrhythmias, myocardial ischemia, and stroke. These patients are generally young and present with multiple episodes of loss of consciousness.

Differentiating Syncope from a Seizure Episode[3]

Syncope	Seizure
Convulsions may be present but not as violent as in seizures	Convulsions, if present, are usually violent
Tongue biting is absent	Tongue biting may be present[4]
No post ictal phase	Post ictal phase associated with confusion and weakness
No bladder or bowel incontinence	Loss of bowel and bladder control during the episode may be present

How to approach the history

We will approach a case of loss of consciousness by taking a detailed history using the mnemonic DOCTOR AID @ PM. Many studies suggest that a focused history and physical examination can help diagnose the cause of syncope in almost 50% of the cases.[5]

Duration

Often patients cannot quantify how long they were out of consciousness. This question may be answered by the accompanying partner or family member.

If the duration was more than five minutes, it could be likely that the patient had a seizure or other causes of loss of consciousness.

Onset

Sudden onset syncope without any associated symptoms may suggest cardiac arrhythmias.[6]

Character or continuous

Waxing and waning syncope suggests either an arrhythmia, delirium, or a psychogenic cause.

Time of the day

Syncope during the early morning while rising from bed could suggest orthostatic hypotension, whereas sudden palpitation followed by loss of consciousness while outdoors (grocery shopping, walking in the park, etc.) may suggest an arrhythmia.

Occasion

- Q: "What were you doing when you lost consciousness?"

Change in position, like getting up from lying down to standing, can cause LOC in a case of orthostatic hypotension.

Long standing, emotional, painful, or stressful stimuli or sight may cause vasovagal syncope.

Situational syncope can occur during urination, defecation, coughing, or swallowing.

Rate of progression

- Q: "Is it getting worse?"
- Q: "How many episodes of loss of consciousness have you had?"

Associated symptoms

Symptoms associated with loss of consciousness help us to evaluate the possible etiology. They can also help us to evaluate for life threatening conditions.

- Chest pain- acute coronary syndrome, pulmonary embolism
- Palpitations- arrhythmias
- Shortness of breath- pulmonary embolism, heart failure
- Facial weakness, spasticity, loss of vision, speech or gait abnormality- stroke, CNS pathology
- Severe headache- subarachnoid hemorrhage
- Warmth, pallor, nausea, vomiting, light headedness before the loss of consciousness- vasovagal or neurocardiogenic

Increasing factors

- Q: "Is there anything in particular that makes it worse?"
- Excessive exertion can worsen cardiac disease and predispose to arrhythmias and may cause syncope and death.

Decreasing factors

- Q: "Is there anything that makes it better?"
- Q: "Have you done something to prevent it?"

Previous history of similar symptoms

✓ Q: "How many episodes of fainting have you had in the past?"

A previous history of syncope can help associate the LOC with a triggering factor. A recurrent episode may suggest carotid sinus hypersensitivity. Multiple episodes in a short time interval may also suggest episodes of arrhythmias.

Medication

Certain antihypertensive medications may cause orthostatic hypotension and syncope. Antipsychotics can prolong QT interval in genetically predisposed patients, leading to dysrhythmias and LOC.

Family History

A family history of similar episodes or sudden death may predispose a hereditary cardiac disease such as Brugada syndrome or hereditary prolonged QTc syndrome, etc.

Physical Examination

One should take a mini mental examination to assess for residual symptoms. It is important to examine the cardiovascular and neurological systems in every case of syncope, because, if the diagnosis is missed, it may be lethal for the patient.

Bibliography

1. Bassetti, C. L., Transient loss of consciousness and syncope. *Handb Clin Neurol* **2014**, *119*, 169-91.
2. Freeman, R.; Wieling, W.; Axelrod, F. B.; Benditt, D. G.; Benarroch, E.; Biaggioni, I.; Cheshire, W. P.; Chelimsky, T.; Cortelli, P.; Gibbons, C. H.; Goldstein, D. S.; Hainsworth, R.; Hilz, M. J.; Jacob, G.; Kaufmann, H.; Jordan, J.; Lipsitz, L. A.; Levine, B. D.; Low, P. A.; Mathias, C.; Raj, S. R.; Robertson, D.; Sandroni, P.; Schatz, I.; Schondorff, R.; Stewart, J. M.; van Dijk, J. G., Consensus statement on the definition of orthostatic hypotension, neurally mediated syncope and the postural tachycardia syndrome. *Clin Auton Res* **2011**, *21* (2), 69-72.
3. Sheldon, R.; Rose, S.; Ritchie, D.; Connolly, S. J.; Koshman, M. L.; Lee, M. A.; Frenneaux, M.; Fisher, M.; Murphy, W., Historical criteria that distinguish syncope from seizures. In *J Am Coll Cardiol*, United States, 2002; Vol. 40, pp 142-8.
4. Benbadis, S. R.; Wolgamuth, B. R.; Goren, H.; Brener, S.; Fouad-Tarazi, F., Value of tongue biting in the diagnosis of seizures. *Arch Intern Med* **1995**, *155* (21), 2346-9.
5. Linzer, M.; Yang, E. H.; Estes, N. A., 3rd; Wang, P.; Vorperian, V. R.; Kapoor, W. N., Diagnosing syncope. Part 1: Value of history, physical examination, and electrocardiography. Clinical Efficacy Assessment Project of the American College of Physicians. *Ann Intern Med* **1997**, *126* (12), 989-96.
6. Calkins, H.; Shyr, Y.; Frumin, H.; Schork, A.; Morady, F., The value of the clinical history in the differentiation of syncope due to ventricular tachycardia, atrioventricular block, and neurocardiogenic syncope. In *Am J Med*, United States, 1995; Vol. 98, pp 365-73.

Approach to Dizziness

Dizziness is a nonspecific term that may have a different meaning, varying from patient to patient.

To simplify the understanding of this symptom, we have used the **funnel approach.** Dizziness is a very vague complaint and involves various pathologies in various organs. In our funnel approach, we start broad and then narrow down to a few disease processes on the basis of history. Furthermore, using targeted investigations, we narrow down our long list of differentials to a specific diagnosis.

In various outpatient, inpatient, and community settings[1-3], the following causes were found to be more common:

- ✓ Inner ear, 40%
- ✓ Central brain stem lesions, 10%
- ✓ Syncope/Presyncope, 25%
- ✓ Psychiatric disorder, 15%
- ✓ Uncertain diagnosis, 10%

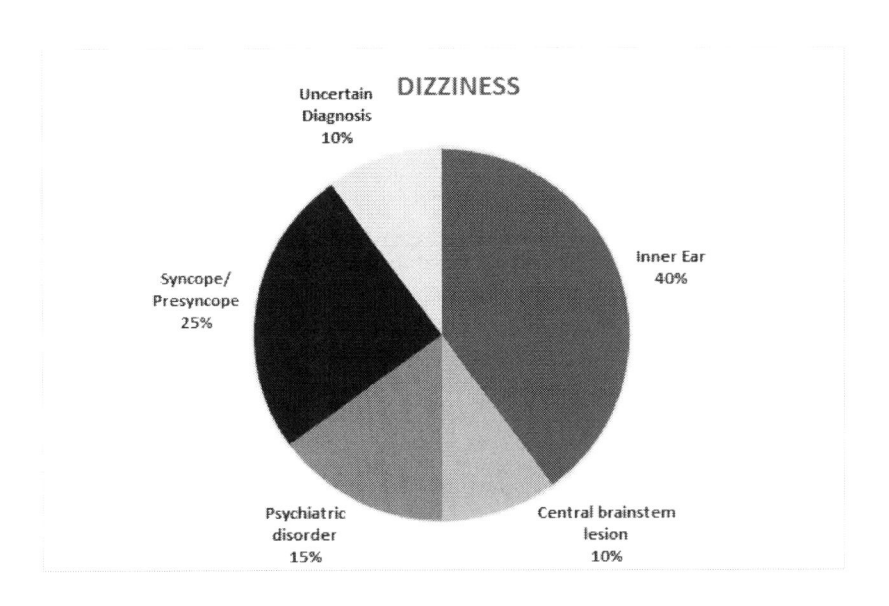

Why is this picture important?

In these settings, inner ear and central brain lesions caused 50% of the dizziness. Asking one question, "Are the surroundings spinning around you or vice versa?" will help you to evaluate the source of the dizziness. However, this is not a precise method. One should still have an open mind to evaluate for inner ear pathology by asking other questions about hearing loss, tinnitus, etc.[4,5]

In order to approach the case on the basis of history and physical examination, it is important to have a clear concept of the possible organs involved. We will discuss how to differentiate light-headedness from vertigo and how history taking should proceed in order to arrive at the diagnosis.

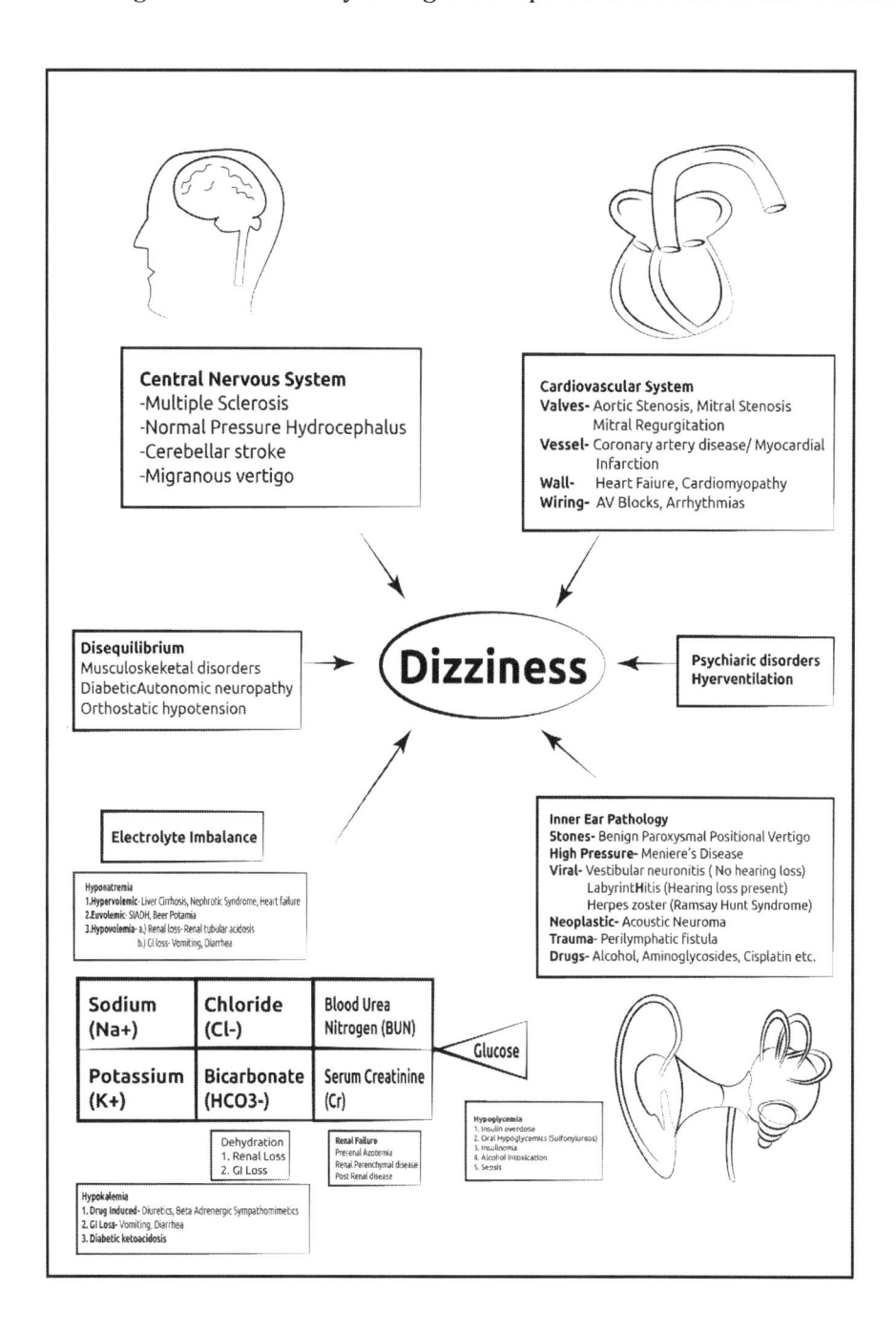

Central Nervous System
-Multiple Sclerosis
-Normal Pressure Hydrocephalus
-Cerebellar stroke
-Migranous vertigo

Cardiovascular System
Valves- Aortic Stenosis, Mitral Stenosis
       Mitral Regurgitation
Vessel- Coronary artery disease/ Myocardial Infarction
Wall- Heart Faiure, Cardiomyopathy
Wiring- AV Blocks, Arrhythmias

Disequilibrium
Musculoskeketal disorders
DiabeticAutonomic neuropathy
Orthostatic hypotension

Psychiaric disorders
Hyerventilation

Inner Ear Pathology
Stones- Benign Paroxysmal Positional Vertigo
High Pressure- Meniere's Disease
Viral- Vestibular neuronitis (No hearing loss)
       LabyrintHitis (Hearing loss present)
       Herpes zoster (Ramsay Hunt Syndrome)
Neoplastic- Acoustic Neuroma
Trauma- Perilymphatic fistula
Drugs- Alcohol, Aminoglycosides, Cisplatin etc.

Electrolyte Imbalance

Hyponatremia
1.**Hypervolemic**- Liver Cirrhosis, Nephrotic Syndrome, Heart failure
2.**Euvolemic**- SIADH, Beer Potamia
3.**Hypovolemia-** a.) Renal loss- Renal tubular acidosis
           b.) GI loss- Vomiting, Diarrhea

Sodium (Na+)	Chloride (Cl-)	Blood Urea Nitrogen (BUN)
Potassium (K+)	Bicarbonate (HCO3-)	Serum Creatinine (Cr)

Glucose

Dehydration
1. Renal Loss
2. GI Loss

Renal Failure
Prerenal Azotemia
Renal Parenchymal disease
Post Renal disease

Hypoglycemia
1. Insulin overdose
2. Oral Hypoglycemics (Sulfonylureas)
3. Insulinoma
4. Alcohol Intoxication
5. Sepsis

Hypokalemia
1. **Drug Induced-** Diuretics, Beta Adrenergic Sympathomimetics
2. **GI Loss-** Vomiting, Diarrhea
3. **Diabetic ketoacidosis**

Differentiating Vertigo from Light-headedness and Disequilibrium

Vertigo may be caused either by a vestibular pathology or by a central brain stem lesion. The inner ear is divided into a vestibular component that deals with balance, motion, and acceleration, and a cochlear component that is responsible for hearing.

On the other hand, light-headedness can be due to postural, vascular, metabolic, and cardiovascular disorders. The inability to balance oneself can also present as dizziness. Disequilibrium can be caused by poor coordination, weakness in limbs, or peripheral neuropathy.

Asking the patient all components of a basic history can reveal a lot of information. We use the mnemonic, DOCTOR AID @ PM, to take a complete history; however, we focus more on duration, onset, character, increasing or aggravating factors, and associated symptoms to reveal maximum useful information.

D-Duration

Asking about the duration of the symptom can help differentiate acute onset disease from a chronic pathology.

- ✓ Q: "For how long has this dizziness being going on?"

O-Onset

As mentioned above, the sudden onset of symptoms takes you to a more acute pathology as compared to a chronic pathology.

Acute- Vestibular neuronitis, stroke, vasovagal syncope.

Recurrent spontaneous- Meniere's disease and vestibular migraine may have a spontaneous precipitation, but they keep recurring in an episodic manner.

Recurrent positional- Benign Positional Paroxysmal Vertigo (BPPV) may occur on changing their head position, e.g., rolling over. The calcium debris (otoconia) gets displaced from one place to another in the semi-circular canal of the vestibule, leading to paroxysmal episodes of vertigo.[6]

- ✓ Q: "Do you get dizzy spells when you roll over while lying in bed?"

C- Character

Ask the patient open ended questions. "Can you describe the dizziness in your own words?" *pause...* If the patient is not able to express clearly, you may then ask leading questions like these:

- ✓ Q: "Did you feel like passing out?"

This suggests a vasovagal or orthostatic phenomenon rather than a vertiginous one.

- ✓ Q: "Do you feel the surroundings are spinning around you?"

This is more classic of vertigo.

- ✓ Q: "Do you find it difficult to balance yourself?" *pause...* "Do you have frequent falls?" This may suggest a lesion causing disequilibrium, such as cerebellar lesions, musculoskeletal disorders, or peripheral neuropathies.

> **Action Box:**
>
> For a quick recall of etiologies, an easy way is to remember three symptoms.
>
> If the patient feels like blacking out or feels light headed, think of cardiovascular, orthostatic, or CNS pathologies.
>
> If the patient complains of a spinning sensation, think of inner ear or CNS pathologies.
>
> If the patient complains of frequent involuntary falls, think of peripheral neuropathy, CNS, or musculoskeletal problem.

T-Time of the day

Patients complaining of light-headedness can give an important clue when you ask what **time of the day** they felt light-headed. A person feeling dizzy upon getting up in the morning may be on diuretics and may have orthostatic hypotension. A person sleeping in bed, who suddenly feels light headed with palpitations is more likely having an episode of arrhythmia. A person feeling dizzy when he rolls over in bed at night is more suggestive of BPPV. Therefore, it is important to perform the Epley's maneuver to diagnose this condition and to treat it with the Dix-Hallpike maneuver.

- ✓ The importance lies more in the posture of the person than the diurnal variation.

O-Occasion

- ✓ Q: "What were you doing when this episode of dizziness started?"

R-Rate of progression

The evolution of the symptom can tell you about the pathogenesis and the status of a disease. Vertigo may last for a couple of weeks. It might not be constant or continuous because any inner ear pathology that causes vertigo is sensed by the CNS and appropriate compensation is made, leading to resolution of symptoms. Also, patients might say that they have been experiencing vertigo continuously over months. At this point, it is important to ask them whether the symptoms stay throughout the day or if they occur in episodes. Are the symptoms resolving or are they recurring? This can suggest a vestibular lesion.[7]

A-Associated symptoms

This is the most important clue in history taking.

- ✓ History of hearing loss or tinnitus (buzzing sound) suggests an inner ear pathology.
- ✓ History of weakness on one side, behavioral changes, change in speech, frequent falls or abnormal gait, facial asymmetry, or visual symptoms point to a central pathology.
- ✓ History of palpitation, feelings of warmth, blacking out, sweating, and nausea before the episode may suggest a cardiovascular cause.
- ✓ History of tingling sensations in the legs may suggest diabetes, as it can cause autonomic neuropathy which causes dizziness.[8]

Action Box:

The Dix-Hallpike Maneuver is done to diagnose benign paroxysmal positional vertigo (BPPV).

The test can be carried out in an outpatient office setting.

A. <u>Steps:</u>

- ✓ Ask the patient to sit on the examination table with legs extended.
- ✓ Turn their head by 45 degrees to one side.
- ✓ Ask the patient to lie down with their head in the same position. Always assist the patient.
- ✓ The head should either hang from the table, extended by 20 degrees, or a pillow should be used beneath the upper back to give the neck the desired extension.
- ✓ Observe the patient's eyes for 30 seconds for a nystagmus. Be attentive, as there may be a latency of about 10 seconds before nystagmus appears.
- ✓ If there is no nystagmus, ask the patient to sit up and turn his/her head by 45 degrees in the opposite direction. Repeat the maneuver to look for an abnormality in the opposite ear.

B. <u>Interpretation:</u>

- ✓ A torsional or rotational nystagmus would appear in a patient with BPPV on lying down, however, it is not purely torsional and has a down beating or an up beating component.

- ✓ A positive test would be when the fast component of the nystagmus (look for the top of the eye, whether it moves clockwise or anti-clockwise) determines the affected ear, which is the ear closest to the ground.
- ✓ An up beating torsional nystagmus suggests pathology in the posterior semi-circular canal of the lower ear.
- ✓ A down beating torsional nystagmus suggests pathology in the anterior/superior semi-circular canal of the upper ear (ageotropic).
- ✓ If a horizontal nystagmus appears on turning the head to the opposite side while the patient lies supine, it suggests pathology in the horizontal semi-circular canal. If the nystagmus is towards the upper ear (apogeotropic), it suggests debris fixed to the cupula while a nystagmus towards the lower ear suggests free floating debris.
- ✓ If there is a pure vertical nystagmus, a central nervous system pathology should be considered.
- ✓ Nystagmus has a latency period of 8-10 seconds.

On repetition, the nystagmus decreases in intensity (fatigable).

Given the time constraints in the Step 2 CS exam, do not waste time in performing this maneuver. Instead, you can add it to your list of diagnostic tests in the patient note.

I-Increasing factors

"What started this episode?" look for triggering factors, or, "What makes this worse?" Changing position can cause vertigo in BPPV. Onset of dizziness on suddenly standing from a supine position suggests orthostatic hypotension. Sudden onset dizziness on long standing can be a vaso-vagal episode. Increased dizziness on exertion is usually suggestive of a cardiovascular disease.

D-Decreasing factors

- ✓ "Is there anything that makes it better?"

Previous history of similar symptoms-

- ✓ "Have you noticed any similar episodes in the past?"

M-Medication

- ✓ Asking the patient about medications may reveal the cause of the dizziness.
- ✓ History of alcohol ingestion or past medication like antidepressants or antihistaminics can cause dizziness.
- ✓ Past history of diabetes, stroke, and ear pathology can be very useful to associate the symptoms to a particular disease.

Bibliography

1. Newman-Toker, D. E.; Hsieh, Y. H.; Camargo, C. A., Jr.; Pelletier, A. J.; Butchy, G. T.; Edlow, J. A., Spectrum of dizziness visits to US emergency departments: cross-sectional analysis from a nationally representative sample. In *Mayo Clin Proc*, United States, 2008; Vol. 83, pp 765-75.
2. Neuhauser, H. K.; Radtke, A.; von Brevern, M.; Lezius, F.; Feldmann, M.; Lempert, T., Burden of dizziness and vertigo in the community. In *Arch Intern Med*, United States, 2008; Vol. 168, pp 2118-24.
3. Herr, R. D.; Zun, L.; Mathews, J. J., A directed approach to the dizzy patient. In *Ann Emerg Med*, United States, 1989; Vol. 18, pp 664-72.
4. Newman-Toker, D. E.; Dy, F. J.; Stanton, V. A.; Zee, D. S.; Calkins, H.; Robinson, K. A., How often is dizziness from primary cardiovascular disease true vertigo? A systematic review. *J Gen Intern Med* **2008,** *23* (12), 2087-94.
5. Newman-Toker, D. E.; Cannon, L. M.; Stofferahn, M. E.; Rothman, R. E.; Hsieh, Y. H.; Zee, D. S., Imprecision in patient reports of dizziness symptom quality: a cross-sectional study conducted in an acute care setting. In *Mayo Clin Proc*, United States, 2007; Vol. 82, pp 1329-40.
6. Hall, S. F.; Ruby, R. R.; McClure, J. A., The mechanics of benign paroxysmal vertigo. *J Otolaryngol* **1979,** *8* (2), 151-8.
7. Kerber, K. A.; Baloh, R. W., The evaluation of a patient with dizziness. In *Neurol Clin Pract*, 2011; Vol. 1, pp 24-33.
8. Vinik, A. I.; Erbas, T., Diabetic autonomic neuropathy. *Handb Clin Neurol* **2013,** *117,* 279-94.

Approach to Fatigue

Introduction

Fatigue is one of the most common symptoms with which a patient may present. Given its nonspecific and subjective nature, it poses a diagnostic challenge to the physician. A wide variety of disease processes can cause fatigue due to systemic deconditioning. Fatigue is one of the most important causes of loss of productive work.

In this chapter, we delve into the important causes of fatigue and how to approach a patient on the basis of his/her symptomatic history.

Definition

Clinically, fatigue is defined as **difficulty initiating** (weakness) or **maintaining** (easily tiring) **daily voluntary activities** (mental and physical). It is a subjective symptom of sluggishness and mental (memory, emotions, and concentration) and physical exhaustion.

Epidemiology

Fatigue is a universal symptom found in all populations. Women are more likely to present with fatigue as compared to men.[1,2] Two thirds of patients presenting with fatigue may have an underlying physical or psychiatric illness. In one study, it was found that in patients presenting with chronic fatigue, 74% of the patients had an underlying psychiatric illness and 7% had a physical illness.[3,4]

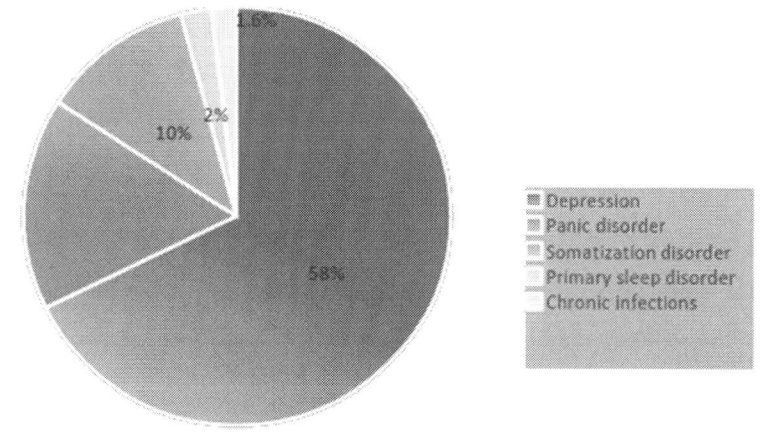

Most common causes of chronic fatigue

Causes of fatigue

Fatigue can be caused by a multitude of disease processes. It may be a subjective feeling or an important presentation of an underlying systemic disease. Fatigue mostly presents with an underlying inflammatory process, decreased metabolic activity, or altered psychological functions. Whenever a patient presents with fatigue, one should start thinking about the possible systems that might be involved or reasons that might be causing the above mentioned causes. The most common etiologies of fatigue are as mentioned below:

VitalSigns.edu-Differential Diagnosis		
Vital Checklist	Areas	Instructions in layman language
V	Vascular	Any cramps in the legs? Now in your mind you should be thinking of arteries or veins. Could the diagnosis be related to electrolytes or muscles?
I	Infections	Any recent infections?
T	Trauma	Any recent accidents?
A	Autoimmune/ Allergies/ Rheumatology	Do you have any problems with your immune system? What is the immune system? The immune system is a self-defense system where your body fights against disease, but in some cases, the body starts fighting against its own cells.
L	Labs-CBC, CMP, Magnesium, Phosphorous, UA, Stools	Any problems with blood work! Any problems with electrolytes!
S	Surgical	Any recent history of surgeries.
I	Inflammation of various body organs	CVS-Heart failure, valves, vessels, walls, wiring Lungs-COPD, restrictive lung disease Brain-Functional versus organic Muscles-Muscle ache Joints- Is there more pain in the morning? *pause*...or in the evening? *pause*... Chronic fatigue syndrome (systemic exertion intolerance disease), fibromyalgia
G	Genetic/GI causes	Celiac disease, IBD
N	Neoplasm	Underlying malignancies and associated paraneoplastic syndromes
S	Stress, Psychiatry or Psychological (go with pronunciation)	Depression, panic disorder, insomnia and sleep disorders Excessive workload, caregiver's fatigue (caring for young children, patient/s, or elderly)

	E	Endocrine	Do you have any thyroid problems? Do you have any vision problems? Do you have any problems with increased urine, increased thirst, and/or increased hunger?
	D	Drugs	Can you please elaborate on your medications? Do you take any OTC medications? Do you take any recreational drugs?
	U	Uterus & Pregnancy related issues	When did you last have your period?

During the exam, it becomes difficult to remember so many causes of fatigue, so an easier way to recall the most common causes is to use the mnemonic- Chronic **FATIGUE**:

Chronic FATIGUE			
Vital Checklist		Areas	Instructions
		Chronic Fatigue	Write your questions here?
	F	Fevers-Infections	
	A	Autoimmune, Anemia, Alcohol	
	T	Tumor, Thyroid, Tobacco	
	I	Insomnia	
	G	Gastrointestinal, Genitourinary (BPH)	
	U	Unknown/idiopathic	
	E	Endocrine, Exertion/caregiver fatigue	

Approach to a case of fatigue

Like other non-pain symptoms, we use our time-tested mnemonic, DOCTOR AID @ PM, to approach the history for a case of fatigue.

D- Duration- Depending on the duration, we can approximate what might be causing the fatigue in the patient.

- ✓ *Recent-* less than one month: infections, neoplasm, sleep disorder, depression, autoimmune disorders.
- ✓ *Prolonged-* more than one month, but less than six months: autoimmune disorder, chronic infections like tuberculosis, hepatitis B, endocrine disorders, and gastrointestinal disorders.
- ✓ *Chronic-* more than six months: chronic fatigue syndrome/systemic exertion intolerance disease/myalgic encephalomyelitis

Sometimes patients may research their symptoms online and inquire about chronic fatigue syndrome (CFS) as a possible cause. It is important to at least know the differentiating features and the diagnostic criteria for CFS.

Diagnostic criteria of CFS according to the U.S Centers for Disease Control and Prevention[5]:

Three criteria for CFS/SEIS/Myalgic encephalomyelitis

A.)
- The individual has severe chronic fatigue for 6 or more consecutive months
- The fatigue is not due to ongoing exertion or other medical conditions associated with fatigue
- The fatigue is not relieved by rest
- The fatigue is of new onset

B.) The fatigue significantly interferes with daily activities and work

C.) The individual concurrently has 4 or more of the following 8 symptoms:
- Post-exertional malaise lasting more than 24 hours
- Unrefreshing sleep
- Significant impairment of short-term memory or concentration (Cognitive dysfunction)
- Muscle pain/Myalgia
- Multi-joint pain/arthralgia without swelling or redness
- Headaches of new types, pattern, or severity
- Tender cervical or axillary lymph nodes
- Frequent or recurring sore throat

O-Onset

Fatigue, being a subjective feeling, is usually noted over a period of time, therefore, it rarely has an acute onset. It mostly has an insidious onset noted over a period of time.

C-Character

It is imperative to differentiate fatigue from muscle aches (myalgias), joint aches, and muscle weakness, as the patient may mistake them for fatigue, and an important clue to a serious disease may be ignored. It is also important to ask whether the patient is short of breath or exhausted. Shortness of breath would point more towards a cardiopulmonary or a hematological etiology as compared to a cause of fatigue.

- "Can you explain your fatigue in your own words?"

In case of a nonspecific reply, ask the patient,

- ✓ "Do you feel fatigued while walking or talking?" *pause...*
- ✓ "Or do you have double vision or droopy eyes?"
- ✓ "Did you ever trip and fall?" *pause...*
- ✓ "Or felt as if you were walking on cotton wool?"

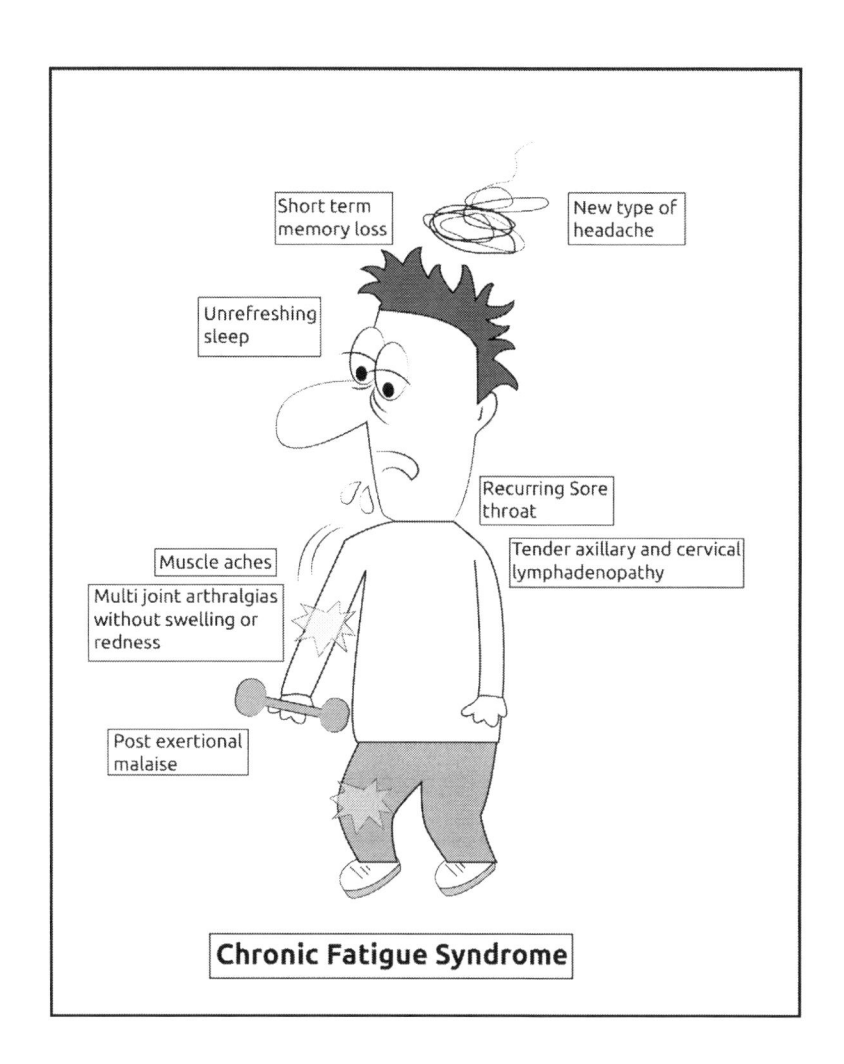

Chronic Fatigue Syndrome

- Short term memory loss
- New type of headache
- Unrefreshing sleep
- Recurring Sore throat
- Tender axillary and cervical lymphadenopathy
- Muscle aches
- Multi joint arthralgias without swelling or redness
- Post exertional malaise

> **Action Box:**
>
> If a patient complains of muscle pain, then think of causes of myalgia.
>
> If a patient complains of fatigue on walking/talking, then dyspnea is more likely. Think of cardiopulmonary causes.
>
> If a patient complains of droopy eyes, double vision, and weakness more in the evening, then think of myasthenia gravis.
>
> Frequent falls and cotton wool sensation while walking suggest sensory neuropathy/CNS disorders.

T-Time of the day

Ask the patient, "What time of the day do you feel more fatigued?"

- ✓ Obstructive sleep apnea/sleep disorders will present with unrefreshing sleep and tiredness in the morning.
- ✓ Muscle weakness or cardiopulmonary causes may cause fatigue with exertion and may be reported more in the evening. Also, patients of myasthenia gravis may present with fatigue that increases as the day progresses.
- ✓ Chronic fatigue syndrome/psychological causes or chronic infections may present with fatigue throughout the day.

O-Occasion

"What were you doing when you started to feel fatigued?" While stress related fatigue can be more during office time, caregiver fatigue can present more in home settings due to the stress of taking care of young children or elderly members.

R-Rate of progression

Progressive fatigue may indicate an underlying inflammatory process or an untreated infection. It may also signify the worsening of a systemic disease.

A-Associated symptoms

These questions are the most important clues for the underlying cause of fatigue. Questions based on the possible etiologies of fatigue can help us redirect our thought process and diagnostic algorithm towards a particular system.

- ✓ If the patient seems depressed or sad, asking about **DIGEST P CAPSULE** to rule out depression may be necessary.
- ✓ History of **fever, chills, cough, burning urination, throat pain, skin rash, headache, and multiple joint aches** can point towards an underlying infection or a rheumatological etiology
- ✓ History of **weight loss, cachexia, anorexia, or low grade fever in the setting of a cough, hemoptysis, change in bowel habits, bloody stools, or urine**, etc., may point to an underlying malignancy
- ✓ **Weight gain, skin changes, brittle hair, constipation, voice changes, or facial morphic** changes may point towards an endocrine pathology such as hypothyroidism, Cushing's syndrome, Addison's disease, or panhypopituitarism. History of **excessive thirst or urination** may suggest diabetes mellitus or diabetes insipidus.

Action Box

It is always a great idea to use the Vital Checklist GHALEN GHULAM (Head to Toe) approach, as this will help us to evaluate for a review of system and cover most of the questions to be asked in associated symptoms.

- ✓ *I-Increasing factors-* "What makes your fatigue worse?"
- ✓ *D-Decreasing factors-* "What relieves your fatigue?"
- ✓ *P-Previous history of similar complaints-* "Have you had similar symptoms in the past?"
- ✓ *M-Medications used for fatigue-* "Did you resort to any medical treatment for your fatigue so far?"

Physical Examination

General examination to look for pallor, icterus, cyanosis, clubbing, edema, and / or lymphadenopathy.

Mental Examination

- ✓ Orientation to time place, person, and situation
- ✓ Intact short term and long term memory
- ✓ Cognitive functions

Systemic Examination would involve-

- ✓ Cardiovascular
- ✓ Respiratory
- ✓ Abdomen
- ✓ Thyroid
- ✓ Extremities

If certain symptoms of a neurological process are evident, a quick neurological exam may also be performed.

Given the scarcity of time in the clinical skills exam, one may have to prioritize which tests to perform. For example, if history suggests a possible endocrine etiology, examination of the thyroid, reflexes, and extremities becomes important. If it is nonspecific, a **mini mental examination** and a quick cardiopulmonary examination may also help you narrow down your diagnosis.

Bibliography

1. Chen MK. The epidemiology of self-perceived fatigue among adults. *Prev Med.* 1986;15:74-81.
2. Ridsdale L, Evans A, Jerrett W, Mandalia S, Osler K, Vora H. Patients with fatigue in general practice: a prospective study. *Bmj.* 1993;307:103-106.
3. Wessely S, Chalder T, Hirsch S, Wallace P, Wright D. Psychological symptoms, somatic symptoms, and psychiatric disorder in chronic fatigue and chronic fatigue syndrome: a prospective study in the primary care setting. *Am J Psychiatry.* 1996;153(8):1050-1059.
4. Manu P, Lane TJ, Matthews DA. Chronic fatigue and chronic fatigue syndrome: clinical epidemiology and aetiological classification. *Ciba Found Symp.* 1993;173:23-31; discussion 31-42.
5. CDC - Diagnosis - Chronic Fatigue Syndrome (CFS). 2015; http://www.cdc.gov/cfs/diagnosis/index.html.

Approach to Hearing Impairment

Hearing loss can be the result of a wide variety of causes. To arrive at the differential diagnosis for hearing impairment in a clinical setup can be a challenge. To help aid this diagnostic dilemma, we have devised a simple step-by-step process (A-SPOT) which will help you to reach the DDx within the 15 minutes allotted during the Step 2 CS exam.

Step		What to do	When
1	A	Note the **A**ge	At the doorway
2	S	Associated **S**ymptoms	During history
3	P	Presence of **P**ain	During history
4	O	**O**totoxic Drugs & Trauma	During history
5	T	Tuning Fork **T**ests: Rinne and Weber	During examination

Step 1: Age
Make sure you note the age of the patient presented at the doorway. Age is the single most important factor that will help you to diagnose the cause leading to hearing impairment in your patient.

Children	Adults	Elderly
Congenital/Genetic causes	Cerumen impaction	Presbycusis
Otitis media	Otitis media	Cerumen impaction
Cholesteatoma and CSOM	Cholesteatoma and CSOM	Meniere's disease (35-60 years)
Foreign body impaction	Otosclerosis	Acoustic neuroma (40-60 years)
Trauma or child abuse	Meniere's disease (35-60 years)	
Keratosis obturans	Otitic barotrauma	
Otitic barotrauma	Acoustic neuroma (40-60 years)	
	Glomus tumor (40-50 years)	

Step 2: Narrow down your DDx: Associated Symptoms

Now ask the patient about the other symptoms experienced along with the hearing loss.

Symptom	Question	Possible Differential Diagnosis
Tinnitus: Unilateral	Q: Have you been experiencing any ringing in your ears? A: Yes, doc, in one ear	Q: Do you also feel dizzy/is the room spinning/are you spinning? A: Yes: ✓ Meniere's disease ✓ Acoustic neuroma ✓ Multiple sclerosis ✓ Glomus tumor ✓ Perilymph fistula A: No: ✓ Cerumen impaction ✓ Infection
Tinnitus: Bilateral	Q: Have you been experiencing any ringing in your ears? A: Yes, doc, in both ears	✓ Otosclerosis ✓ Presbycusis ✓ Ototoxic drugs ✓ Noise induced damage
Fullness in ear	Have you been experiencing fullness in your ear?	✓ Cerumen impaction ✓ Meniere's disease ✓ Sudden sensorineural hearing loss (Emergency!): Only sensorineural hearing loss with ear fullness
Ear discharge	Have you been experiencing ear drainage? Do you have a history of ear infections?	✓ Otitis media ✓ CSOM and cholesteatoma
Vertigo	Have you been feeling dizzy?	✓ Lasting for minutes: Meniere's ✓ Lasting for months: Labyrinthitis
Noise trauma: Occupation, exposure to explosion/gunfire	Were you exposed to a sudden, very loud sound like an explosion or gunfire? What occupation are you involved in?	✓ Acoustic trauma (single, brief exposure to a very intense sound) ✓ Noise-induced hearing loss (chronic exposure)
Tullio phenomenon: Loud sounds produce vertigo	Do loud sounds make you dizzy/produce vertigo?	✓ Syphilitic hearing loss ✓ Meniere's disease
Recruitment/intolerance to loud sounds	Are you unable to tolerate loud sounds?	✓ Meniere's disease
Fluctuating hearing loss	Have you had similar episodes of hearing loss in the past?	✓ Meniere's disease
Paracusis willisii	Do you hear better in noisy environments?	✓ Otosclerosis
Confusion of rhyming words	Do you confuse rhyming words? Like fin/tin?	✓ Presbycusis
Recent travel/underwater diving	Did you go underwater diving or have you travelled in an airplane recently?	✓ Otitic barotrauma/Aero-otitis media

Step 3: Narrow down your DDx: Pain

Now, determine the presence/absence of pain to narrow down your DDx.

Sudden painful loss of hearing	Sudden painless loss of hearing	Gradual painless loss of hearing
✓ Otitis externa ✓ Chronic otitis media (immobile tympanic membrane)	Complete canal occlusion with cerumen (wax swells up when water enters the ear canal during bathing and swimming: sudden loss of hearing)	✓ Middle ear effusion ✓ Otosclerosis ✓ Glomus tumor or vascular anomaly ✓ Cholesteatoma

Step 4: Rule out use of ototoxic drugs and trauma

Ask:

✓ Have you had any accidents/injuries/recent surgery?

If trauma is present	
Conductive	Sensorineural
Trauma to the ossicles leading to disruption of ossicular chain	Trauma to labyrinth or VIIIth nerve, e.g. fractures of temporal bone, concussion of labyrinth, or ear surgery
Perforation of the TM	**Sudden hearing loss**: Head injury, ear operations, noise trauma, barotrauma, or rupture of cochlear membranes

Ask:

✓ What medicines are you currently taking?
✓ Have you received any intravenous antibiotics?
✓ Do you take diuretics?
✓ Do you take pain medications?
✓ Have you taken chemotherapy?

Ototoxic drugs	
Aminoglycoside antibiotics	Streptomycin Gentamycin, Tobramycin Neomycin Kanamycin
Diuretics	Furosemide
Chemotherapy agents	Cisplatin Carboplatin
Analgesics	Salicylates Indomethacin Ibuprofen
Chemicals	Tobacco Marijuana Alcohol
Others	Propranolol Propyl thiouracil

Step 5: Narrow down your DDx: Tuning fork tests

Conductive or Sensorineural:
Perform the clinical tests listed below to determine whether the patient has conductive or sensorineural hearing loss.

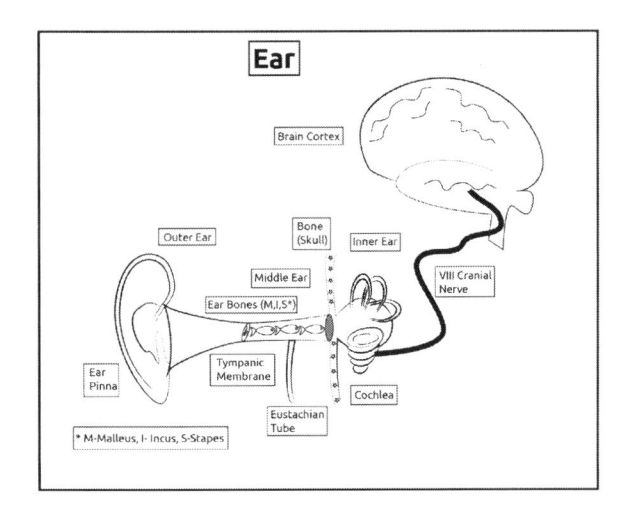

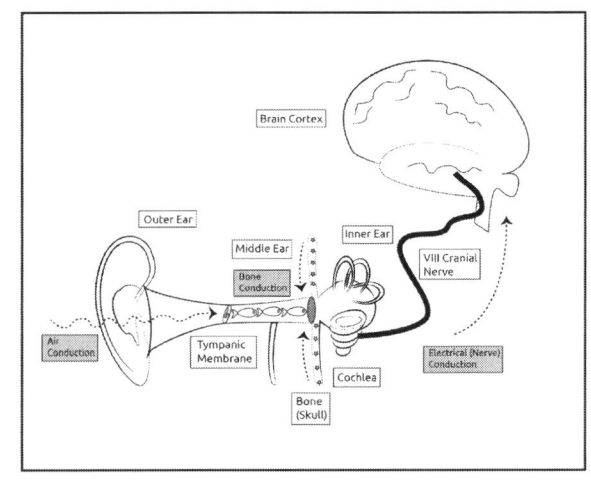

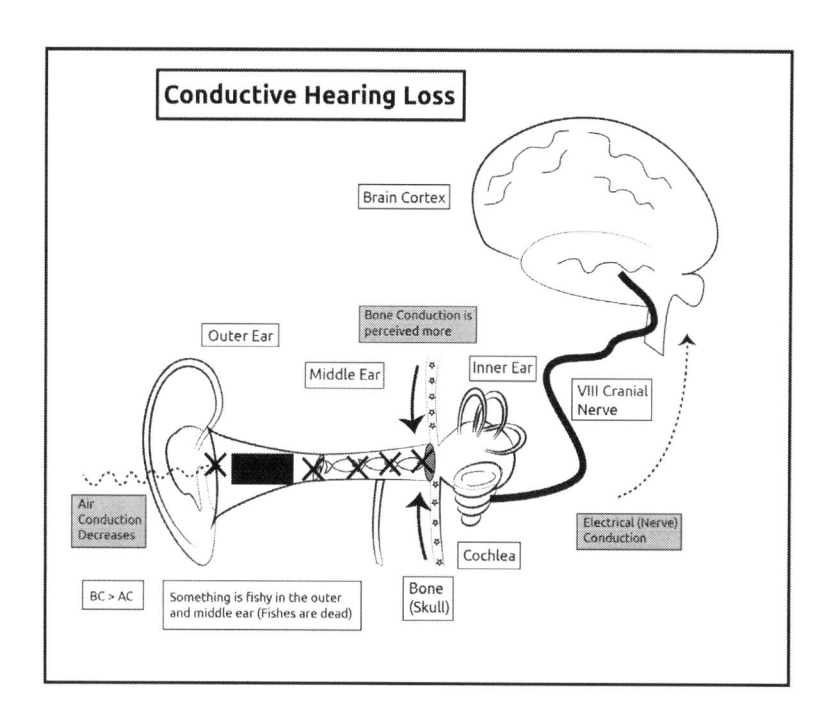

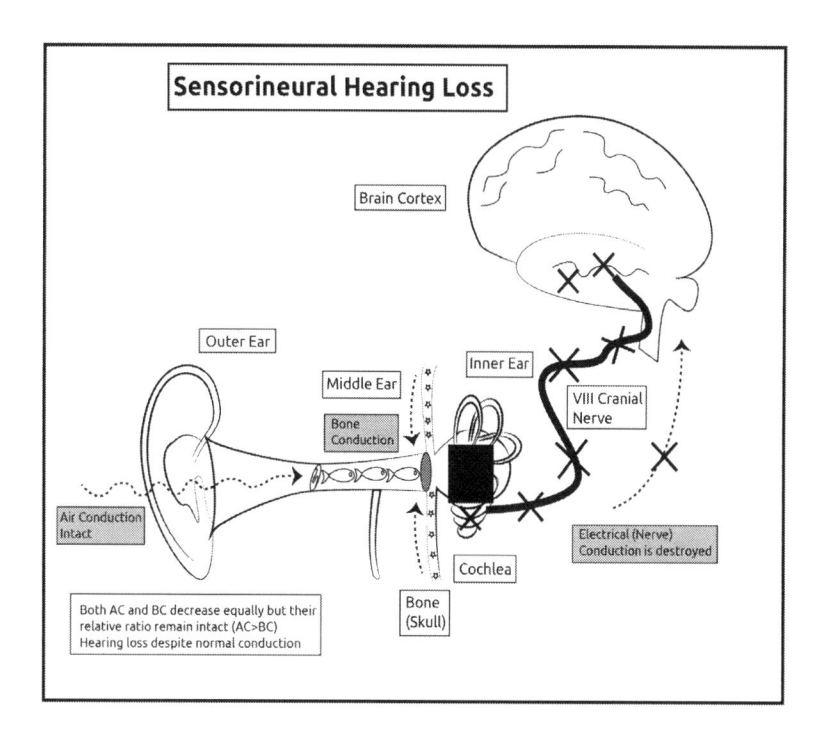

If we know which ear is affected, we can perform the Rinne and Weber tests to determine the type of hearing impairment.

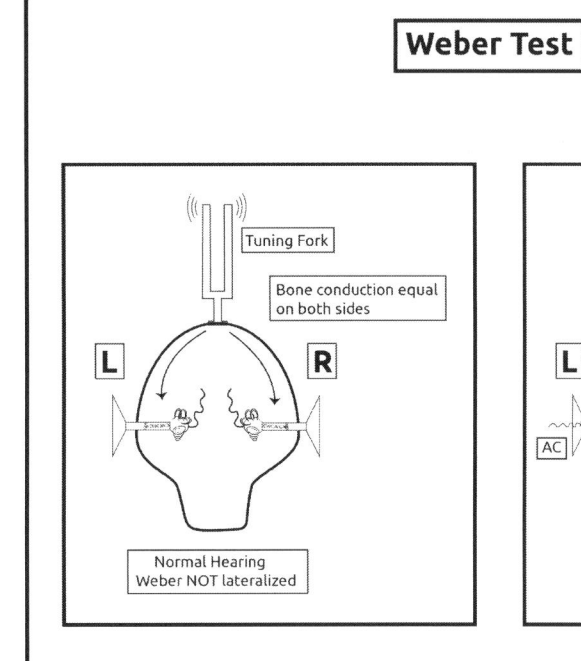

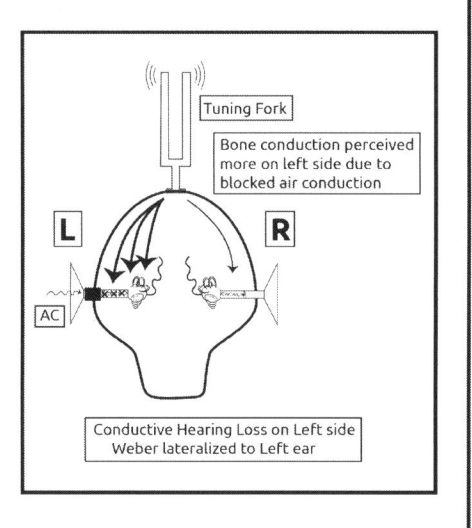

Weber Test

Normal Hearing — Weber NOT lateralized
- Tuning Fork
- Bone conduction equal on both sides

Conductive Hearing Loss on Left side — Weber lateralized to Left ear
- Tuning Fork
- Bone conduction perceived more on left side due to blocked air conduction
- AC

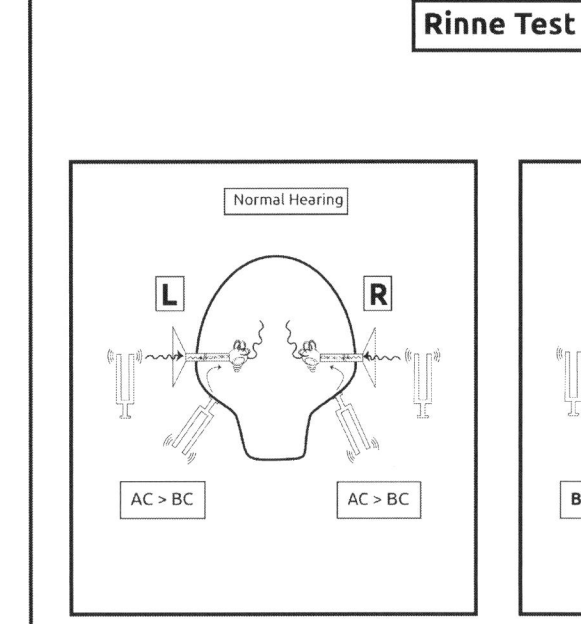

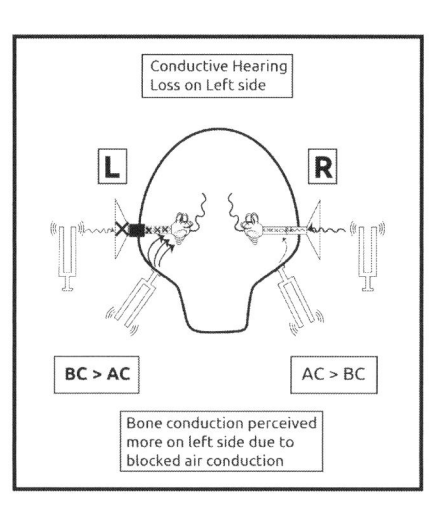

Rinne Test

Normal Hearing
- AC > BC (Left)
- AC > BC (Right)

Conductive Hearing Loss on Left side
- BC > AC (Left)
- AC > BC (Right)
- Bone conduction perceived more on left side due to blocked air conduction

RINNE'S TEST		What to explain to the patient while you are performing this maneuver
WHY	The Rinne test compares air conduction with bone conduction.	"I will now perform a special test using a tuning fork to find out the type of hearing impairment you are experiencing."
HOW	The vibrating tuning fork is placed on the mastoid bone (BC/bone conduction). The patient is asked to indicate when they stop hearing the sound. When the patient stops hearing the sound, the tuning fork is placed in front of the ear canal (AC/air conduction).	"I will place the vibrating tuning fork on the bone at the back of your ear and wait for you to tell me when you stop hearing the sound. You can do this by simply raising your finger to indicate that you have stopped hearing the sound." "I will then bring the tuning fork in front of your ear and ask you if you still hear the sound. Is this alright with you?"
WHAT TO INTERPRET	**Normal hearing/Sensorineural hearing loss (SNHL)**: AC > BC. This means that the sound is still heard when the tuning fork is placed in front of the ear canal. This is called a **Positive Rinne's Test.** In SNHL, AC remains more than BC, but total time of hearing the sound decreases. **Conductive hearing loss**: BC > AC. This means that the sound is not heard when the tuning fork is placed in front of the ear canal. This is called a **Negative Rinne's Test.**	"Thank you for letting me do that. It was really helpful."

WEBER'S TEST		What to explain to the patient while you are performing this maneuver
WHY	Weber's test is lateralized to the ear with conductive hearing loss, as the ambient noise is unable to travel via the ear canal. The only transmission of sound occurs through bone and is, therefore, perceived better.	"I will now perform another simple test with the tuning fork to find out more about your problem."
HOW	First, activate the tuning fork (512-Hz) by striking it gently against your elbow. Then, place it in midline on the patient's scalp or on the forehead. Ask the patient in which ear the sound is heard best.	"I will place the vibrating tuning fork at the center of your forehead. Please tell me in which ear the sound is heard best."
WHAT TO INTERPRET	Normally the sound is heard equally in both ears. If patient has **conductive hearing loss**: the sound will be heard best in the affected ear (lateralization). If the patient has sensorineural hearing loss: the sound will be heard best in the normal ear.	"Thank you for letting me do that. It was really helpful."

What to interpret

Conductive hearing loss	Sensorineural hearing loss
Negative Rinne's Test (BC > AC)	Positive Rinne's Test (AC > BC)
Weber lateralized to the poorer ear	Weber lateralized to better ear

Do Rinne's test Followed by Weber's Test

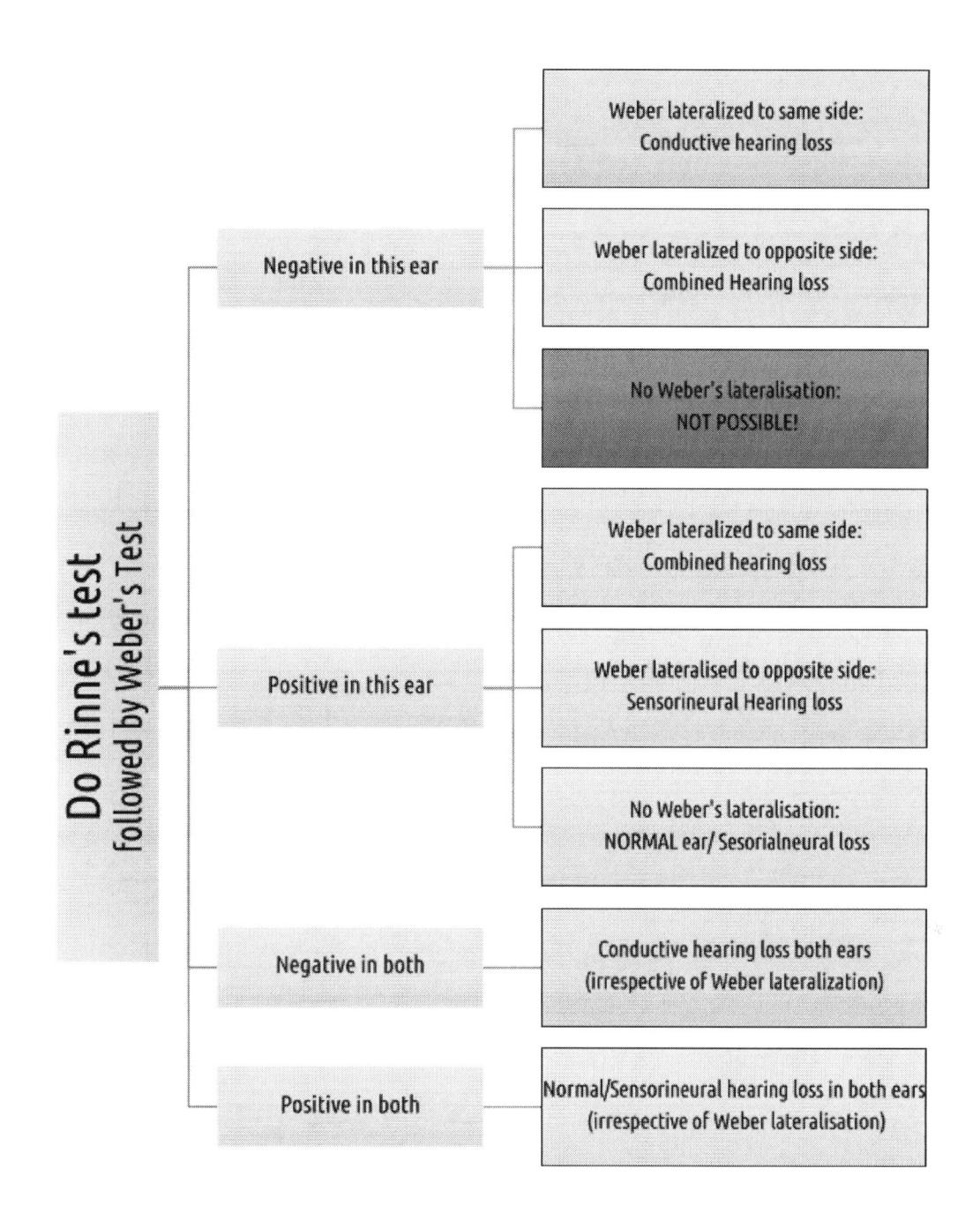

- **Negative in this ear**
  - Weber lateralized to same side: Conductive hearing loss
  - Weber lateralized to opposite side: Combined Hearing loss
  - No Weber's lateralisation: NOT POSSIBLE!

- **Positive in this ear**
  - Weber lateralized to same side: Combined hearing loss
  - Weber lateralised to opposite side: Sensorineural Hearing loss
  - No Weber's lateralisation: NORMAL ear / Sesorialneural loss

- **Negative in both**
  - Conductive hearing loss both ears (irrespective of Weber lateralization)

- **Positive in both**
  - Normal/Sensorineural hearing loss in both ears (irrespective of Weber lateralisation)

Key:
○	Conductive Hearing Loss
○	Sensorineural Hearing Loss
○	Combined Hearing Loss

HOW TO REMEMBER

In the ear under exam:

Rinne's Negative = Conductive Hearing Loss

- ✓ Rinne's negative with Weber lateralized to the same side: Pure conductive hearing loss
- ✓ Rinne's negative with Weber lateralized to the opposite side: Combined (conductive and sensorineural)

Rinne's Positive = Normal ear/Sensorineural hearing loss

- ✓ Rinne's positive with Weber lateralized to the same side: Combined hearing loss
- ✓ Rinne's positive with Weber lateralized to the opposite side: Sensorineural hearing loss

When there is no Weber lateralization:

- ✓ Rinne's negative in this ear: NOT POSSIBLE
- ✓ Rinne's positive in this ear: Normal/sensorineural hearing loss
- ✓ Rinne's negative in both the ears: Conductive hearing loss in both
- ✓ Rinne's positive in both: Normal/sensorineural loss in both

	An easy to remember and hard to forget	
Rinne's negative	Conductive hearing loss	If you **don't** rinse [Rin(ne)'s] your ear, your ear gets blocked, and you get conductive hearing loss, i.e. No rinsing = negative Rinne's = blocked conduction = conductive hearing loss
Weber lateralization	Weber lateralized to the same side in conductive hearing loss	If a spider spins a web [web(ber)] in the ear which you have not rinsed, it will get further blocked. Weber lateralized to same side = web in the ear = conductive hearing loss in this ear.
The other possibilities automatically become easy to remember if you remember the above.		

Now, narrow down your DDx based upon the type of the hearing loss.

Conductive hearing loss		
	Etiology	CAUSES
V	Vascular	Hemotympanum
I	Inflammation	Allergic, CSOM, furuncles, serous otitis media
T	Trauma	Child abuse, violence
A	Autoimmune	
L	Labs	
S	Social & Drugs	Wax impaction due to poor hygiene
I	Infection	Malignant otitis externa, furuncle
G	Genetic	Disruption of ear ossicles Congenital malformation of external ear Cholesteatoma Fused ear ossicles
N	Neurological/Neoplasm	Glomus tumor
S	Systemic	Otosclerosis, tympanosclerosis

Sensorineural Hearing Loss		
Acquired		
	Etiology	CAUSES
V	**V**ascular	✓ Meniere's (endolymphatic hydrops) ✓ CNS infarction/hemorrhage
I	**I**nflammation	✓ Suppurative labyrinthitis ✓ Meningitis (auditory nerve/cochlear damage)
T	**T**rauma	✓ Trauma to labyrinth or VIIIth nerve, e.g. fractures of temporal bone, concussion of labyrinth, or ear surgery
A	**A**utoimmune	
L	**L**abs	
S	**S**ocial & Drugs	✓ Ototoxic drugs
I	**I**nfection	✓ Infections of labyrinth- viral, bacterial, spirochaetal ✓ Mumps (epidemic parotitis) ✓ Measles (auditory nerve damage)
G	**G**enetic	
N	**N**eurological/**N**eoplasm	✓ Acoustic neuroma ✓ CNS tumor ✓ Multiple sclerosis
S	**S**ystemic	✓ Systemic disorders: DM, hypothyroidism, kidney disease, blood disorders
	Others	✓ Presbycusis ✓ Noise induced hearing loss ✓ Sudden hearing loss

Tests/Investigations

Hearing evaluation:

- ✓ Whispering test
- ✓ Test of hearing at a distance

Tuning Fork Tests:

- ✓ Rinne's Test
- ✓ Weber Test

Do the external examination by inspection and palpation. Examine for the presence of swelling and observe the size and contents. Rule out malignant otitis externa caused by pseudomonas in elderly diabetics/immunosuppressed patients.

Perform an otoscopy. Look for the following with regards to the TM:

Color:

- ✓ Pearly white: Normal
- ✓ Red and congested: Acute otitis media
- ✓ Bluish: Secretory otitis media, hemotympanum
- ✓ Chalky plaque: Tympanosclerosis

Light reflex

Position:

- ✓ Retracted: Tubal occlusion, retraction pockets in the attic and posterosuperior region
- ✓ Bulging: Acute otitis media, hemotympanum

Surface:

- ✓ Perforation: AOM, CSOM
- ✓ Vesicles/bullae: Herpes zoster, myringitis bullosa

Mobility: Pneumatic otoscopy:

- ✓ Mobile: Normal
- ✓ Restricted: Fluid or adhesions in the middle ear

Examination of mastoid: Look for obliteration of retroauricular groove/swelling/fistula/scar. Tenderness is present in mastoiditis.

Diagnostic tests to order:

For conductive hearing loss:

- ✓ Examination under otoscope (to look for evidence of blockage)
- ✓ Audiologic testing (audiometry)

For sensorineural hearing loss:

- ✓ Examination under otoscope
- ✓ Audiologic testing
- ✓ Radioimaging of temporal bone (X-ray/CT scan)
- ✓ Serology for syphilis
- ✓ Thyroid function tests
- ✓ CBC
- ✓ Blood sugar

How to report an ENT examination in a patient note:

"Nasal turbinates erythematous but not hypertrophied. Oral cavity examination unremarkable. MMM. Oropharynx examination shows 3+ tonsillar hypertrophy bilaterally. No pooling of secretions in the posterior oropharynx and no post-nasal drip. Left ear examination shows normal external auditory meatus, TM with positive LR, landmarks clearly visible. No discharge. Right ear examination shows normal external auditory meatus, TM with positive LR, landmarks clearly visible. No discharge."
(Here MMM: Mucous Membranes Moist)

"No erythema or tenderness of auricle, periauricle, or external auditory meatus. Cerumen not seen. TMs with light reflex, no stigmata of infection, no lymphadenopathy, oropharynx normal. Weber test revealed no lateralization; Rinne's test is positive (revealed air conduction > bone conduction)."

Approach to Insomnia

Insomnia is one of the most common complaints increasingly being reported in daily medical practices. It is very likely that you may get a case of insomnia in conjunction with a systemic disease in your USMLE Step 2 CS exam.

Insomnia is the inability to fall asleep, maintain sleep, or waking too easily or too early in the morning **despite adequate time to sleep**. The most important components to insomnia are the associated daytime symptoms due to poor sleep.

These symptoms include:

- ✓ **Fatigue**
- ✓ Daytime sleepiness
- ✓ Poor concentration
- ✓ Irritability and mood lability
- ✓ Reduced energy
- ✓ Increased chances of accidents or mistakes
- ✓ Reduced performance in work or education

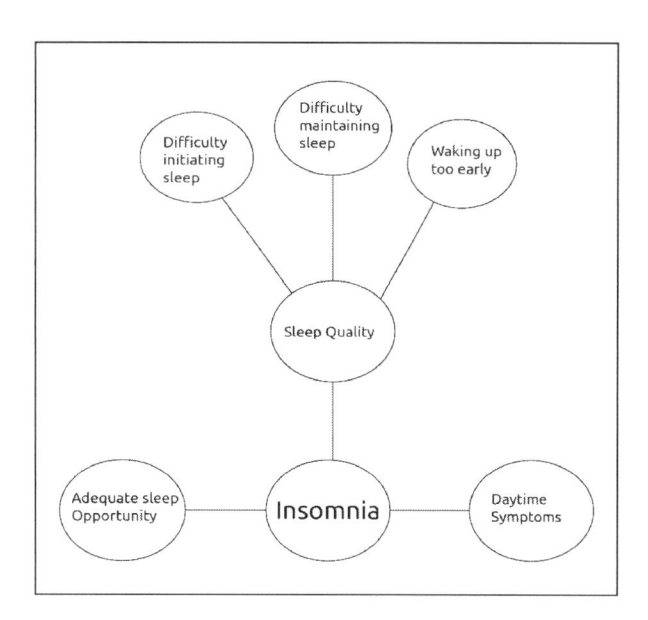

E.g. A nightshift worker who works through the night and comes to the doctor with complaints of inability to sleep will not qualify as having insomnia, because he is not getting an adequate **sleep opportunity**. After months of night shifts when his schedule changes, if the patient is still unable to sleep at night even though he has the time and opportunity, it is then considered insomnia.

Fatigue is one of the most closely associated symptom to insomnia. Just like a history of 'shortness of breath' in a patient presenting with 'chest pain' is indispensable, a history of fatigue needs to be asked in a case of insomnia and vice versa.

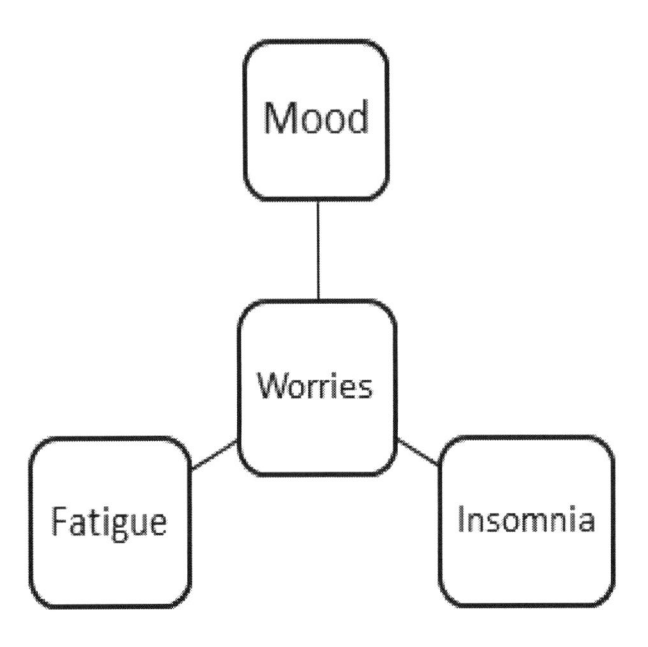

```
           Mood
            |
         Worries
          /    \
    Fatigue    Insomnia
```

Action Box:

If a patient presents with insomnia, fatigue, or mood changes, the patient is obviously worried, and at this point, you must take a moment to empathize.

Advise the patient to write their worries on paper and discuss them indetail. Expressive writing serves many fruitful purposes.[1] First, it helps the patient to express themselves completely, giving them a lighter feeling and reducing stress. Secondly, it gives the patient an opportunity to reflect on their worries and to subconsciously devise solutions. Lastly, it improves the patient's working memory capacity, thus improving their functionality.[2]

[1]. A new reason for keeping a diary. **2015**.
[2]. Klein, K.; Boals, A., Expressive writing can increase working memory capacity. *Journal of Experimental Psychology: General* **2001**, *130* (3), 520.

Insomnia may present with or without an underlying psychiatric or systemic disease. If it persists despite complete treatment of the underlying disease, insomnia must be considered an independent entity.

In this chapter, we will discuss how to approach a patient with sleep disturbances.

To understand the causes of insomnia easily, we can divide them according to the age of the patient. This will help you narrow down from the vast list of differentials to very specific and most likely causes.

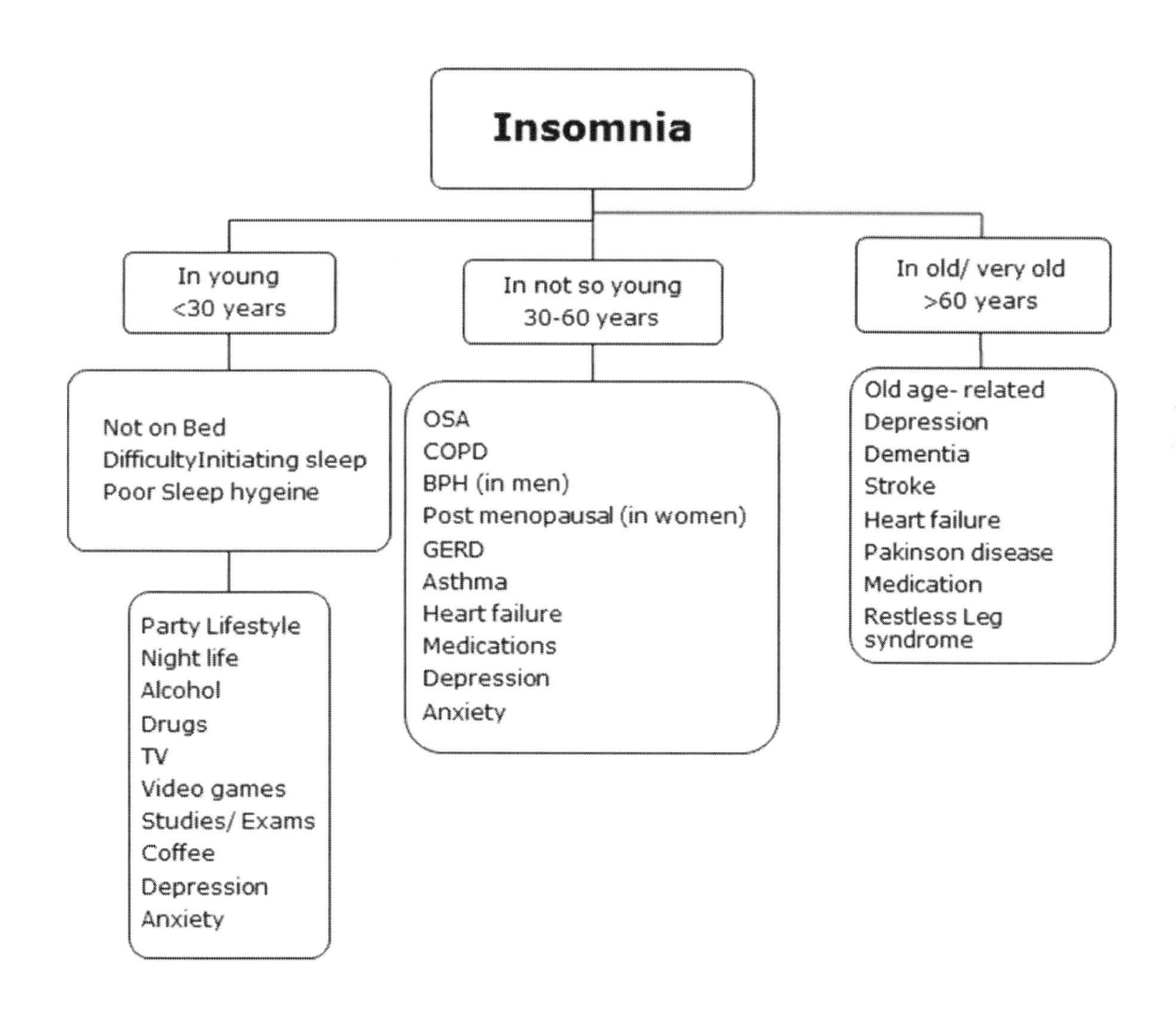

Insomnia

In young <30 years
- Not on Bed
- Difficulty Initiating sleep
- Poor Sleep hygeine

- Party Lifestyle
- Night life
- Alcohol
- Drugs
- TV
- Video games
- Studies/Exams
- Coffee
- Depression
- Anxiety

In not so young 30-60 years
- OSA
- COPD
- BPH (in men)
- Post menopausal (in women)
- GERD
- Asthma
- Heart failure
- Medications
- Depression
- Anxiety

In old/ very old >60 years
- Old age- related
- Depression
- Dementia
- Stroke
- Heart failure
- Pakinson disease
- Medication
- Restless Leg syndrome

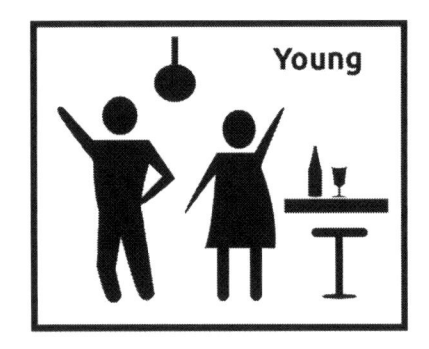

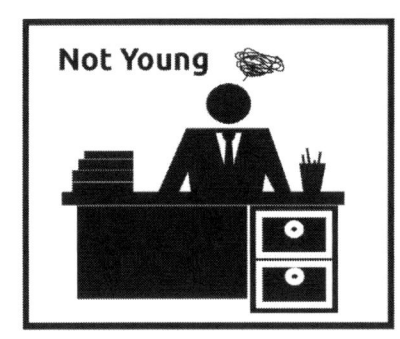

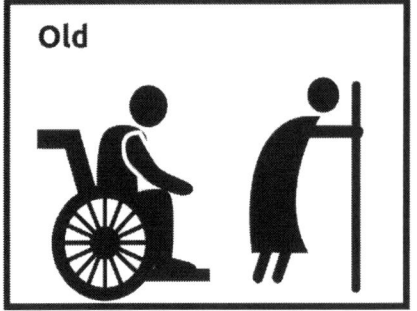

In young patients

In younger age groups, the most common causes of sleep disturbances are usually 'difficulty initiating sleep' or 'not being on the bed.'

A younger person is more likely to have an active nightlife, consume alcohol and abuse drugs, work at night, or undergo stress due to examinations or studies. Poor sleep hygiene is also a very common cause of insomnia in young patients. Watching TV until late at night and spending hours on laptops or phones while in bed destroy sleep initiation, causing trouble falling asleep.

Therefore, it becomes imperative to ask young patients about their sleep habits and what they like to do before or after retiring to bed.

In not so young patients

As you grow older, lifestyle diseases, age-specific diseases, work related stress, social and financial stress, and psychiatric problems like depression or anxiety start to affect your quality of sleep. Frequent night time awakening due to increased urinary frequency and urgency in benign prostatic hyperplasia, an episode of breathlessness in patients of COPD, and asthma or heart failure can affect sleep significantly.

Work, social, and financial stress can cause a lot of anxiety, leading to poor sleep quality. Obese individuals may suffer from obesity hypoventilation syndrome (Pickwickian syndrome) or obstructive sleep apnea (OSA), causing snoring and poor sleep. This may also cause significant daytime symptoms, leading to decreased energy levels, decreased motivation, irritable mood, increased chances of motor vehicle accidents, and lower performance at work.

Medications causing insomnia

- ✓ Beta blockers
- ✓ Bronchodilators
- ✓ Steroids
- ✓ CNS stimulants
- ✓ CNS depressants

> **Action Box:**
>
> "Do you wake up in the middle of the night to urinate?" *pause...* "How many times do you wake up?"
>
> Nocturia is waking up at night to void. One episode per night is considered normal, but if there are more episodes, it may be associated with daytime symptoms. Also, it is considered a symptom of obstructive sleep apnea and other systemic disorders. It is usually seen in elderly patients.
>
> Enuresis/bedwetting is the involuntary loss of urine while asleep. The patient does not wake up during this episode and it may not be associated with significant daytime symptoms. This is usually seen in young children.

In old and very old patients

With normal aging, REM sleep decreases and the latent period for sleep onset increases. Therefore, older individuals usually have poor sleep.

The most common causes in older patients are related to neurological problems.

Depression, dementia syndromes, strokes, Parkinson disease, etc. may cause poor sleep.

Systemic diseases like decompensated heart failure, late stage COPD, and BPH may also affect sleep significantly.

Vital Checklist trivia
Insomnia in depression versus anxiety

In depression, the patient has an increased REM sleep in initial hours and a decreased sleep latency, leading to normal or ease in falling asleep, but poor sleep quality, resulting in early morning awakening. In atypical depression, patients may have hypersomnia.

In anxiety, however, the sleep latency is increased, leading to difficulty falling asleep. Patients may lie on the bed for hours before actually falling asleep.

Our approach to insomnia should be similar to any non-pain symptom. Using the mnemonic **DOCTOR AID @ PM** can be very useful to reach the right diagnosis and rule out a lot of etiologies.

D – Duration

- ✓ Q: "For how long has this problem been going on?"

O- Onset

- ✓ Acute? (Jet lag, trauma, tragedy) or chronic (psychiatric or systemic?)
- ✓ Q: "Did the problem start suddenly?" *pause*... "Gradually?"

C- Characteristic

- ✓ Inability to sleep, or other symptoms obstructing sleep?
- ✓ Q: "Are you not able to sleep? Or do you get up in the middle of the night?"

T- Time of the night

- ✓ Initially falling asleep or early morning? (depression vs anxiety)
- ✓ Q: "Do you wake up early in the morning?"
- ✓ Q: "Are you sad?"

O- Occasion

- ✓ Marriage, party, exam time?
- ✓ Q: "What were you doing during the period when you started having sleep troubles?"

R- Rate of Progression

- ✓ Q: "Do you think this is getting worse?"

A-Associated symptoms

- ✓ Fatigue, daytime symptoms; disease specific symptoms may narrow the diagnosis. (breathlessness to COPD or heart failure; frequency and urgency for BPH; **D.I.G.E.S.T P CAP**sule for depression, etc.)

I-Increasing factors

- ✓ Q: "Any stress? *pause*... "Any medications? Any lifestyle habit at night?"
- ✓ Q: "What do you think is making your sleep troubles worse?"

D-Decreasing factors- Any lifestyle changes? Yoga? Medication? Treatment of primary disease?

- ✓ Q: "What are you doing to make it better?"

P-Previous medical history of similar symptoms

M-Medications

- ✓ Q: "What medications are you taking for your insomnia?"

Approach to Joints and Extremities

There will be cases on your Step 2 CS examination where the patient may present with a myriad of complaints related to the musculoskeletal system. These complaints can range from a vague muscular pain to a more serious presentation suggestive of joint infection or autoimmune diseases like rheumatoid arthritis, etc.

As with all cases, the most important aspect is the history, which comprises of more than 50% of your diagnosis. The rest is comprised of the physical examination and the 'coaching' of the patient.

Overview
We need to approach these cases in a systematic way for which we propose this checklist: **"ChInA SPADE"**

Ch – Chronology

Ask the patient about the duration of his/her symptoms.

- More than 6 weeks – chronic conditions requiring complete medical evaluation
- Less than 6 weeks – acute conditions, usually bacterial or viral infection or autoimmune reactions
- Bacterial – Salmonella, Shigella, Campylobacter, Tropheryma whipplei, Yersinia, Chlamydia, Neisseria gonorrhoeae
- Viral – Parvovirus

In – Inflammation

Check for signs of inflammation.

- Rubor – redness over the joint
- Calor – elevated temperature of the skin overlying the joint
- Dolor – painful joint movements
- Tumor – swelling of the joint
- Functio laesa – loss of function, restricted movements

A – Aspirate

> **Action Box:**
> In the Step 2 CS exam, it is very important to mention arthrocentesis/joint aspirate in your diagnostic test list if you suspect an inflamed joint, as your management will solely depend on it. Additionally, if antibiotics are prescribed before a diagnostic arthrocentesis, it spoils the clinical picture and makes the management more difficult.
>
> A joint aspirate (arthrocentesis) can be diagnostic for inflammatory conditions of the joint.

Findings in joint aspirate[1]					
Findings	Normal	Non inflammatory	Gout/ pseudogout	Septic	Traumatic/ hemorrhagic
Color	Transparent	Transparent	Opaque/ Turbid	Opaque/ Turbid	Red/bloody
WBC count	<200	0-2000	2000-100,000	15,000-100,000	200-2000
% of Polymorpho-nuclear WBCs/mm^3	<25%	<25%	>50%	>75%	50-75%
RBCs	Nil	Nil	Few	Few	Many
Culture	Negative	Negative	Negative	May be positive	Negative
Crystals	Negative	Negative	Positive	Negative	Negative

[1]Horowitz, D. L.; Katzap, E.; Horowitz, S.; Barilla-LaBarca, M.-L., Approach to Septic Arthritis - American Family Physician. **2015**.

Characteristics of various joint diseases						
	RA	SLE	OA	AS	PA	Fibromyalgia
Symmetry	Present	Present	+/-	Present	+/-	Present
Pattern	Small & large joints	Small & large joints	Small & large joints	Large Joints	Small & large joints	Diffuse
Axial	+	--	+	+	+	+

Action Box:
RA, OA, AS, PA, and Fibromyalgia have the letter "A" in their name. Axial also starts with "A." You can use this to remember that these pathologies have axial involvement.

The bones which are involved in the axial skeleton are the skull, hyoid bone, vertebra, sternum, and ribs. Basically, all the bones that are oriented vertically are part of the axial skeleton.

Distributions	F>M	F>M	F=M	M>F	F=M	F>M
Extra-articular Manifestations	See below					

RA,- Rheumatoid Arthritis; SLE,- Systemic Lupus Erythematosus; OA,- Osteoarthritis; AS,- Ankylosing Spondylitis; PA,- Psoriatic Arthropathy; Fibro,- Fibromyalgia.

Action Box:

An easier way to remember joint examination is through the following mnemonic:

- ✓ **I Promote Mr. SP Sp**
- ✓ **I** – Inspection
- ✓ **Promote** – Palpation
- ✓ **M** – Motor reflexes
- ✓ **r.** – Range of motion
- ✓ **S** – Sensory examination
- ✓ **P** – Pulses
- ✓ **Sp** – Specialized tests

Disease	Extra-articular manifestation
Rheumatoid Arthritis	✓ **Eyes**: Scleritis, episcleritis ✓ **Skin**: Leg ulcers, rheumatoid nodules ✓ **Neurological**: Polyneuropathy ✓ **Respiratory**: Pulmonary fibrosis, pleural disease, Caplan's syndrome ✓ **CVS**: Pericardial disease, valvulitis, myocardial fibrosis ✓ **Kidneys**: Nephropathy ✓ **Liver**: Hepatomegaly
Systemic Lupus Erythematosus	✓ Malar rash ✓ Discoid rash ✓ Serositis ✓ Oral ulcers ✓ Photosensitivity ✓ Neurologic involvement ✓ Hematologic involvement ✓ Immunologic abnormality ✓ Renal involvement
Ankylosing Spondylitis	✓ Aortic insufficiency ✓ Iritis ✓ Tendinitis (Never give levofloxacin or ciprofloxacin to these patients, as it can lead to Achilles tendon rupture)
Psoriatic Arthropathy	✓ Sausage-shaped tendinitis ✓ Skin manifestation
Osteoarthritis	✓ None
Fibromyalgia	✓ Tender points ✓ Myalgia ✓ Irritable bowel syndrome

Examination of Joints

You should always examine and document the joints under the following headings:

- ✓ Inspection
- ✓ Palpation
- ✓ Range of motion
- ✓ Motor reflexes
- ✓ Sensory examination
- ✓ Distal pulses
- ✓ Specialized tests

Shoulder Joint Examination

Inspect

- ✓ Scars, sinuses, surgical marks
- ✓ Redness
- ✓ Abnormal contour

Palpate

- ✓ Effusion – boggy swelling
- ✓ Crepitus – crunchy feeling of subcutaneous air
- ✓ Tenderness

Range of motion

- ✓ Ask the patient to raise his/her arm above 90° - if they are able to do so, the supraspinatus muscle is intact.
- ✓ Perform the Neer's shoulder test to check for rotator cuff impingement.
- ✓ Perform the Hawkin's test to check for rotator cuff impingement or to check function of the long tendon of biceps brachii.
- ✓ Perform the 'Empty Can' test.
- ✓ Ask the patient to touch his/her shoulder with the opposite hand. This results in internal rotation and any pain during this maneuver indicates subscapularis muscle pathology.
- ✓ Perform the Apley's Scratch Test
- ✓ Ask the patient to make a complete arc with the hand. If there is pain in the movement, it is termed as the 'painful arc sign,' and indicates pathology of the rotator cuff muscles.

Motor reflexes

- ✓ Always compare the reflexes with the opposite normal side
- ✓ Check for the following reflexes:
  - ✓ Biceps reflex
  - ✓ Triceps reflex
  - ✓ Supinator reflex

Sensory examination

- ✓ Perform a complete sensory examination of the affected limb
- ✓ This helps in ruling out any nerve entrapment

Pulses

- It is important to examine the pulses of the limb arteries so as to pick up any arterial entrapment
- Check for the following pulses:
    - Radial pulse
    - Brachial pulse

Specialized tests

- As mentioned in the range of motion examination
- Perform the Spurling's maneuver to rule out cervical radiculopathy
- Perform Adson maneuver to evaluate for cervical rib

Elbow Joint Examination

Inspect

- Scars, sinuses, surgical marks
- Redness
- Abnormal contour

Palpate

- Effusion – boggy swelling
- Crepitus – crunchy feeling of subcutaneous air
- Tenderness

Range of motion

- Check the flexion and extension movements
- Check both active and passive range of motion
- Also check for supination and pronation

Motor reflexes

- Always compare the reflexes with the opposite normal side
- Check for the following reflexes:
    - Biceps reflex
    - Triceps reflex
    - Supinator reflex

Sensory Examination

- ✓ Perform a complete sensory examination of the affected limb
- ✓ This helps in ruling out any nerve entrapment

Pulses

- ✓ It is important to examine the pulses of the limb arteries so as to pick up any arterial entrapment
- ✓ Perform the Allen's test in case of doubtful arterial patency
- ✓ Check for the following pulses:
    - ✓ Radial pulse
    - ✓ Ulnar pulse
    - ✓ Brachial pulse

Specialized tests

- ✓ Cozen's test for lateral epicondylitis
- ✓ Tinel's sign for carpal tunnel syndrome and other nerve entrapments

Knee Joint Examination

Inspect

- ✓ Scars, sinuses, surgical marks
- ✓ Redness
- ✓ Abnormal contour

Palpate

- ✓ Effusion – boggy swelling
- ✓ Crepitus – crunchy feeling of subcutaneous air
- ✓ Tenderness

Range of motion

- ✓ Check the flexion and extension movements
- ✓ Check both active and passive range of motion

Motor reflexes

- ✓ Always compare the reflexes with the opposite normal side
- ✓ Do not attempt to check for reflexes in a tender knee
- ✓ Check for the following reflexes:
  - ✓ Knee jerk
  - ✓ Ankle jerk

Sensory Examination

- ✓ Perform a complete sensory examination of the affected limb
- ✓ This helps in ruling out any nerve entrapment and neurological deficits

Pulses

- ✓ It is important to examine the pulses of the limb arteries so as to pick up any arterial entrapment of rupture
- ✓ Check for the following pulses:
  - ✓ Femoral pulse at the groin
  - ✓ Popliteal pulse at the popliteal fossa
  - ✓ Dorsalis pedis and posterior tibial pulses

Specialized tests

- ✓ Anterior drawer test for anterior cruciate ligament tear
- ✓ Posterior drawer test for posterior cruciate ligament tear
- ✓ McMurray's test for meniscal injuries

Examination of other joints

Students are advised to follow a similar **'I Promote Mr. SP Sp'** approach for any joint they need to examine. We have discussed the shoulder, elbow, and knee joint as representative examples above. Kindly refer to the individual cases for more details about the other joints.

Tests

TESTS FOR THE MUSCULOSKELETAL SYSTEM

- ✓ **NAME OF TEST**
- ✓ **WHAT TO DO**
- ✓ **INFERENCE**

Shoulder
Empty Can Test
Neer Test
Hawkins-Kennedy Test
Apleys Scratch Test
Painful Arc Test
Spurling's Test
Adson's Test
Lift Off Test (Gerber's Test)
Drop-Arm Test
Cross-Arm Test

Elbow
Cozan's Test

Wrist
Allen's Test
Tinel's Test
Finkelstien Test
Phalen's Test

Knee
Mcmurray's Test
Lachman's Test
Posterior Drawer Test
Anterior Drawer Test

Patellofemoral Tests
Patellofemoral Grind Test (Clarke's Test)
Patellar Apprehension Test

Ankle
Inversion Stress Test
Eversion Stress Test
Squeeze Test
Anterior Drawer Test
Posterior Drawer Test
Patrick's Test

Hip
Patrick's Test

Spine
Log-Roll Maneuver

Lumbar
Straight Leg Raise Test
Waddels Signs
Babinski's Sign
Hoffman's Sign
Homan's Test
Cerebellar Signs

Special Tests
Test For Trochanteric Bursitis
Ober's Test
Test For Lateral Femoral Cutaneous Nerve Entrapment

SHOULDER

EMPTY CAN TEST

Structures involved:

Supraspinatus tendon and muscle

How it is done:

- ✓ In the standing or sitting position, stabilize the shoulder to be tested
- ✓ Move the arm to 90 degrees forward flexion and 30 degrees abduction
- ✓ Internally rotate the arm until the thumb points downwards, as if emptying a beer cup
- ✓ With your other hand, apply downward pressure on the superior aspect of the distal forearm and ask the patient to resist

Inference: Pain or weakness elicited while performing the maneuver is considered a positive result and shows supraspinatus tendinitis, injury, or inflammation. Actual weakness is more reliable than pain alone. However, it may be kept in mind that the accuracy of this test has been reported to be questionable, as pathology of other structures in the area may also present with similar effects.

NEER TEST

Structures involved:

Supraspinatus tendon
Infraspinatus tendon

Tendon of the long head of the biceps

How it is done:

- ✓ In the standing position, the patient is asked to relax his/her arm by his/her side with the elbow fully extended
- ✓ Internally rotate the arm and forcefully flex it until full range is attained or the patient reports pain

Inference: The test is considered positive if pain is elicited in the anterior-lateral aspect of the shoulder.

HAWKINS-KENNEDY TEST

Structures involved:

Supraspinatus tendon

Tendon of the long head of the biceps
Acromioclavicular joint

How it is done:

- ✓ In the seated position, place the arm in 90 degree flexion with the elbow flexed at 90 degrees
- ✓ Forcefully rotate the shoulder internally until full range or pain is elicited

Inference: Pain elicited in the superior-lateral position is considered positive for strain on the supraspinatus (most commonly). However, it may be noted that the test is considered less sensitive than the NEER test.

APLEYS SCRATCH TEST

Structures involved:

Rotator cuff

How it is done:

- ✓ The patient touches the superior and inferior aspects of the opposite scapula

Inference: Loss of range of motion shows a pathology with the rotator cuff.

PAINFUL ARC TEST

Structures involved:

Subacromial structures between the coraco-acromial arch and the humerus

How it is done:

- ✓ In the sitting or standing position, abduct the arm in the scapular plane
- ✓ If pain begins, continue until 120 degrees of abduction
- ✓ Once at 120 degrees, start reversing the motion back to the starting position

Inference: Pain that exists between 60 and 120 degrees is considered to be pathognomonic for subacromial impingement syndrome.

SPURLING'S TEST

Structures involved:

Cervical radiculopathy due to cervical nerve root compres-sion

How it is done:

- ✓ Standing behind the seated patient, interlock your fingers and rest the volar aspect of both hands on top of the patient's head
- ✓ Laterally flex the neck 30 degrees to the affected side and apply a downward pressure, making sure not to flex any further

Inference: If the pain that arises in the neck radiates down the ipsilateral dermatome, cervical radiculopathy is confirmed.

ADSON'S TEST

Structures involved:

This is a test for thoracic outlet syndrome

How it is done:

- ✓ With the patient seated, extend, abduct, and externally rotate the affected arm, all while palpating the radial pulse
- ✓ Ask the patient to inspire and hold his/her breath at the height of inspiration
- ✓ Ask the patient to extend and rotate his/her head towards the affected side

Inference: Disappearance or decrease in the radial pulse demonstrates a positive test.

LIFT OFF TEST (GERBER'S TEST)

Structures involved:

Subscapularis

How it is done:

- ✓ Ask the patient to stand with the dorsum of the hand at the mid-lumbar spine Raise the dorsum of the hand while maintaining or increasing the internal rotation and extension at the shoulder

Inference: Inability to lift the dorsum of the hand implies pathology with the sub-scapularis.

DROP-ARM TEST

Structures involved: Supraspinatus

How it is done:

- ✓ With the patient seated, abduct the shoulder to 90 degrees
- ✓ Release the arm and ask the patient to slowly lower it

Inference: Inability to lower the arm is considered a positive result and is usually a sign of supraspinatus pathology.

CROSS-ARM TEST

Structures involved:

This is a test for acromioclavicular joint dysfunction.

How it is done:

- ✓ The patient is seated and then raises the affected arm to 90 degrees.
- ✓ The arm is made to be actively adducted causing the acromion to be forced into the distal end of the clavicle.

Inference: Pain in the area of the acromioclavicular joint suggests acromioclavicular dysfunction.

ELBOW

COZAN'S TEST

Structures involved:

Lateral epicondylalgia (tennis elbow)

How it is done:

- ✓ Stabilize the patient's elbow in 90 degrees flexion while palpating over the lateral epicondyle
- ✓ Now, position the patient's hand into radial deviation and forearm pronation
- ✓ Ask the patient to resist wrist extension

Inference: A positive test shows pain or reproduction of symptoms in the region of the lateral epicondyle.

WRIST

ALLEN'S TEST

Structures involved:

The wrist is usually supplied by two arteries: the radial and the ulnar. Allen's test serves to evaluate if the blood flow to the hand is normal.

How it is done:

- ✓ Apply pressure on the arteries supplying the wrist (namely the radial ad ulnar) for several seconds
- ✓ Once the palm is cool and pale due to the lack of blood supply, slowly release the pressure on one artery
- ✓ The palm should slowly regain its color

Inference: The return of color to the palm signifies that only one artery is usually necessary to maintain blood flow to the palm.

TINEL'S TEST

Structures involved:

At the wrist-median nerve compression (carpel tunnel syndrome). Tinel's test usually shows irritated nerves.

How it is done:

- ✓ Lightly tap over the nerve suspected to be irritated

Inference: The presence of pain or a 'pins and needles' sensation over the area distributed by the nerve signifies nerve entrapment or pressure neuropathy.

FINKELSTIEN TEST
Structures involved:

This is a test for de Quervain's tenosynovitis

How it is done:

- ✓ With the patient seated, make the patient form a fist around the thumb and perform ulnar deviation.

Inference: A positive test is pain over the first extensor compartment.

PHALEN'S TEST

Structures involved:

This is a test for carpal tunnel syndrome

How it is done:

- ✓ Have the patient place his/her elbows on the table
- ✓ Make the patient hold the position of maximum flexion of the palms for at least one minute.

Inference: Symptoms experienced with carpal tunnel syndrome are elicited with a positive test.

KNEE

MCMURRAY'S TEST

Structures involved:

Medial and lateral meniscus of knee

How it is done:

- ✓ The patient should be in a supine position with knee fully flexed
- ✓ Hold the sole of the foot with one hand and palpate the medial or lateral aspect of the tibio-fibular joint
- ✓ If testing the medial meniscus, start in internal rotation. For the lateral meniscus, use an externally rotated leg
- ✓ For medial meniscus: Palpate the postero-medial aspect of the knee during extension of the knee and external rotation of the tibia.
- ✓ For lateral meniscus: Palpate the postero-lateral aspect of the knee during extension of the knee and internal rotation of the tibia.

Inference: To be considered positive, pain must be elicited, or a click must be heard by the examiner.

LACHMAN'S TEST

Structures involved:

Anterior cruciate ligament

How it is done:

- ✓ With the patient supine, flex the knee to 20-30 degrees with external rotation
- ✓ Place one hand on the tibia and one on the patient's thigh with thumb on the tibial tuberosity
- ✓ Pull anteriorly on the tibia

Inference: A positive test will show forward translation of the tibia.

POSTERIOR DRAWER TEST

Structures involved: Posterior cruciate ligament

How it is done:

- ✓ The patient should be in supine position with knees bent to approximately 90 degrees
- ✓ Sit on the toes of the knee to be tested and grasp the proximal lower leg
- ✓ Translate the lower leg posteriorly

Inference: To be considered positive, a lack of end-feel or excessive posterior translation must be noted.

PATELLOFEMORAL TESTS

PATELLOFEMORAL GRIND TEST (CLARKE'S TEST)

Structures involved:

This is a test for patellofemoral pain syndrome.

How it is done:

- ✓ With the patient seated or supine, extend the knee
- ✓ Place the first web space of the hand over the patella and apply pressure
- ✓ Ask the patient to contract the thigh

Inference: Presence of pain constitutes a positive test.

PATELLAR APPREHENSION TEST

Structures involved:

This is a test for lateral patellar instability

How it is done:

First step:

- ✓ Place the knee in full extension
- ✓ Apply lateral force to the patella with thumb
- ✓ Maintain the pressure and flex the knee to 90 degrees, then return to extended position

Second Step:

- ✓ Repeat the previous steps with a medially directed force

Inference: For a positive test, there will be an orally expressed apprehension or apprehensive thigh movement on the first step, and absence of these symptoms in the second step.

ANKLE

INVERSION STRESS TEST

Structures involved:

Calcaneofibular ligament, talofibular ligament

How it is done:

- ✓ With the patient seated and legs hanging off the table, hold the heel with one hand and the tibia and fibula with the other
- ✓ Push the calcaneus and talus inward and lower leg laterally
- ✓ Repeat with the leg flexed

Inference: Pain and excessive range of motion of the talus may be noted on the affected side.

EVERSION STRESS TEST

Structures involved:

Deltoid ligament

How it is done:

- ✓ With the patient seated and legs hanging off the table, hold the heel with one hand and the tibia and fibula with the other
- ✓ Push the calcaneus and talus into eversion and lower leg medially
- ✓ Repeat with the leg flexed

Inference: Pain and excessive range of motion of the talus may be noted on the affected side.

SQUEEZE TEST

Structures involved:

Talofibular syndesmotic injury

How it is done:

- ✓ In the supine position, compress and release the patient's calf

Inference: To be considered positive, pain is elicited in the region of syndesmosis.

ANTERIOR DRAWER TEST

Structures involved:

Anterior talofibular ligament, anteromedial capsule

How it is done:

- ✓ With the knee flexed at 90 degrees and slight plantarflexion, place one hand on the tibia and exert a posterior force
- ✓ Place the other palm on the posterior aspect of the calcaneus and bring the calcaneus and talus forward

Inference: To be considered positive, pain or increased joint laxity is noted.

POSTERIOR DRAWER TEST

Structures involved:

Posterior talofibular ligament

How it is done:

- ✓ With the knee flexed at 90 degrees and slight plantarflexion, place one hand on the tibia and exert an anterior force
- ✓ Place the other palm on the anterior aspect of the calcaneus and bring the calcaneus and talus backward

Inference: To be considered positive, pain or reduction in range of motion must be elicited.

HIP

PATRICK'S TEST

Structures involved:

Hip, lumbar and sacroiliac region. Patrick's or FABER's test (Flexion, Abduction, External Rotation)

How it is done:

- ✓ The patient should be in the supine position
- ✓ Place the leg in the figure-4 position (hip flexed and abducted with the lateral ankle resting on the contralateral thigh just above the knee)
- ✓ Stabilize the opposite side of the pelvis at the anterior superior iliac spine
- ✓ Apply a posterior force with external rotation and abduction to the ipsilateral knee until you reach the end of the range of motion

Inference: To be considered positive, pain or reduction in range of motion must be elicited.

SPINE

LOG-ROLL MANEUVER

Structures involved:

Spine. This is used to move the patient without flexing the spinal column. (This test is for only educational purposes. You might not be expected to perform this test in your step 2 CS exam)

How it is done:

- ✓ Four people are needed to perform a log roll
- ✓ The first person stands at the head end and stabilizes the neck
- ✓ The second and third individuals place themselves on the side to which the patient is to be turned and hold the patient at the opposite shoulder, hip, and knee, while interlocking their hands
- ✓ On the count of three by the first person, the patient is turned to the side of individuals two and three
- ✓ The fourth person now presses down on the exposed spinal segments, evaluating for pain
- ✓ Once done, the patient is shifted back to the normal position on the count of three by the person at the head-end

Inference: Pain during the test over spinal segments shows spinal injury.

LUMBAR

STRAIGHT LEG RAISE TEST

Structures involved:

Lumbar disc herniation

How it is done:

- In the supine position, hold the posterior aspect of the foot of the patient and raise the leg until pain is elicited
- Perform the same test with the normal leg

Inference: To be considered positive for lumbar disc herniation, pain should be produced in between 30-70 degrees.

WADDELS SIGNS

Waddels signs are generally used to diagnose non-organic causes of pain

How it is done:

- Non-anatomic tenderness (crossing normal anatomical boundaries expected)
- Pain on stimulated rotation (pressing down on the head or on rotation of the neck)
- Positive straight leg raise test that is non-consistent
- Hyperasthesia

Inference : A positive result usually leads the examiner to look for non-organic causes to pain.

BABINSKI'S SIGN

Structures involved:

Upper motor neuron lesion

How it is done:

- In the supine position, run a pointed object along the plantar aspect of the patient's foot

Inference: Up-going of the toes is usually considered a positive test.

HOFFMAN'S SIGN

Structures involved:

Upper motor neuron lesion

How it is done:

- ✓ Flip the dorsal aspect of the middle finger

Inference: A positive test will elicit a reflex contraction of the thumb and index finger, signifying an upper motor neuron lesion.

HOMAN'S TEST

Structures involved:

Deep venous thrombosis

How it is done:

- ✓ In the supine position, place the knee in extension and the foot in dorsiflexion
- ✓ Palpate the belly of the calf

Inference: Pain elicited on palpation is considered positive for DVT.

CEREBELLAR SIGNS

These tests are done to evaluate cerebellar function and presence of these signs indicates a lesion in the cerebellum.

Dysdiadochokinesia: Ask the patient to pat one palm on the other in rapid, alternating movements. A patient with a cerebellar lesion will not be able to complete this task.

Romberg's test: Ask the patient to stand with legs spaced closely together. Then have he/she hold out both hands with open palms, as if holding a plate. Next, the patient will look up and close his/her eyes. A patient with cerebellar lesions will lose his/her balance.

Finger-nose test: Ask the seated patient to touch his/her nose with his/her index finger. Now ask him/her to stretch his/her hand and touch your index finger. Ask him/her to perform these movements in quick succession. If lesions are present in the cerebellum, the index finger will not be able to touch your finger perfectly and will, instead, shoot past it (a phenomenon known as past-pointing). This is also known as dysmetria.

Knee-heel test: Ask the supine patient to place the heel of one leg on the other knee in a cross fashion. Stand at the foot end of the patient and place your index finger well above the legs. Now, ask him/her to trace the heel along the leg until he/she meets the toes and then raise it to meet the index finger. A patient with cerebellar lesions will past-point with the index finger.

Graphesthesia: With the tip of a closed pen, trace letters on the patient's palm with his/her eyes closed. A healthy individual will be able to recognize the letters traced. A patient with cerebellar signs, however, will not.

Stereognosis: Ask the patient to close his/her eyes and place a well-known object (E.g. an apple, a pencil) in his/her palm and ask him/her to recognize it. A deficiency in identification is noted in those with cerebellar lesions.

Cerebellar gait: One of the best tests to diagnose cerebellar diseases is to make the patient walk in a straight line with the toes of one leg touching the heel of the other (also known as tandem walking). A patient with cerebellar disease will have a wide based gait, veering to one side with the imminent danger of falling and irregularity of steps.

SPECIAL TESTS

TEST FOR TROCHANTERIC BURSITIS

This is conducted in two parts.

- ✓ First, observe the patient's gait for any abnormalities. Any asymmetry, tilt, or preference for a particular side may be due to underlying pathologies or weakness of certain muscle groups.
- ✓ Second, check the range of motion of the joint.

OBER'S TEST

Structures involved:

This is a test to check for iliotibial band syndrome or inflamed tensor fascia lata

How it is done:

- ✓ Make the patient lie on his/her unaffected side with the hip and knee flexed at 90 degrees
- ✓ Forcefully adduct the extremity to be tested until the full range of motion is achieved in the hip

Inference: A positive test will elicit a lack of adduction and a lateral knee pain.

TEST FOR LATERAL FEMORAL CUTANEOUS NERVE ENTRAPMENT

Being a pure sensory nerve, compared to other disorders, there will be a conspicuous lack of reflexive or motor disorders. A sensory deficit will be noted below and slightly medial to the anterior superior iliac spine. Also, there may be tingling, numbness, or burning sensation present in the lateral aspect of the thigh, the region supplied by the lateral femoral cutaneous nerve.

Approach to Urinary Incontinence

Definition: The involuntary loss of urine.

How does normal continence work?

- ✓ The empty bladder gradually fills with urine from the ureters.
- ✓ As the bladder fills, its walls relax to allow more urine in (this is called compliance).
- ✓ As the bladder reaches capacity, the pressure against the bladder wall rises.
- ✓ The pressure in the bladder is communicated to the spinal cord (lumbosacral).
- ✓ In babies, the spinal cord triggers a bladder contraction without input from the conscious brain, triggering urination (involuntary voiding).
- ✓ "Toilet-trained" children and adults learn to suppress the spinal cord voiding reflex for a little while until they can make it to the bathroom (voluntary voiding).
- ✓ The external urinary sphincter is a muscle that wraps around the urethra. It can be voluntarily tightened long enough to get to a bathroom.
- ✓ The reason you can maintain continence without realizing it is a second sphincter in the neck of the bladder that stays tight while your bladder is filling.
- ✓ As a general rule – the bladder generates pressure, the sphincter creates resistance. If the pressure is greater than the resistance, you leak.

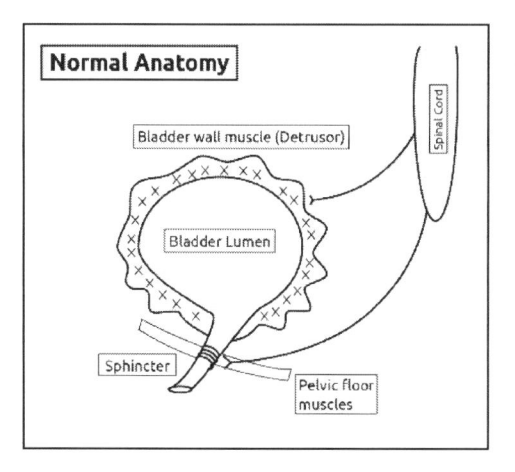

Why does incontinence happen?

BLADDER PRESSURE > SPHINCTER RESISTANCE

Types of incontinence

STRESS INCONTINENCE

- ✓ Bladder pressure is normal.
- ✓ Sphincter resistance is low.

You LEAK

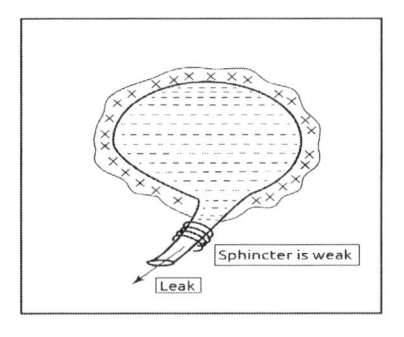

URGE INCONTINENCE (**U R G**oing **E**mergently to the bathroom)

- ✓ Bladder muscles are hyperactive (overactive detrusor).
- ✓ Bladder pressure is high.
- ✓ Sphincter resistance is normal.

You LEAK

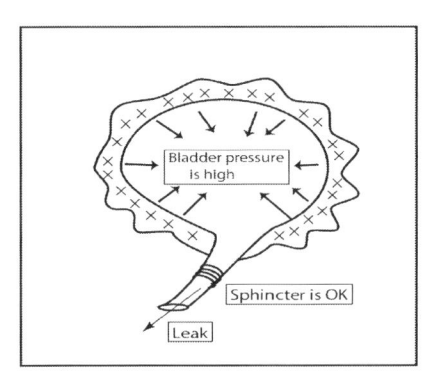

MIXED INCONTINENCE

- ✓ Bladder pressure is normal or high.
- ✓ Sphincter resistance is normal or low.
- ✓ Patient often has BOTH STRESS AND URGE INCONTINENCE.

You LEAK

NEUROGENIC INCONTINENCE

- ✓ Bladder pressure is often high.
- ✓ Sphincter doesn't work correctly because nerves aren't controlling it correctly.

You LEAK

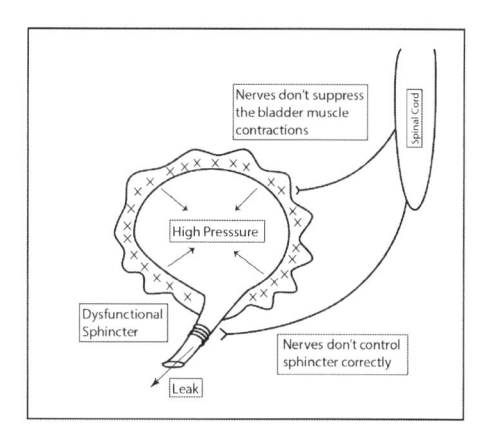

OVERFLOW INCONTINENCE

- ✓ Bladder is very full. Pressure may be normal or high, however, patient is not emptying the bladder. Urine keeps filling into the bladder and it simply overflows.
- ✓ Sphincter is usually weak, gets overwhelmed, and urine overflows.

The patient with overflow incontinence is typically ELDERLY, with DEMENTIA, LIMITED MOBILITY, often bedridden or wheelchair bound, and usually CONTINUOUSLY VOIDS WITH INCONTINENCE INTO DIAPERS. They often don't realize that they are leaking.

In overflow incontinence, the bladder is often continuously full. A bladder scan will show that the patient is in urinary retention.

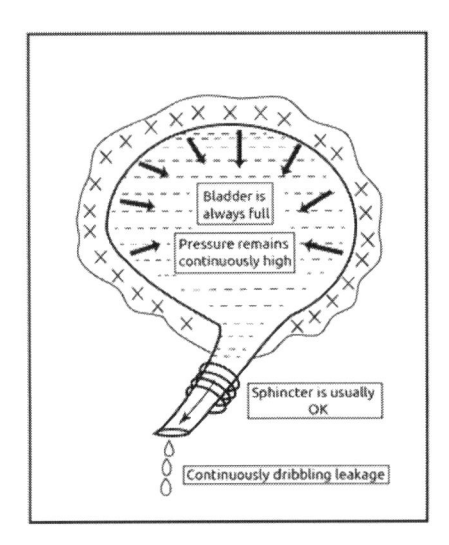

Points on history:

STRESS INCONTINENCE

- ✓ The patient leaks when they cough, sneeze, or laugh.
- ✓ The patient leaks when they exercise.
- ✓ The patentis usually dry when he/she is sitting still.
- ✓ Usually affects women, especially after childbirth.
- ✓ Usually, more childbirths = more stress incontinence
- ✓ Men rarely get stress incontinence UNLESS they have had prior prostate surgery or injury to the nerves of the sphincter.

REMEMBER: Stress incontinence is caused by anything that weakens the sphincter, e.g. pregnancy, childbirth, pelvic injury, and pelvic surgery.

Things to find out:

- ✓ Find out about prior pregnancies
- ✓ Were there any complications from childbirth?
- ✓ Find out about prolapse (do you feel a lump or bulge in the vagina, do you feel like something is bulging out of the vagina?)
- ✓ Men – Have you had prior prostate surgeries?
- ✓ Urethral surgeries?
- ✓ Any injuries to the perineum, scrotum, or pelvis?

URGE INCONTINENCE
- ✓ I get a sudden urge to pee, but I can't get to the restroom fast enough.
- ✓ I leak on my way to the bathroom.
- ✓ I can't get my pants down fast enough.
- ✓ Associated symptoms: I wake up at night to pee. I pee very often during the day.
- ✓ I drink 6 cups of coffee and 2 liters of Pepsi daily.
- ✓ I leak without any warning.

REMEMBER: Urge incontinence is caused by anything that increases bladder pressure, e.g. hyperactive urinary bladder, drinking too much coffee/tea/soda/alcohol, holding urine for too long, certain medications, urinary tract infections, kidney stones, recent urinary tract surgery, and menopause in women.

Things to find out:

- ✓ Do you drink coffee, tea, or soda?
- ✓ Do you drink alcohol?
- ✓ Recent UTI?
- ✓ Recent urinary tract infection or surgery?
- ✓ Changes in medications?

MIXED INCONTINENCE

Features of STRESS INCONTINENCE and URGE INCONTINENCE.

NEUROGENIC INCONTINENCE

- ✓ Very similar to URGE INCONTINENCE.
- ✓ There is always a history of NEUROLOGICAL ILLNESS.
- ✓ Examples of neurological illness that cause neurogenic incontinence:
    - ✓ Parkinson's disease
    - ✓ Stroke
    - ✓ Dementia
    - ✓ Multiple sclerosis
    - ✓ Spinal cord injury
    - ✓ ANY NERVE DISORDER CAN CAUSE NEUROGENIC INCONTINENCE

Remember: Always find out about neurological illness in a patient with incontinence.

PHYSICAL EXAMINATION FOR INCONTINENCE:

- ✓ Incontinence does NOT REQUIRE special testing to diagnose.
- ✓ Incontinence is diagnosed by HISTORY and PHYSICAL EXAM.

Stress incontinence: Patient dribbles or sprays urine when asked to cough.

- ✓ BLADDER SCAN post void residual is MANDATORY.
- ✓ URINALYSIS is MANDATORY.
- ✓ Cystoscopy is necessary in some cases.

IMPORTANT TIPS ABOUT INCONTINENCE:

- ✓ Get a complete medication history.
- ✓ Get a bladder scan and urinalysis.
- ✓ Get a prior pregnancy history.
- ✓ Get a complete surgical history.
- ✓ Think about underlying neurological illness.
- ✓ The diagnosis is obvious with history and a physical in most cases.

CASE HISTORY

Case 1

65-year-old female reports that she has been leaking urine for 20 years. The leakage has worsened in the last 2 years. She would like treatment for her leakage.

History

- ✓ She has had 6 pregnancies: 1 miscarriage, 5 vaginal deliveries.
- ✓ She leaks with coughing and sneezing. She typically needs 1 pad per day.
- ✓ Over the last year, her doctor recommended that she lose weight, and she started an exercise program at the local gym. Her leakage is now much worse and she soaks through her gym clothes. She can no longer exercise.
- ✓ She urinates every 3-4 hours during the day and once at night. She can usually make it to the bathroom in time.

Physical Examination

- ✓ Pelvic examination: Weak pelvic floor muscles.
- ✓ When she is asked to cough, she sprays urine.
- ✓ Bladder scan: 0ml. She empties her bladder.
- ✓ Urinalysis: normal.

Diagnosis

- ✓ STRESS INCONTINENCE – the diagnosis is clear with just history and a physical exam.

Treatment:

- ✓ Options available are physical therapy, Kegel exercises, surgical repair, and bulking agent injections.

CASE HISTORY

Case 2

68-year-old male has had urinary incontinence for 3 months.

History

- ✓ He has congestive heart failure. He has difficulty walking due to swollen legs and he moves very slowly. Three months ago, his doctor started him on Lasix, a diuretic, which gives him a stronger urge to urinate frequently. (Note the importance of a medication history)
- ✓ Since he cannot walk quickly to the bathroom, he leaks urine before he gets there.
- ✓ He wears 2 pads per day.
- ✓ He is up 3-4 times per night to urinate.
- ✓ He has had no prior surgeries.
- ✓ He drinks 4 cups of coffee daily and he drinks a beer in the evenings.

Physical Examination

- ✓ Urological exam: Normal. Mildly enlarged prostate.
- ✓ Does not leak urine with coughing or sneezing.
- ✓ Bladder scan is 35ml, normal. He empties his bladder well.
- ✓ Urinalysis is normal.

Diagnosis

- ✓ URGE URINARY INCONTINENCE – caused by diuretic therapy and limited mobility. His enlarged prostate may be contributing.

Treatment

VERY DIFFICULT

- ✓ Patient needs a diuretic for congestive heart failure and cannot stop taking it.
- ✓ Can try anticholinergic medicines (ditropan, enablex, etc.) to reduce bladder pressure and calm the urges to urinate.
- ✓ Can try urinating on a schedule (timed voiding every 2 hours) to keep his bladder from getting full (similar to how young children's bladders are trained).

CASE HISTORY

Case 3:

93-year-old patient wears diapers for incontinence. He is now soaking 4 diapers per day.

History

- ✓ He is bedridden.
- ✓ He wears a diaper full time and soaks 4 diapers per day.
- ✓ He is often agitated and confused.
- ✓ He never really asks to use the bathroom. He dribbles urine continuously into his diapers.
- ✓ He has had worsening Alzheimer's dementia for the last 10 years.

Physical Examination

- ✓ Urological exam: large prostate. Groin and perineal skin has a red "diaper rash" due to chronic wetness. The urine has a strong, "infected" smell.
- ✓ His lower abdomen is firm and distended (enlarged and full bladder).
- ✓ Urinalysis: Large WBCs and bacteria (chronic retaining of urine in the bladder leads to chronic infection of the urine with bacteria or yeast).
- ✓ Bladder scan: 1200 ml – consistent with urinary retention.

Diagnosis

- ✓ OVERFLOW URINARY INCONTINENCE.

Treatment

- ✓ A catheter is required – straight catheter, Foley's catheter, or suprapubic tube.
- ✓ Some male patients may be candidates for prostate surgery to relieve the blockage of urine flow.

CASE HISTORY

Case 4

26-year-old healthy female college athlete suddenly leaked a large amount of urine during basketball practice. She discussed this with her doctor who asked her to not drink energy drinks, coffee, and soda. In spite of this, she has had 3 more large leakage episodes in the last 1 month.

History

- ✓ She has to urinate every hour during the day.
- ✓ She wakes up 3-4 times a night to urinate.
- ✓ Her leakage is unpredictable – sometimes none, sometimes 3 times a day.
- ✓ She has been having VISION problems in the last 3 months.
- ✓ Her legs sometimes feel numb and weak.
- ✓ She has lost her balance a few times during practice.
- ✓ She gets shooting pain in her neck.
- ✓ She has had trouble holding a pen and has found it difficult to write properly over the last 3 months.
- ✓ She has never been pregnant, takes no medications, and has had no prior surgeries.

Physical Examination

- ✓ Pelvic exam: normal.
- ✓ Neurological exam: weakness of the lower extremities, weak hand grip, and decreased hand strength.
- ✓ Bladder scan: normal. Urinalysis normal.

Diagnosis

- ✓ NEUROGENIC INCONTINENCE is strongly suspected. She may have a neurological disorder such as Multiple Sclerosis.

Treatment

- ✓ Diagnose and treat the underlying neurological disease.
- ✓ Referral to a neurologist is appropriate.
- ✓ Could use anticholinergic therapy to decrease bladder pressure.
- ✓ Dietary changes – avoid coffee, tea, soda, alcohol, and energy drinks.

Approach to Headache

Headache is one of the most common presenting complaints in a clinical setting. A clear understanding of the most likely etiology of the headache and how to approach a patient with headache is very crucial to attain an accurate differential diagnosis.

In this chapter, we will first look at the most common causes of headache and then use our 'Funnel Approach' to narrow down our differentials.

Pain sensitive structures in the head

Whenever a patient comes with a headache, a physician must think of the following pain sensitive structures in the head as a probable source[1]:

Extracranial structures

- Skin
- Fascia and muscles of head and neck
- Blood vessels outside the cranium
- Trigeminal nerve
- Periosteum of the skull

Intracranial structures

- Large arteries near the circle of Willis
- Parts of the Dura Mater
- Dural venous sinuses
- Dural arteries
- Cranial nerves

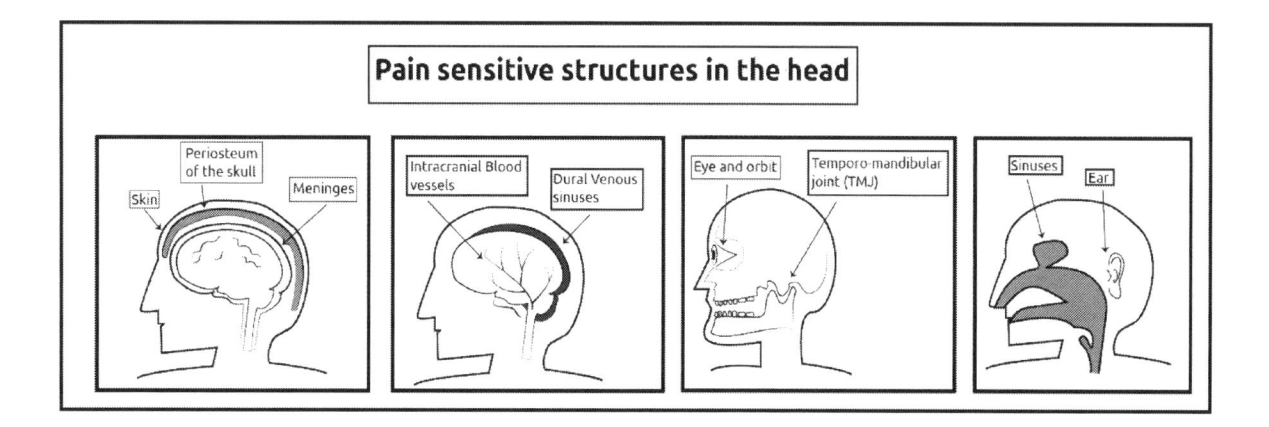

Pain sensitive structures in the head

Periosteum of the skull, Skin, Meninges, Intracranial Blood vessels, Dural Venous sinuses, Eye and orbit, Temporo-mandibular joint (TMJ), Sinuses, Ear

Most Common causes of headache

Headaches can be classified into *primary headaches* and *secondary headaches*.

Primary headaches

These are headaches due to an unclear etiology and are considered disorders in themselves.

- ✓ Tension headache (most common)[2]
- ✓ Exertional headache
- ✓ Cluster headache (least common, but most severe)[3]
- ✓ Migraine
    - ✓ With aura
    - ✓ Without aura

Secondary headaches

These are headaches with clear cut etiologies originating from various pain sensitive structures in the head.

- ✓ **Skin**- Herpes zoster
- ✓ **Muscles and joints**- Chronic myositis, TMJ dysfunction, muscle spasm, cervical arthritis
- ✓ **Blood vessels**- Giant cell arteritis
- ✓ **Eye and orbit**- Glaucoma, orbital cellulitis, orbital fractures
- ✓ **ENT**- Sinusitis, inflammation and infections of ear and nose
- ✓ **Dura Mater**- Meningitis, meningoencephalitis, encephalitis
- ✓ **Dural vessels**- Intracranial venous sinus thrombosis
- ✓ **Great vessels near the circle of Willis**- Subarachnoid hemorrhage, intracranial hemorrhage, intracranial/mycotic aneurysm
- ✓ **Nerves**- Trigeminal neuralgia, glossopharyngeal neuralgia, cranial neuritis
- ✓ **Mass lesion**- Brain tumors, tuberculoma, neurocysticercosis, CNS lymphoma (in HIV patients)

Characteristics of headache signifying life threatening conditions

Easy to remember, hard to forget mnemonic for life threatening headaches is: **NEWBIE H**ead **A**che

	Clinical features	Possible etiology
1.	**N-** Neurological signs Severe headache with loss of consciousness or focal neurological signs	Hypertensive emergency or intracranial hemorrhage
2.	**E-** Early morning headaches or sleep disturbance due to headache	Space occupying lesion (brain tumor), CO_2 retention (COPD, obstructive sleep apnea), and increased intracranial pressure
3.	**W-** "Worst headache of my life"	Subarachnoid hemorrhage (SAH)
4.	**B-** Bending/postural Headache worsening on change in head position, particularly on bending forward	Pseudotumor cerebri/raised ICP
5.	**I-** Illness Headache with fever and signs of sepsis	Meningitis/encephalitis/brain abscess
6.	**E-** Elderly Onset after 55 years of age	Intracranial neoplasm
7.	**Head-**Headache associated with local tenderness on the temples and blurring/loss of vision	Giant cell arteritis or carotid artery atherosclerosis
8.	**Ache-** Awakens the patient at night	Cluster headache

How to approach the history for a case scenario of headache

Once we have a clear understanding of what structures in the head can be possible sources of the pain, we should try and use our approach to history with 'Life Isn't Good DOCTOR AID@PM,' and arrive at a few provisional diagnoses. After narrowing down our spectrum, we can do a focused examination and direct our investigations towards that particular cause.

Location

- ✓ Q: "Where is it hurting the most?" pause... "Is it on one side or both sides of the head?"

Unilateral headaches can be migraines or cluster headaches. A migraine can also present as bilateral headache in some patients, therefore, one must be attentive to the patient's complaint. Giant cell arteritis, or carotid artery atherosclerosis, can present with a unilateral headache with blurring of vision.

Severe retro-orbital pain can occur in certain viral fevers (Ebola virus, dengue fever).
Pain occurring on the occiput should raise suspicion of a cervical spondylosis or muscle strain.

Grade

- ✓ Q: "Can you grade your pain from 0 to 10, with 10 being the worst pain you have ever had?" Worst headache of life may suggest subarachnoid headache, orbital cellulitis, or venous sinus thrombosis.

Duration

- ✓ Q: "How long have you been having this headache?"
- ✓ New onset headaches in a cancer patient should raise suspicion for a brain metastasis. In an HIV patient, think of toxoplasmosis or CNS lymphoma.
- ✓ Headache occurring over a few days to a week with early morning symptoms in an elderly person (age>50 years) should raise suspicion for a brain tumor.
- ✓ Chronic headaches can be due to chronic migraines, chronic cluster headaches, and chronic tension type headaches. It would suggest a benign ongoing pathology as compared to a life threatening condition.

Onset

- ✓ Q: "How does the headache start?" *pause*… "Is it sudden or gradual?"
- ✓ **Sudden** onset severe headache can be due to a subarachnoid hemorrhage, an intracranial bleeding, or a venous sinus thrombosis. These sudden onset headaches are called thunderclap headaches, since they are usually explosive in nature with severe headache. It is recommended that serious causes be ruled out using a CT scan of the head in such cases. It can also be trigeminal neuralgia if it starts suddenly and lasts only a few seconds with certain stressors like shaving, cold breeze, and brushing or washing the face.
- ✓ **Gradual**- Migraine and cluster headaches (15-180 minutes) may start gradually over the day and worsen in a few minutes to hours, lasting anywhere between 4 hours to 72 hours.

Character

- ✓ Q: "What is the nature of the headache?" *pause*… "Can you describe it in your own words?"
- ✓ Throbbing/pulsating headache is usually a migraine or a cluster headache.
- ✓ Dull/tightening headache may occur in tension type headaches.
- ✓ Sharp/shooting pain may be a cluster headache, and if it is lasting only a few seconds, it may be trigeminal neuralgia.
- ✓ Deep, heavy pain may occur from a space occupying lesion in the brain.

Time of the day

- ✓ Q: "What time of the day does the headache usually occur?"
- ✓ Early morning headaches may suggest an intracranial tumor or raised intracranial pressure. It is usually associated with nausea and vomiting.

- ✓ In case of a patient with COPD or chronic lung disease, early morning headaches may suggest hypercapnia or type II respiratory failure.
- ✓ Headaches in the evening may suggest tension type headaches, and they are usually stress induced.

The diagnostic criteria for episodic and chronic tension type headache disorder, given by the **International classification of headache disorders 3rd edition** are as follows:

Episodic Tension Type Headache[4]	Chronic Tension Type headache[5]
At least 10 episodes lasting 30 minutes to a week with:	Headache for hours to days, occurring on more than 15 days of a month for more than 3 months in a year with:
At least two of the following:	
✓ Bilateral headaches ✓ Non-pulsating/tightening type headache ✓ Mild to moderate severity ✓ Not aggravated by daily physical activities like walking, running, or jumping	
Plus the two following:	
✓ Not more than a single episode of photophobia or phonophobia ✓ No associated nausea or vomiting	

Occasion

- ✓ Q: "What were you doing when the headache started?" Headache waking up a patient from sleep may be a cluster headache. Headache while shaving or brushing may suggest trigeminal neuralgia. Headache over the weekends may suggest a stress induced headache.

Radiation

- ✓ Q: "Does the headache move anywhere apart from the current location?" Pain radiating down the back of the neck may suggest cervical spondylosis. Pain radiating in the trigeminal/dermatomal distribution is suggestive of trigeminal neuralgia or herpetic neuralgia.

Associated symptoms

Associated symptoms are important diagnostic clues for the etiology of the headache. Lacrimation, rhinorrhea, and autonomic symptoms on one side of the face with unilateral headache suggests cluster headaches. Signs of fever, chills, seizures, and other neurological signs may indicate an infectious pathology such as meningitis, encephalitis, or a brain abscess. Associated nausea and vomiting can occur in severe migraine and also in increased intracranial pressure, due to a space occupying lesion. Unilateral headache with focal tenderness in the region of superior temporal artery and blurring of vision should raise suspicion for giant cell arteritis (GCA) or carotid atheroma and must be handled emergently to prevent permanent loss of vision. An ESR >100 would suggest a possible GCA, and must be managed with high dose steroids before other diagnostic procedures can be carried out.

Increasing factors

- ✓ Q: "What makes your headache worse?" Postural changes may worsen the headache in case of a raised ICP or intracranial SOL. Chocolates, wines, OCPs, and cheese may precipitate an attack of migraine. The patient may become sensitive to light (photophobia) and noise (phonophobia) in cases of migraine, cluster headache, and meningitis.

Decreasing factors

- ✓ Q: "What makes your headache better?" Medications and lying in a peaceful and dark room usually decrease the severity of many headaches, and are most likely to be answered by the patient.

Previous history of similar symptoms

- ✓ Q: "Have you had any similar symptoms in the past?" New onset headaches, especially in an elderly patient, a cancer patient, or an immunocompromised patient should raise suspicion of intracranial malignancy, metastasis, or opportunistic infections, such as toxoplasmosis respectively. Chronic recurring headaches would suggest tension type headache or migraine headache.

Medications used to alleviate the headache

- ✓ Q: "Did you take any medications for the headache?" pause… "Did they help?" Mild forms of migraine or tension headaches resolve easily with acetaminophen (Tylenol) or NSAIDs.

Physical Examination

In every patient presenting with headache, it is imperative to do a quick neurological assessment to rule out serious irreversible causes.

The following systems must be examined:

- ✓ **General examination** for pallor, icterus, cyanosis, clubbing, lymphadenopathy, or edema. Also comment on the patient's build and nutrition.
- ✓ **Mini mental assessment** of orientation to time, place, person, and situation. Alertness, memory, and cognitive functions should also be assessed.

- ✓ **Head and neck examination** with inspection, palpation, and eye movement and vision should also be performed.
- ✓ **Neurological examination** would include cranial nerves examination, quick muscle strength and reflexes in all four limbs, and plantar reflex.
- ✓ **Cardiovascular and pulmonary examination** may be done if enough time is available. In real life practice it is strongly advised to examine all integral systems, but in a clinical skills examination, the physical assessment should be focused and limited to the specific system.

References

1. Bigley, G. K., Table 54.1, Pain Sensitivities of Structures in the Head - Clinical Methods - NCBI Bookshelf. **1990**.
2. Schwartz, B. S.; Stewart, W. F.; Simon, D.; Lipton, R. B., Epidemiology of tension-type headache. In *JAMA*, United States, 1998; Vol. 279, pp 381-3.
3. Sjaastad, O.; Bakketeig, L. S., Cluster headache prevalence. Vaga study of headache epidemiology. In *Cephalalgia*, England, 2003; Vol. 23, pp 528-33.
4. Society, I.-I. H., IHS - International Headache Society» Infrequent episodic tension-type headache |2.1|G44.2. **2015**.
5. Society, I.-I. H., IHS - International Headache Society» New daily-persistent headache (NDPH) |4.8|G44.2. **2015**.

Approach to a Pediatric Case

The USMLE Step 2 CS exam, or the pediatric clerkship, may include a pediatric encounter.

During Step 2 CS, these encounters are different from the other encounters, as the pediatric patient is usually not physically present in the exam. It will either be the child's mother in person or phone call.

Doorway Information

Like all encounters, these begin with the doorway information.
Important information that must be noted:

- ✓ The child's, as well as the mother's name
- ✓ The child's age
- ✓ The chief complaint
- ✓ The legal guardian

Upon entering the patient encounter room:

Telephone encounter

Sit down at the desk and begin by studying the parent's last name. Ascertain how to address the parent by checking the salutation as well. Push the yellow speaker button to dial the phone. This will connect the line to the parent. Don't touch any other buttons on the phone, including numbers, as this may disconnect the line. The call is only permitted once, so don't hang up until all the necessary information is gathered.

Since a physical examination cannot be performed due to absence of the patient, utilize all 15 minutes in taking a detailed history, counseling the patient's parent in detail, reinforcing and reassuring often. Never give false hope and always request to bring the patient to the hospital for a complete physical examination. Perform a full closure. Counsel them about any siblings. Be kind and considerate and don't be in a hurry to leave the room. Utilize all of the time given to show personal skills.
At the end of the call, press the same speaker button above the yellow dot to disconnect.

(Read more about this encounter on Page 8 of this information manual: http://www.usmle.org /pdfs /step-2-cs/cs-info-manual.pdf)

Parent encounter

Just like a telephonic case scenario, you do not have to perform a physical examination in a pediatric patient since the parent or caregiver will come with the complaint; therefore, it is advised to spend more time on history taking, counseling, empathy, and closure to score maximum points.

Draw diagrams on the patient education sheet and engage the parent fully. (If parent is present in the room) Also, counsel them about their own life and coping with an ill child, or a special child (e.g. a child with Down's syndrome or a sibling with Down's syndrome, etc.). Counsel them about immunizations, vaccinations, and the need to bring the child back for a follow up.

After the Encounter

Write a full patient note and mention that the **historian** was the patient's parent/caregiver. Leave the **physical examination** section of the history blank, since it was not performed. Leave the sections for **supporting physical findings** blank since there was no physical examination. In the **diagnostic work up** section, make sure that the first thing mentioned is 'Physical Examination.'

Aids for Pediatric History Taking

Remember that children are not just miniature adults, but they have their own special needs and concerns. The history to be obtained for pediatric cases won't be the same as that obtained for adults. To score more points with the parent, always use the child's name, e.g. "Does little John have a fever?" This adds a personal touch to the conversation and makes the parent/caregiver more comfortable in discussing the problem with you.

Use the same mnemonic that was used for the physical examination:

Skin				
G	General	G	Glands	
H	Heart (Cardiovascular)	H	HEENT	
A	Abdomen	U	Urogen	
L	Lungs	L	Lymph node	
E	Extremities	A	Anemia and GI bleeding	
N	Neurological	M	Musculoskeletal	
Psychiatric				

1. *General:*

   ✓ "How is the child looking?"
   ✓ "Is the child irritable?"
   ✓ "Does the child have a fever?"
   ✓ "Is the child awake and responsive?"
   ✓ "Does the child's skin look yellow to you? What about the child's eyes?"
   ✓ "Has this yellow discoloration progressed?"

2. Heart:

- ✓ "Does the child turn blue?"
- ✓ "Does the color of the child's lips look blue to you?"
- ✓ "Does the child stop mid-way while breastfeeding and start sweating?"
- ✓ "Have you noticed the child having cycles of suck-rest-suck while breastfeeding?"
- ✓ "Does the child get tired very soon while playing?"
- ✓ "Does the child rest before continuing to walk or run?"

3. Abdomen:

- ✓ "Have you noticed any appetite changes?"
- ✓ Ask about the hydration status: "Is he/she drinking well?"
- ✓ "Does he/she have a dry mouth?"
- ✓ "Does he/she have sunken eyes?"
- ✓ "Is there a sunken soft spot over his/her head?"
- ✓ "Does the child have nausea/vomiting" Ask details about the vomit.
- ✓ "Does the child complain of any abdominal pain?"
- ✓ "What are the child's usual eating habits?"
- ✓ "Are you breastfeeding the child?"
- ✓ "What kind of food does the child receive?"
- ✓ "How many meals does the child receive during the day?"
- ✓ "Do you get up to feed the child at night?"
- ✓ "Which formula milk are you using?"
- ✓ "What special diet has been prescribed for this child?"
- ✓ "Any supplements?"
- ✓ "Vitamins/Calcium?"

If the clinical scenario is of dehydration, fever, diarrhea or vomiting, an examinee must counsel the parent about increasing the fluid intake--Pedialyte and water. Never suggest soda or pop.

4. Lungs:

- ✓ "Does the child have shortness of breath?"
- ✓ "Is the child breathing too fast?"
- ✓ "Is the child breathing irregularly?"
- ✓ "Does he/she cough?" Ascertain the characteristics of the cough and rule out whooping cough.

5. Extremities:

- ✓ "Does the child complain of cramps in the legs?"
- ✓ "Does the child fall a lot?"
- ✓ "Is the child growing well?"

6. Neurological:

- ✓ "Is the child cheerful and playful like before?"
- ✓ "Have you noticed any seizures?"
- ✓ "Is the child listless?"

- ✓ "Does the child have a vigorous or a weak cry?"
- ✓ "Do you think the child is crying inconsolably?"
- ✓ "Has the child achieved milestones comparable to other children of the same age?"

7. *Glands:*

- ✓ "Have you noticed any neck swelling?"
- ✓ "Does the child have cold intolerance?
- ✓ Does the child have heat intolerance?"
- ✓ "Does the child complain of a sore throat?"

8. *HEENT:*

- ✓ "Does the child's head look abnormally big to you?"
- ✓ "Does the child have ear pulling/ear tugging?"
- ✓ "Any ear discharge?"
- ✓ "Does the child have a runny nose?"
- ✓ "Is the child having difficulty swallowing?"
- ✓ "Does the child have any hearing problems?"
- ✓ "Does the child have any vision problems?"

9. *Urogenital:*

- ✓ Inquire about any changes in urinary habits.
- ✓ "Is there any change in urine color or smell?"
- ✓ "How many wet diapers does the child normally make? How many is the child currently making?"
- ✓ "Is the peeing well?"
- ✓ "Does the child cry while passing urine?"
- ✓ "Is he/she still using diapers?"
- ✓ "Have there been any bed-wetting accidents?"

10. *Lymph Nodes:*

- ✓ "Have you noticed any swollen glands or lumps anywhere on the child?"

11. *Anemia and GI/Bowel Problems:*

- ✓ "Has there been any change in bowel habits or in stool color or consistency?"
- ✓ "How frequent are his/her bowel movements?"
- ✓ "Is there any blood in the stool?"
- ✓ "Is there any relationship between bowel movements and oral intake?"
- ✓ "Have you noticed any changes in the child's poop?"
- ✓ "Is the child pooping well?"
- ✓ "Does the child have loose stools?"
- ✓ "Does the child have constipation?"

12. *Musculoskeletal:*

- ✓ "Is the child playful and running around?"

✓ "Does the child prefer to sit at one spot instead of running around during play?"

13. Skin

✓ "Does the child have rashes anywhere on the body?"
✓ "Can you describe the rash for me?"
✓ "When did you notice the rash? Is it spreading or fading?"
✓ "Does he/she have any diaper rash?"
✓ "You said he/she has a history of eczema. Has it worsened? Is it the same?"

14. Psychiatric:

✓ Inquire about the child's sleeping habits.
✓ "Does the child sleep well?"
✓ "Does the child wake up screaming at night?"
✓ "Have there been any accidents of bed-wetting or urinating in clothes?"
✓ "Is the child inattentive and/or restless?"
✓ "Have there been any environmental changes?"
✓ "Any stressful event in the family?"

15. Other important history to be elicited for children:

✓ **Ill Contacts**
✓ **Daycare/School**
✓ **Siblings**
✓ **Birth History**:
✓ Type of delivery (vaginal/C-section), indication for C-section, term/preterm/post-term, and any complications after the delivery.
✓ "Was the child admitted to the hospital after birth, and for how long?"
✓ "Did the child cry immediately at birth?"
✓ "Do you know what resuscitation measures were taken?"
✓ "Was the child put on a ventilator?"
✓ **Vaccinations**
✓ **Last Check Up**
✓ Child weight/height at last check up: ("Was it in normal range according to your doctor?")
✓ Current medications
✓ Past medical history/past surgical history
✓ Drug allergies

This can be followed by eliciting maternal history based on the mnemonic:

"What IF PAM'S Family SHOUTS? Vaccinate 'em!"

What IF PAM'S FAMILY SHOUTS? Vaccinate 'em!		
What	Worries	"Are you worried about your child" "Does this worry you?"
I	Insomnia	"Have you had sleepless nights because of this?"
F	Fatigue/Fever	"Do you think this is tiring you and you are unable to handle this?"
		"Do you think you need our social worker's help to be able to handle this better?
P	Past Medical History	
A	Allergies	
M	Medications	
S	Surgeries	
Family	Family History	
S	Social History	(Tobacco, Alcohol, Recreational Drugs)
H	Hospitalization	
O	Obstetric and Gynecological (LPGA) History	
U	Urogenital and Bowel Problems	
T	Travel History	
S	Sick Contacts and Sexual History	
Vaccinate	Vaccination History	
em	Empathy to be shown	

Approach to a Case of Muscle Weakness

In this chapter, we aim to provide an easy manual to muscle weakness. With the checklist, we aim to educate the student in the different etiologies of muscle weakness. The chart has to be read as muscle weakness plus any one of the following symptoms will lead to the following etiology. For example, muscle weakness plus sudden and severe headache may be stroke if accompanied by vomiting, dizziness, or altered consciousness.

Patient presents with muscle weakness

(Distinguish true weakness from functional weakness)

Based on history: True weakness symptoms

S

- ✓ **Sudden and Severe Headache**
- ✓ **Stroke**: Sudden and severe headache accompanied by vomiting and dizziness/altered consciousness
- ✓ **SAH:** "Worst headache of life" (thunderclap headache)
- ✓ **Intracranial Headache (epidural and subdural headache)** : Headache after a blow-out injury with/without lucid interval
- ✓ **TIA**: Sudden headache that lasts a few minutes
- ✓ **Meningitis**: Severe headache with stiff neck and high fever
- ✓ **Migraine**: Pulsating, throbbing headache that is usually one sided; associated with/without aura
- ✓ **Tension Headache**: Dull, aching headache that gets worse by the end of the day
- ✓ **Slurred/Strange Speech**
- ✓ **Stroke:** Slurred speech/difficulty understanding speech
- ✓ **TIA**: Slurred/garbled speech that lasts a few minutes
- ✓ **Brain Tumor**: Slurred Speech
- ✓ **Multiple Sclerosis**: Scanning speech-normal melody or speech pattern is disrupted with abnormally long pauses between words or individual syllables of words. Also, some people may have nasal speech
- ✓ **ALS**: Thick speech and difficulty in projecting the voice as muscles for breathing weaken; becomes more difficult for individuals to speak loudly enough to be understood
- ✓ **Guillain Barre Syndrome**: Facial nerve often becomes involved, causing slurred speech
- ✓ **-Myasthenia Gravis**: Slurred speech due to in coordination or muscle weakness. Muscles of the tongue, palate, and larynx/jaw do not function properly

- ✓ **Parkinson's Disease**: Monotone speech with reduced volume (hypophonia) and difficulty with articulation of sounds/syllables

T

- ✓ **Topple Over/Dizziness/Vertigo**
- ✓ **Multiple Sclerosis**: People with MS may feel off balance or lightheaded. Mostly they have the sensation that their surroundings are spinning (vertigo)
- ✓ **Brain Tumor**: Metastatic tumors are the most common cause of dizziness
- ✓ **Parkinson's Disease**: Dizziness/dizzy spells due to orthostatic hypotension that may occur associated with the disease or as a complication of medication
- ✓ **Cerebellar Ataxia**: Inability to coordinate balance, gait, and extremity and eye movements
- ✓ **Migrainous Vertigo**: Vertigo may occur spontaneously provoked by head motion/visual stimuli
- ✓ **Post-Traumatic Vertigo**: The vestibular system can be disturbed following blunt trauma to the head and neck region leading to BPPV, post-traumatic Meniere's syndrome, and perilymphatic fistula/labyrinthine concussion

R

- ✓ **Raise Your Arms/Legs (Weakness in Arms/Legs)**
- ✓ **Stroke**: Sudden numbness, weakness, or paralysis in face, arm, or leg, especially on one side of the body
- ✓ **TIA**: Sudden weakness/numbness on one side of the body, but it lasts only few minutes
- ✓ **Multiple Sclerosis**: Numbness or weakness in one or more limbs that typically occurs on one side of the body at a time or the legs and trunk
- ✓ **Myasthenia Gravis**: Muscle weakness (mostly in voluntary muscles) that worsens as the affected muscle is used repeatedly (usually more pronounced weakness by the end of the day)
- ✓ **Guillain Barre Syndrome**: Ascending weakness following days or weeks after a respiratory or digestive tract infection
- ✓ **Parkinson's Disease**: Slowness of movement (bradykinesia), short steps while walking, and difficulty getting out of the chair in addition to difficulty with eye/facial movements
- ✓ **ALS**: Disease frequently begins in hands and feet/limbs and then spreads to other parts of the body. Muscles become progressively weaker as the disease advances
- ✓ **Todd's Paralysis**: Brief, temporary paralysis (weakness of limbs) that follows a seizure

O

- ✓ **Orientation to Time, Place, Person, and Situation**
- ✓ **Head Injury**: A head injury could be an injury to the brain, skull, or scalp. Many patients have altered mental status
- ✓ **Stroke/TIA**: Damage to the brain after a stroke can cause cognitive problems

- ✓ **SAH**: Many patients have confusion in subarachnoid hemorrhage
- ✓ **Meningitis**: Inflammation of meninges can cause a change in mental status
- ✓ **Encephalitis**: Viral infection causing inflammation of brain tissue. In severe cases the patient can present with confusion
- ✓ **Basilar Migraine**: It can also present with confusion

K

- ✓ **(K)onfusion**
- ✓ **Stroke:** Patients can get disoriented to surroundings
- ✓ **Alzheimer's Disease**: Short term memory loss with increasing age, due to the formation of tau proteins in the brain
- ✓ **Vascular Dementia**: Confusion due to vascular damage to the brain with an Hx of DM/HTN/hyperlipidemia
- ✓ **Norma Pressure Hydrocephalus**: Confusion/memory loss in addition to gait disturbances and loss of bladder control
- ✓ **Intracranial Hematoma**: Rupture of blood vessels within the brain or between the skull and brain, most likely have Hx of head trauma
- ✓ **Seizure**: Confusion in post ictal stage
- ✓ **Lewy Body Dementia**: Cognitive problems such as confusion, reduced attention span, and eventually memory loss

E

- ✓ **Blurry Vision/Facial Weakness**
- ✓ **Stroke**: Facial nerve palsy leading to facial droop and blurred vision
- ✓ **Multiple Sclerosis**: Blurred vision/double vision
- ✓ **INO** (internuclear ophthalmoplegia)
- ✓ **Myasthenia Gravis:** Ptosis and diplopia (which may be horizontal or vertical). In addition, weakness of the face and throat muscles leading to difficulty in speaking / swallowing / chewing
- ✓ **Migraine**: Blurred vision/tunnel vision/seeing spots/flashes of light

Approach to a Case of Edema

While edema usually does not come as a primary diagnosis but accompanies other cases, it is beneficial to know its causation and differential diagnosis.

The word edema comes from the Greek word 'oidein,' which means 'to swell'. Also known as 'dropsy,' or 'hydrops,' edema is not a new phenomenon. Sumerian, Babylonian, Egyptian, and Greek texts describe the disfigurement caused by edema and its management. However, it was John Blackall and Richard Bright in the early nineteenth century who described a possible renal and cardiac etiology for edema.[1]

PATHOPHYSIOLOGY

The compartments in the body can be broadly divided into two: the extracellular space and the intracellular space.[2] The extracellular space (outside the cell) is comprised of intravascular space (inside the blood vessel) and interstitial space. The extracellular space consists of proteinaceous and non-proteinaceous material, required for the normal functioning of the cell.[3] The interstitial space contains interstitial fluid, which is a solution that bathes and surrounds the cells of organisms. An abnormality in the mechanisms, maintaining homeostasis in the interstitium, leads to edema.[4]

There are six forces that lead to edema[5]:

1) Increased hydrostatic pressure in the blood vessels
2) Reduced oncotic pressure in the blood vessels
3) Increased tissue oncotic pressure
4) Increased permeability of the vessel wall
5) Reduced clearing of the lymphatic channels
6) Changes in the water retaining properties of the tissues

QUESTIONS TO BE ASKED IN AN EDEMA CASE (SYMPTOMATOLOGY AND DIAGNOSIS)

Edema is a pretty straightforward diagnosis. Its mere presence indicates a pathology. The treatment involves resolution of the cause. Asking questions in a systematic manner helps identify the pathology and inciting cause.

Is it present in both legs?

Here we try to elicit the location of the pathology. In most cases, a bilateral edema precipitates in a cause of central origin, mostly from the thorax or the abdomen. Some examples are:

- ✓ **Cardiac origin:** A congestive heart failure exerts back pressure along the veins, leading to an increased hydrostatic pressure in the veins and this pushes water into the interstitium.

The edema may be accompanied by signs of heart failure, such as dyspnea, orthopnea and paroxysmal nocturnal dyspnea.

- ✓ **Pulmonary origin:** Pulmonary hypertension usually causes pulmonary edema, but may precede by causing bilateral pedal edema due to venous congestion and stasis.[5] Sleep apnea may also lead to edema.

- ✓ **Hypothyroidism:** Thyroid disorders may cause myxedema. There is deposition of mucopolysacharides in the skin, giving it a waxy texture and subsequent edema. The study published by Montenegro, et al in the 'American Journal of Kidney Diseases' also suggests that hypothyroidism may lead to renal impairment and hyponatremia, leading to edema.[8]

- ✓ **Hepatic origin:** Liver failure causes reduced formation of albumin. These reduce the oncotic pressure of the blood, thus leading to extravasation of fluid and edema. Ascites is a common associated feature. Other signs of cirrhosis, such as spider angiomas, jaundice, alopecia, gynecomastia, and palmar erythema may be present.

- ✓ **Renal origin:** Renal failure leads to increased loss of proteins from the blood via glomerular filtration. The subsequent reduced oncotic pressure of the blood favors edema.

Some medication may cause edema due to fluid retention, e.g. pioglitazones.[10]

When present unilaterally, edema has limited causes.

- ✓ **Local lymphatic involvement:** In cases of local lymph node enlargement or blockage of lymphatic drain, the resulting back pressure leads to edema. If this occurs before confluence of the lymphatic channels from both legs, it may lead to unilateral edema, e.g. filariasis - the microfilaria invade the lymph channels of the leg and cause blockage, leading to unilateral edema and, later, elephantiasis.[5]

- ✓ **Venous insufficiencies:** In older individuals and those with increased dependent pressure, such as pregnant women, the constant venous stasis may lead to varicosities, and in later stages, edema.

- ✓ **DVT:** The venous system of the foot may be divided into superficial, deep, and perforator veins. The superficial veins drain in to the deep via the perforators. If there is a blockage here, it may lead to edema due to increased backpressure.[5]

- ✓ **Cellulitis:** The inflammation ensued may result in edema due to increased vascular permeability. It is commonly seen with necrotizing fasciitis, a disease with rapid subcutaneous spread of infection.[12]

Is the edema pitting or non-pitting?

Edema can be pitting or non-pitting. It is evaluated by pressing over the medial malleolus for 30 seconds. The resultant indentation will revert slowly.

- ✓ **Pitting edema:** Most edema is pitting. It shows the excess of fluid present in the interstitium, e.g. edema due to chronic venous insufficiency.

- ✓ **Non-pitting edema:** Only local causes lead to non-pitting edema. It is mostly found in cellulitis, myxedema, and causes of lymphatic origin.

How long has the edema persisted?

The timing since the onset gives us an idea of the nature of the pathology. Most cases of edema are due to increased positioning of legs in the dependent position. This will have an acute etiology. Chronic diseases, however, have a slow mode of onset and gradual progression.[14]

Has the extent of edema increased?
Increased edema demonstrates an ongoing pathology.

Is there sacral edema?
Edema always occurs in the dependent position. In bed-ridden patients, the sacral region must always be evaluated for edema, being the most dependent position.[5]

INVESTIGATIONS

Thorough investigations as to the cause of edema must be made. Treatment always depends on eliminating the inciting factor.[20]

- ✓ History and physical exam are paramount
- ✓ CBC with differential
- ✓ Basic metabolic panel, beta natriuretic peptide
- ✓ Urinalysis (for nephrogenic proteinuria)
- ✓ EKG
- ✓ Echocardiagram (to rule out CHF)
- ✓ Serum albumin
- ✓ Liver function tests
- ✓ Renal function tests
- ✓ Ultrasound
- ✓ Lymphoscintigraphy (to evaluate lymph flow)

TREATMENT

The treatment of edema may be summarized as:

Symptomatic treatment: The fluid in the interstitial space may be absorbed back into the bloodstream by using diuretics. This increases the elimination of water by the kidney, creating a hyperosmolar environment in the vessels, thus promoting motion of fluid from the interstitium to the vessel.

Diuretics exert their effect on various sites in the kidney.[15] For example, loop diuretics, like Lasix, block $NA^{+}/-K^{+}/-2Cl^{-}$ channels in the ascending Loop of Henle.[16] These drugs are highly bound to albumin.[15]

Treatment of the cause:

- ✓ *Chronic venous insufficiency:* Mechanical therapies, such as limb elevation and compression stockings, have shown to be of use.[17] The study by Trayes, et al in 'American Family Physician' showed that local skin care with emollients also provide relief.[18]

- ✓ *Lymphedema:* Complex decongestive physiotherapy involving manual lymphatic massage and multi-layer bandages have been shown to be of effect. The study by Sierakowski, et al in 'Lymphology' show that compression stockings provide a socially acceptable and effective means of control during early lymphedema management.[19] Surgical options may also be explored (debulking surgery).[17]

- ✓ *DVT:* Treat DVT with the conventional fibrinolytics, such as heparin and warfarin. Use of compression devices on bed ridden patients after surgery is also indicated.

- ✓ *Medication induced edema:* Stop offending medication.

REFERENCES

1. EKNOYAN, G. A history of edema and its management. Kidney Int Suppl, v. 59, p. S118-26, Jun 1997. ISSN 0098-6577 (Print)0098-6577. Disponível em: < http://dx.doi.org/ >.
2. Extracellular Space by Gene Ontology database (EMBL-EBI)
3. Didangelos, A.; Yin, X.; Mandal, K.; Baumert, M.; Jahangiri, M.; Mayr, M. (2010). "Proteomics Characterization of Extracellular Space Components in the Human Aorta". *Molecular & Cellular Proteomics* 9 (9): 2048–2062. doi:10.1074/mcp.M110.001693. PMC 2938114. PMID 20551380..
4. Marieb, Elaine N. (2003). *Essentials of Human Anatomy & Physiology* (Seventh ed.). San Francisco: Benjamin Cummings
5. Kumar, Abbas, Fausto (1999). *Pathologic Basis of Disease, 7th edition*. Elsevier Saunders. p. 122. ISBN 0-7216-0187-1
6. DAO, Q. et al. Utility of B-type natriuretic peptide in the diagnosis of congestive heart failure in an urgent-care setting. J Am Coll Cardiol, v. 37, n. 2, p. 379-85, Feb 2001. ISSN 0735-1097 (Print)0735-1097. Disponível em: < http://dx.doi.org/ >.
7. MONTENEGRO, J. et al. Changes in renal function in primary hypothyroidism. Am J Kidney Dis, v. 27, n. 2, p. 195-8, Feb 1996. ISSN 0272-6386 (Print)0272-6386. Disponível em: < http://dx.doi.org/ >.
8. SHEAR, L.; CHING, S.; GABUZDA, G. J. Compartmentalization of ascites and edema in patients with hepatic cirrhosis. N Engl J Med, v. 282, n. 25, p. 1391-6, Jun 18 1970. ISSN 0028-4793 (Print)0028-4793. Disponível em: < http://dx.doi.org/10.1056/nejm197006182822502 >.
9. BELTOWSKI, J.; RACHANCZYK, J.; WLODARCZYK, M. Thiazolidinedione-induced fluid retention: recent insights into the molecular mechanisms. PPAR Res, v. 2013, p. 628628, 2013. ISSN 1687-4757 (Print). Disponível em: < http://dx.doi.org/10.1155/2013/628628 >.
10. OKHOVAT, J. P.; ALAVI, A. Lipedema: A Review of the Literature. Int J Low Extrem Wounds, Oct 17 2014. ISSN 1534-7346. Disponível em: < http://dx.doi.org/10.1177/1534734614554284 >.
11. PESSA, M. E.; HOWARD, R. J. Necrotizing fasciitis. Surg Gynecol Obstet, v. 161, n. 4, p. 357-61, Oct 1985. ISSN 0039-6087 (Print)0039-6087. Disponível em: < http://dx.doi.org/ >.

12. SUBRAMANYAM, P.; PALANISWAMY, S. S. Lymphoscintigraphy in unilateral lower limb and scrotal lymphedema caused by filariasis. Am J Trop Med Hyg, v. 87, n. 6, p. 963-4, Dec 2012. ISSN 0002-9637. Disponível em: < http://dx.doi.org/10.4269/ajtmh.2012.12-0422 >.
13. TRAYES, K. P. et al. Edema: Diagnosis and Management - American Family Physician. 2015. Disponível em: < http://www.aafp.org/afp/2013/0715/p102.html >.
14. Ellison DH. Diuretic drugs and the treatment of edema: from clinic to bench and back again. *J Kidney Dis*. 1994;23:623–43.
15. Wittner M, Di Stefano A, Wangemann P, Greger R. How do loop diuretics act? *Drugs*. 1991;41(suppl 3):1–13
16. FELTY, C. L.; ROOKE, T. W. Compression therapy for chronic venous insufficiency. Semin Vasc Surg, v. 18, n. 1, p. 36-40, Mar 2005. ISSN 0895-7967 (Print)0895-7967. Disponível em: < http://dx.doi.org/ >.
17. TRAYES, K. P. et al. Edema: diagnosis and management. Am Fam Physician, v. 88, n. 2, p. 102-10, Jul 15 2013. ISSN 0002-838x. Disponível em: < http://dx.doi.org/ >.
18. SIERAKOWSKI, K.; PILLER, N. Pilot study of the impact of sporting compression garments on composition and volume of normal and lymphedema legs. Lymphology, v. 47, n. 4, p. 187-95, Dec 2014. ISSN 0024-7766 (Print)0024-7766. Disponível em: < http://dx.doi.org/ >.
19. SUGA, K. et al. Assessment of leg oedema by dynamic lymphoscintigraphy with intradermal injection of technetium-99m human serum albumin and load produced by standing. Eur J Nucl Med, v. 28, n. 3, p. 294-303, Mar 2001. ISSN 0340-6997 (Print)0340-6997. Disponível em: <

NOTES -

Section E

The Art of Challenging Questions

Section E - The Art of Answering Challenging Questions

Challenging questions can produce a range of emotions for the medical students and physicians taking the Step 2 CS Exam or in real life. These challenging questions require one to be calm, composed, and sincere towards the patient. There needs to be a systematic approach, so as not to create a negative impact on the patient. I have devised an approach to answer all challenging questions put forth by the standardized patients. This has been tested by me with my real life patients. I have not invented universal theories, but adapted and modified to make one theory of empathy--'**L.U.C.K.Y Touch.**'

We have used the **L.U.C.K.Y Touch** principles to answer the challenging questions empathetically.

Step 1 – Label the emotion

When faced with a challenging question, the first step is to recognize and **label the patient's emotion.**

Is the patient happy? Is he/she sad? Is he/she concerned? Is he/she feeling lonely? Sometimes, patients will be lying on the examination table writhing in pain, and an emotion still has to be discerned. If a patient is crying, offer a tissue and support them. The patient may be feeling anything at the moment. It is the doctor's responsibility to recognize and label it.

The various emotions that a patient may be expressing are, but not limited to:

- ✓ Happiness
- ✓ Sadness
- ✓ Nervousness
- ✓ Frustration
- ✓ Embarrassment
- ✓ Pride
- ✓ Fear
- ✓ Love
- ✓ Anxiety
- ✓ Loneliness

Try to understand the facial expressions and behavior of the patient and label it accordingly.

Mirror Neurons have been recognized to play a major part in empathy. Recent studies have shown the activity in these neurons to be responsible for generating and recognizing facial expressions and pain. These neurons are thought to be present in the insula and anterior cingulate gyrus of the brain cortex. As a physician, I have adopted this theory by Dr. V.S Ramachandran, to **label** the patient's emotion each time they have been sad, depressed, anxious, and fearful.

I have asked ask them a very simple question, complementing it with a tap on the shoulder or a gentle touch on their hand to show support and win confidence,

- ✓ Q: "You seem to be sad. Is something bothering you?"

My mirror neurons have adapted to this, and now every time I see a patient in emotional dilemma, I immediately understand their emotions and responding subconsciously in a compassionate manner. Using this approach I have won the trust of many people.

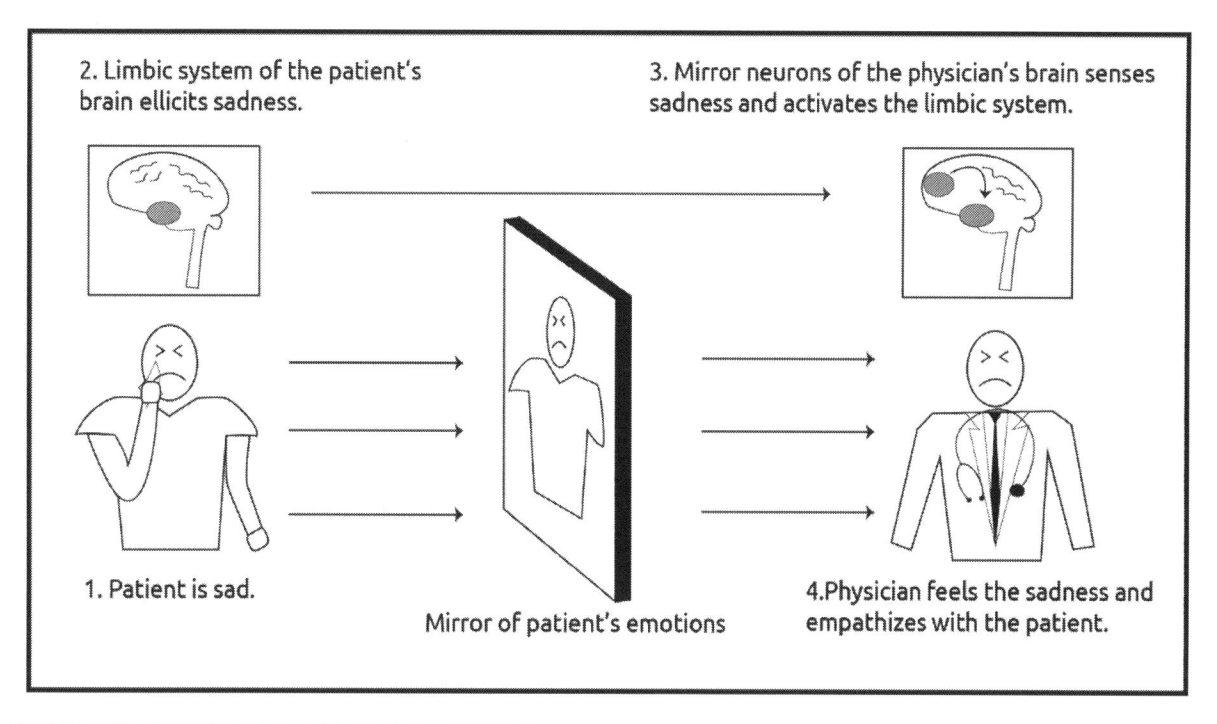

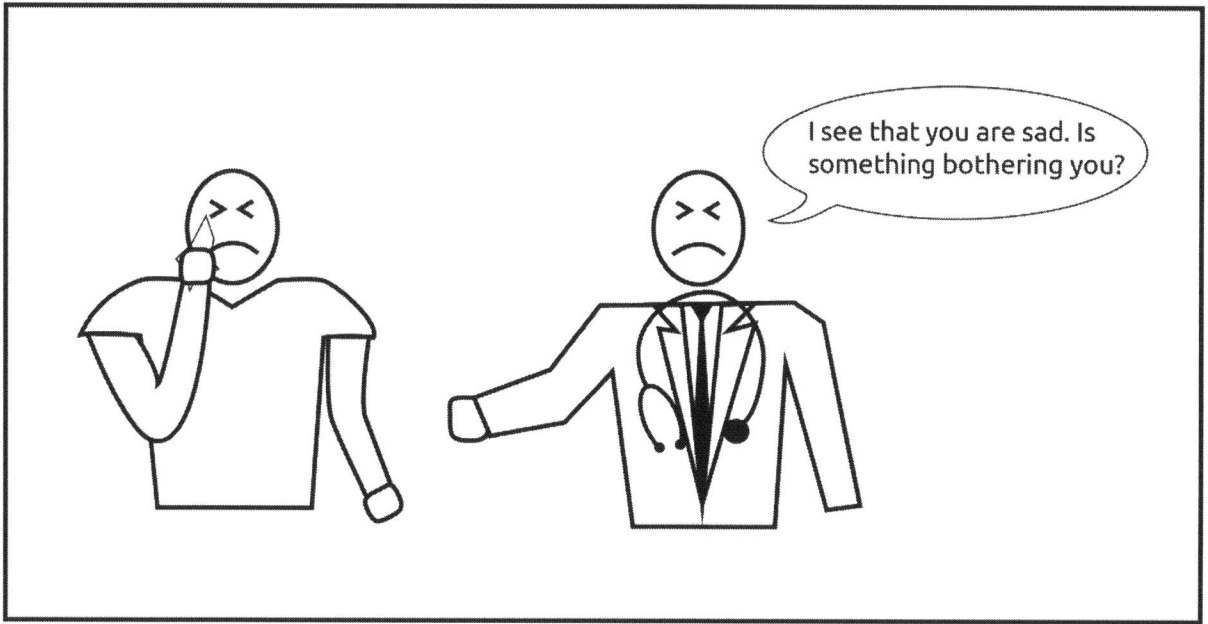

- Q: "I see that you are sad! Is everything ok?" "No," replies the patient. Move to the next step.

Step 2 – Understand the background of the emotion

Steven Covey, in his book The Seven Habits of Highly Effective People, explains the habit of seeking to understand and then to be understood. Don't listen to reply, but listen to understand the patient's feelings.

Let's say the examiner enters the room and sees that the standardized patient is pacing and acting very stressed out. This is how one should proceed:

- ✓ Q: "I see that you are very stressed out. I am a physician in this hospital, and I am here to help you. "
- ✓ "Let me ask some questions to understand your concerns, and then I will address your needs. Before we proceed, do you have any questions?"

Always adapt and modify.

Step 3 – Commend-Recommend-Commend the patient

We have adopted this principle from Dale Carnegie to always give a sincere compliment at first, followed by a practical recommendation, and more praising at the end.

The patient says, "Doc, I have had multiple sexual encounters outside my marriage and my wife does not know about it. I am worried that I have contracted a sexually transmitted infection."

The doctor replies, "I appreciate you being honest and upfront with me (**Commend**). This information will be strictly confidential between us, however, we will do some tests after the examination to evaluate for any STIs. In case we find something significant, we will sit again and discuss the treatment plan. Meanwhile, I would strongly encourage you to share this information with your wife first (**Recommend**). *pause...* Again, I am really glad that you were honest about your concerns (**Commend**)."

Step 4 – Keep it *simple* and *supportive* for the patient

After labeling the patient's emotions and understanding the root cause and appreciating him/her for sharing it, it is now time to reinforce the empathy and provide support to the patient. Just remember to **keep it simple!** Don't try to explain hardcore medical terminology to the patient and make him/her more nervous. Simply explain the situation to him/her and offer support. We have modified the K.I.S.S principle from Keep it Simple and Stupid to **Keep it Simple and Supportive.**
Offer a tissue to a crying patient. A cup of water to a patient who is coughing would be a great idea, however, be mindful of abdominal pain. If the patient has abdomenal pain, do not give them water, as it is likely to interfere with your examination findings. Pat the shoulder of a patient who is in distress and needs support. All of these are simple measures of expressing empathy and supporting the patient.

"Doc, do you think I have cancer?"

The doctor replies, "I can see a mass on this MRI, however, until and unless we do a biopsy of this, we cannot prove if this is cancer or not….As you know, tissue is the issue."

Step 5 – Start with why (or start with 'Y')

Encourage the patient to elaborate (Why-How-What approach to elaborate the problem)

This step involves encouraging the patient to share their history, to express his/her concerns, and to come to a diagnosis as a team. Encourage the patient to continue with treatment and be compliant with the doctor's advice; encourage them to come for regular follow-ups. First ask 'why' to gain more insight on the problem. Second, ask 'how,' and last, ask 'what.' This Simon Sinek's "Start with Why" approach has helped me to win patients and family caregivers.

Step 6 -- TOUCH

"*Cure sometimes, treat often, comfort always.*"-- Hippocrates

Last, but not the least, is **Touch**. With the advent of technology, the physical exam is becoming obsolete. However, the worst mistake a practitioner can make in the physical exam is to not touch the patient and to just discuss the labs or radiology tests. Touch sensitizes the pacinian receptors sensitive corpuscles, which reduces stress by activating the Vagus nerve. Touching the patient helps to release Oxytocin--the cuddle hormone, thus increasing trust.

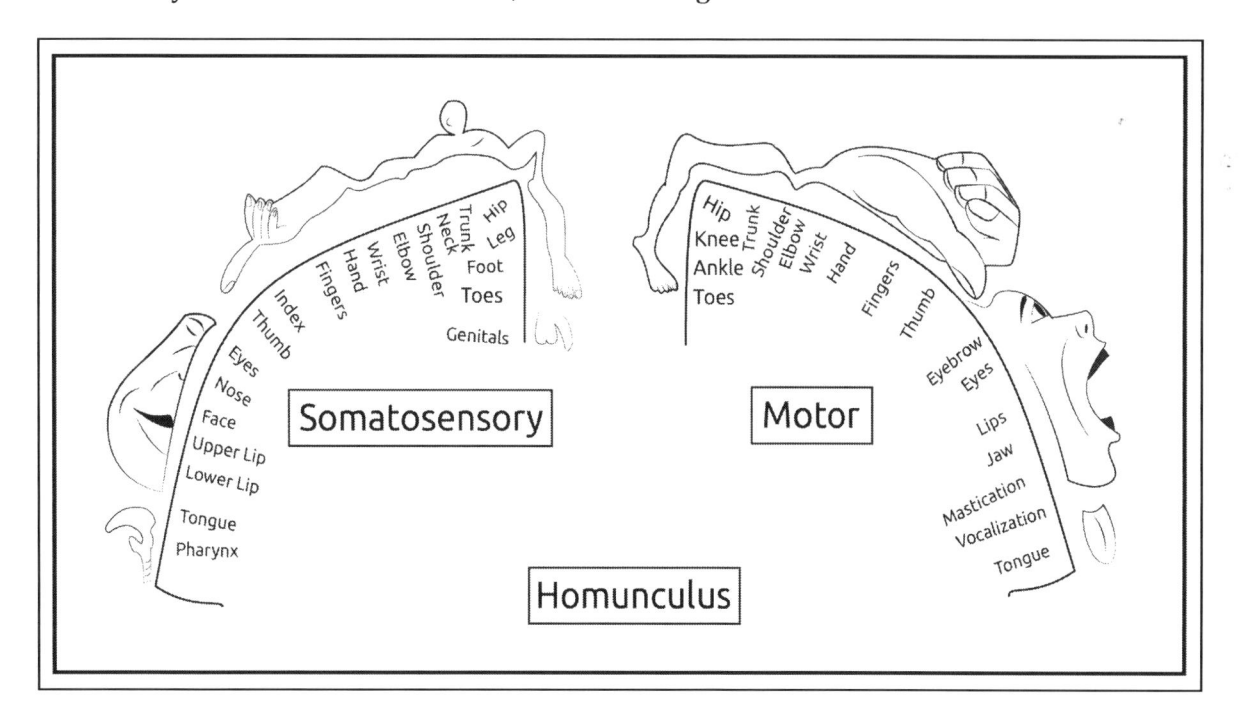

THE 'LUCKY' TOUCH

The *'LUCKY Touch'* approach can be used for challenging questions. It will surely get a student lucky on the exam!

PRACTICE SHEETS

Next are some commonly encountered challenging questions. Please go through them and use the LUCKY approach to answer them.

Practice Question 1

A 56-year-old lady, Mrs. Morrison, comes to Dr. Smith's office for a hypertension follow-up. She has been under Dr. Smith's care for the past 15 years, but you are covering for Dr. Smith today. However, she insists on seeing Dr. Smith only.

How would you manage the situation?

Label the Emotion

- ✓ "Mrs. Morrison, I notice that you are stressed out today."

Understand the Background

- ✓ "I am covering for Dr. Smith, and I assure you that I am completely aware of all your past medical history from the electronic medical records. Can you please tell me what is going on?" (If the patient says that she doesn't want to see you, but only Dr. Smith, then go to the next step-Commend)

Commend-Recommend- Commend the Patient

- ✓ "I appreciate you being upfront about this and assure you that I will take excellent care."

Keep it Simple & Supportive to the Patient

- ✓ "I am here to help you in every way."
- ✓ "I am a well-qualified physician and I assure that we will take good care of you. I will also update Dr. Smith about your visit today when he comes back."
- ✓ "I am here to support you."
- ✓ "I will give my 100%."
- ✓ "I just want you to relax and know that we are here to help."

(You may use any variation of these lines depending on the clinical scenario)

Start with 'Y'
(Encourage the patient to elaborate using the why-how-what approach)

- ✓ "Let me explain the why of the problem to you" (Explain with the help of a simple line diagram). "Before I prescribe any meds, can you show me if you are maintaining a logbook for your blood pressure? How is your blood pressure control? I am going to prescribe a refill for you and I want you to take your medications as you are doing. Do you have any questions for me?"

Practice Question 2

A poor patient comes in for surgery, but refuses, as he cannot afford it. The patient is in severe pain and only wants a pain prescription.

Label the Emotion

- ✓ "I see that you are worried about the cost of treatment because you don't have insurance yet."

Understand the Background

- ✓ "I also understand that your major concern is the pain and you want some relief so that you can leave the hospital."

Commend-Recommend- Commend the Patient

- ✓ "I appreciate you for being upfront with me regarding your concerns."

Keep it Simple & Support the Patient

- ✓ "Let me assure you that I am here to help you. This surgery is very important for your health and there might be serious complications if this is not performed right away. I can send in my social worker to help you with your financial concerns, and I assure that we can provide the best treatment for you by working together."

Start with 'Y'
(Encourage the patient to elaborate using the why-how-what approach)

- ✓ "Let me explain the disease process and you will understand the importance of surgery for your condition" (Explain with the line diagrams if possible).
- ✓ "Any there any other questions for me?"

Practice Question 3

A 52-year-old lady comes to your office complaining of racing of the heart. The patient starts crying and says, "It keeps me awake all night. Is something bad going to happen to me?"

Label the Emotion

- ✓ "It seems that you are worried about your heart racing. Is that right? *pause*...Is there anything else that is troubling you?"
- ✓ Once you have labelled the emotion, you will win the patient's confidence and you might be able to uncover an underlying cause of her worry, for example, a physically abused elderly woman.

Understand the Background

- ✓ Offer her a tissue.
- ✓ Tap gently on the shoulder.
- ✓ Encourage the patient to speak. "Tell me more about your problems."
- ✓ Understand the background of her concerns.

Commend-Recommend-Commend the Patient

- ✓ "I appreciate you sharing your concerns with me."
- ✓ "We will sit together as a team to devise a plan to diagnose and treat your disease."
- ✓ "I really admire you for coming out with your problem and sharing it with me."

Keep it Simple & Support the Patient

- ✓ "But please don't worry. I am here to help you. Let me ask you some simple questions and then we can discuss what this might be."

Start with 'Y'
(Encourage the patient to elaborate using the why-how-what approach)

- ✓ Explain to the patient in the layman language what possible causes could be the reason for her racing heart.
- ✓ Explain what investigations you are going to perform and how you plan to treat her.
- ✓ Please refer to the d/d tables and understand the why-how-what of palpitations.

Practice Question 4

A female patient comes to your office and you suspect her to have a sexually transmitted disease. She asks you, "Should I tell my partner about this?"

What would you advise her?

Label the Emotion

- ✓ "I see that you are confused about telling your partner about this."

Understand the Background

- ✓ "I know that this is a difficult decision for you. Can you explain what difficulty are you facing in telling your partner about the disease?"
- ✓ When you gain the patient's confidence, she might tell you that she had been having extramarital affairs with other men.

Commend-Recommend- Commend the Patient

- ✓ "I appreciate you for sharing your concern with me."
- ✓ "I recommend that you follow safe sexual practices in future. I would suggest that you inform your husband about your disease, as he might contract it from you. I praise your genuine honesty and concern for your troubles."

Keep it Simple & Support the Patient

- ✓ "Let me assure you that I am here to help you. I assure you that whatever we discuss is confidential and that I am always there to help you."

Start with 'Y'
(Encourage the patient to elaborate using the why-how-what approach)

- ✓ "This disease is transmitted by sexual intercourse and your partner may be at risk to get this disease too. It is important that he gets a similar checkup and treatment soon so that we can put a stop to the transmission of this disease. I would like you to tell him about this and bring him to the clinic so that we can discuss and plan the management appropriately."

Practice Question 5

A 35 year old lady, Ms. Laura Kurtis comes to your office complaining of excessive weight gain. She has gained over 30 lbs. in the past 4 months. She is worried about her appearance and also about the complications of obesity. You measure her BMI as 32. She asks you if she could have joint problems because of her weight. How do you counsel her?

Label the emotion

> ➢ I see that you are concerned about your weight and how it is affecting your appearance and health.

Understand the background

> ➢ "What do you know about obesity and its complications?"
> ➢ Patient might say, "Umm, nothing!" or "Maybe, heart attack."
> ➢ Based on her answer, you can point out other complications and assess her knowledge about her disease.
> ➢ This will help you to understand the patient's point of view.
> ➢ "What is bothering you about your appearance?"

Commend the patient

> ➢ I appreciate you for discussing your problems with me. I would recommend you to follow a healthy lifestyle. Also, we will do some tests to rule out any complications of obesity.

Keep it simple & support the patient

> ➢ Obesity can affect your joints, due to excessive weight. Also, lack of exercise can cause weak muscles around the joints and early arthritis.

Start with 'Y' - Encourage the patient to elaborate Why-how-what approach

> ➢ Explain to her in simple language, the pathogenesis and complications of obesity and how she can lose weight.

Practice Question 6

A 65 year old male with a history of prolapsed intervertebral disc presents to you with severe back pain. He tells you, "Doc, my back really hurts. Please give me some morphine as the regular pain meds are not working anymore." How would you counsel this patient?

Label the emotion

- It seems that you are in a lot of pain.

Understand the background

- Back pain can sometimes be really troublesome.
- Can you explain the nature of your pain and which medications are you taking for pain? Do you have bowel and urine incontinence?
- Have you been using narcotics for you pain before?

Commend the patient

- Thank you for letting me know about your previous medications and your pain. I would suggest that we first examine you and then do some tests to evaluate any complications of your disease.

Keep it simple & support the patient

- (This can be the part of third step-commend-recommend-commend)

Start with 'Y' - Encourage the patient to elaborate Why-how-what approach

- I can assure you that you are in good hands. We will work on your pain and help you with it.

Practice Question 7

Mr. Hansen, a 54 year old Caucasian gentleman comes to your office complaining of a long term cough and shortness of breath. He has smoked two packs per day for the last two years. He wants to quit smoking but is unable to do so. How do you counsel him?

Label the emotion

➢ "I see that you are having trouble in quitting smoking. Is that right Mr Hansen?"

Understand the background

➢ "Can you please elaborate on the difficulties you are facing in quitting smoking."

Commend the patient

➢ "Mr Hansen, I must commend you on the decision you have taken to quit smoking and I appreciate you coming in today for help."

Keep it simple & support the patient

➢ Let me assure you that I am here to help you in every possible way I can. You do not need to get disheartened. From nicotine patches to smoking cessation groups, we have various methods that we can try and see which one helps you the most to quit smoking.

Encourage the patient to elaborate Why-how-what approach

➢ I guarantee you that if we work as a team, you will be able to quit soon. Do you have any other concerns or questions for me?

Practice Question 8

You enter the office and see that the patient, Mr. Clark, is coughing excessively. He is in distress and is coughing into his hand. What would be your approach?

Label the emotion

- ➢ "Mr. Clark, I can see that the cough is really troubling you.
- ➢ Let me hand you some tissues."

Understand the background

- ➢ "Once you are comfortable, we can start with some questions to get to the root cause of this problem."

Commend the patient

- ➢ It is not important to finish all the steps in LUCKY Touch approach.
- ➢ It should become your second nature, once you have practiced enough. You must respect the patient's values, culture and then praise. Never be judgemental. Never force things.

Keep it simple & support the patient

- ➢ "Let me explain to you with simple diagrams why cough happens."
- ➢ Refer to the chapter on "approach to cough."
- ➢ I am here to help you and I assure you that you will not go back home dissatisfied. I would like to run a few blood tests and do a few investigations to have a better understanding of your problem.

Start with 'Y' - Encourage the patient to elaborate Why-how-what approach

- ➢ Explain with a few line diagrams the probable reasons for the cough.
- ➢ Remember to talk in layman language.
- ➢ Then ask if the patient has any other questions for you.

Practice Question 9

A 17 year old girl comes to your office complaining of feeling obese. Her BMI is 17 kg/m². She admits to using practices like self- induced vomiting, laxatives and herbal drugs. She says "Doc, I am too fat. My friends are so slim and sexy. I want to lose weight. Please give me some pills to get rid of the fat." How do you counsel this girl?

Label the emotion

- ➢ "I see that you are very concerned about your weight and appearance."

Understand the background

- ➢ "I understand that you have tried various means for losing weight. What is it that worries you about your weight? Tell me more about your concerns."

Commend the patient

- ➢ "I respect you for coming forward with your concerns. I would like to ask you a few more questions to understand your problem better."

Keep it simple & support the patient

- ➢ "People at your age have various concerns about their appearance. Let me assure you that I would do my best to help you regain confidence and resort to a healthy living and lifestyle. I would also like to fix an appointment with a counsellor to help you deal with this situation better."

Encourage the patient to elaborate Why-how-what approach

- ➢ Explain to the patient in simple language how Anorexia Nervosa can adversely affect her health and fertility. It may increase risk of fracture, various nutritional deficiencies, inability to conceive, poor hair and skin and other complications.
- ➢ Explain the various investigations you want to do to check for electrolyte abnormalities and other deficiencies and hormone imbalances.
- ➢ Ask if the patient has any more questions.

Practice Question 10

You enter your office to see the patient, Ms. Jenny, weeping. She looks like she has been abused at home. When you try to strike a conversation with her, she ignores you and refuses to answer any question. How do you continue this encounter?

Label the emotion

- "Ms. Jenny I can see that you are anxious and concerned. "

Understand the background

- "Ms. Jenny, whatever we discuss in this room, will be confidential between you and I. If there is something that is bothering you, please let me know. I will try my best to find a good solution to it."
- "I can assure you that the information you provide will not be discussed with anyone without your permission and is only for me to help you."

Commend the patient

- "I commend you for seeking this appointment and visiting my office."

Keep it simple & support the patient

- "I want you to be assured that I am only here to help you. I am worried about domestic abuse at your home. Your wellness and safety is of utmost importance to me. Please let me ask few more questions so that I can understand the situation better and involve our social service department."

Start with 'Y' - Encourage the patient to elaborate Why-how-what approach

- "We have social support groups and women's shelter to give you support should you be a victim of domestic abuse. I can send in my social worker after this to help you with that information."

Practice Question 11

Mrs. Ginny, a 38 year old lady comes to your office complaining of fatigue, depression and constipation for the last three weeks. She reports that she lost her husband and little girl in a car accident three weeks earlier. Suddenly she breaks down crying and says "Doc, I want to die right now. I can't take it anymore". How do you approach her now?

Label the emotion

- "Mrs Ginny, I am terribly sorry for your loss. I can see that losing your family has deeply upset you."
- Act and offer her Kleenex.
- Once the patient stops crying and is calm, proceed further.

Understand the background

- "Tell me more about what is going on in your mind."
- Gently tap on the shoulder of the patient to show empathy and compassion.
- Let the patient speak and be a patient listener.(*Use your ears and tongue in the ratio of 2:1*)

Commend the patient

- "I know it is a very trying phase for you Mrs Ginny. I really appreciate you for coming in today to talk and discuss about your concerns. Let me tell you that you are a very strong woman and we will do everything possible to help you."

Keep it simple & support the patient

- "Let me assure you that whatever we speak about is purely confidential and will stay between the both of us. I would like to ask you a few more questions."
- Ask specific questions to rule out depression (DIGEST P CAPSULE)
- "Have you ever thought of hurting yourself?"

Encourage the patient to elaborate Why-how-what approach

- "Mrs Ginny, it seems like losing your husband and daughter has affected you a lot. It is normal to feel depressed and cry. We have highly qualified counsellors at the hospital and I would suggest you to set up an appointment with the counsellor at the front desk who can help you to deal with this situation. Let's do some basic blood work to evaluate your condition. Do you have any other questions for me?"

Practice Question 12

Upon entering the room, you see the patient Mr. Dorothy holding his head with both his hands, due to severe headache. As soon as he sees you, he asks you to turn down the lights. How do you react?

Label the emotion

- FIRST dim the lights!

Understand the background

- "Mr. Dorothy, I have turned down the lights as I can understand that it is bothering you. Are you feeling better now?"
- Gently tap on the shoulder of the patient to reassure him that you are there to take care of him and his concerns.
- Once the patient seems more cooperative, proceed further.
- "Can you tell me more about your pain please?"

Commend the patient

- "I appreciate your cooperation despite such intense headache."

Keep it simple & support the patient

- "I can see that you are in pain. Please let me know if I can do anything else to make you more comfortable. Let me assure you that I am here to help you. I would like to ask you a few more questions to get a better understanding of this problem."

Start with 'Y' - Encourage the patient to elaborate Why-how-what approach

- "So let me explain to you with simple drawings the various causes that might be causing your headache. Then, I would like to examine you and order a few tests to diagnose your condition. Is that okay Mr. Dorothy?"
- Refer to the chapter "Approach to headaches" for the causes and explanations.

Practice Question 13

Mr. Jack, a 47 year old male patient comes to your office complaining of frequent urination, weight loss and increased thirst for the past few months. He denies having any fever, depression or bowel complaint. He asks you "Doc, my mother had diabetes, do you think that's what I have now?" How do you counsel him?

Label the emotion

- "Mr Jack, I can see that you are worried if you have diabetes since your mother had it too. Am I right?"

Understand the background

- "I can understand you are distressed. Can you tell me more about what is worrying you?"
- Follow the 2:1 principle here.

Commend the patient

- "You have a very valid question and I appreciate you bringing it up to me."

Keep it simple & support the patient

- "The symptoms that you have do point towards diabetes, especially because you have a family history of it but there are other diseases too that can present with the same symptoms. Mr Jack, let me assure you that I am here to help you and we will get to the bottom of this problem. But before that, I would like your cooperation to answer a few questions for me. Is that okay?"

Start with Y - Elaborate Why-how-what approach

- Explain with a few diagrams about the types of Diabetes Mellitus, how diabetes happens and the various complications associated with it. (blurring of vision, dizziness, numbness and tingling in extremities, changes in libido, etc)
- "I would like to order a few blood tests and a few imaging studies before I can comment on the diagnosis. Once the results are out, I would be at a better place to discuss the problem and plan the management. Do you have any other questions for me?"

Practice Question 14

You are about to see a patient, Ms. Grey, who is visiting you for severe abdominal pain. Just as you enter the room she tells you rudely "Can you not see that I am writhing in pain here? Give me a painkiller immediately!" What do you do?

Label the emotion

- "Ms. Grey I see that you have severe belly pain. "

Understand the background

- "However, I need to understand the cause of your belly pain before I can give any pain medication. I will be very quick in asking questions and doing examination. As soon as I am done, I will ask my nurse to help you out."

Commend the patient

- "I appreciate your patience at this time until I figure out the cause. After your examination, we will plan the appropriate investigation and treatment as quickly as possible to relieve your pain sooner."
- "I admire you for your strength to bear with us while in severe pain."

Keep it simple & support the patient

- "We are here to help you and we will provide best medical management."

Encourage the patient to elaborate Why-how-what approach

- "Let me explain the 'why, how and what' of your belly pain and what we plan to do for it."
- Refer to D/D table.

Practice Question 15

Ms. Iguila Jules, a 45 year old lady comes to your clinic with complaints of sleeping problems for the last six months. Upon asking her questions, she tells you that she drinks 4-5 cups of coffee during the day, she also watches TV until 10pm because she can't get to sleep. It takes her two hours in bed to fall asleep. She says "Doc, please give me some sleeping pills. This is really disturbing my activities and job" How do you counsel her?

Label the emotion

Understand the background

Commend the patient

Keep it simple & support the patient

Encourage the patient to elaborate Why-how-what approach

Practice Question 16

The patient today is a 17 year old girl, Susan Brown, who is accompanied by her mother, Ms. Brown, for complaints of vaginal discharge. The girl is showing reluctance in answering your questions in front of her mother. What will you do?

Label the emotion

- "Susan, I see that you are uncomfortable in answering my questions right now. Is that right?"

Understand the background

- (*Talking to the mother*) "I can understand Ms. Brown, that you are very concerned about your daughter's health and I appreciate it. Susan seems a little reluctant to talk about her problem in front of you. It would be very kind of you, if you could give me a few minutes to enquire Susan in person about her complaints. Thank you Ms. Brown."

Commend the patient

- (Sometimes, in such scenarios you can commend the patient while trying to understand the background, as it becomes easier and more communicative to assess and empathize with the patient)

Keep it simple & support the patient

- "I assure you that whatever you tell me would be strictly confidential and will not be shared with anyone without your permission. "

Encourage the patient to elaborate Why-how-what approach

- "We will work together to get you relieved of this problem as soon as possible."

Practice Question 17

Mr. Peter Angelhart, an 87 year old gentleman comes to the ER complaining of sudden loss of hearing in his right ear. He reports feeling dizzy and hearing bells in his right ear before he lost hearing completely. He has no history of trauma or falling. As soon as you are about to start the physical examination he says "Will I be able to hear again doc? I really don't want to lose my hearing at this age. Please do something." How do you proceed?

Label the emotion

Understand the background

Commend the patient

Keep it simple & support the patient

Encourage the patient to elaborate Why-how-what approach

Practice Question 18

You have received a call from Ms. Gordon, a mother of a three year old girl Jane, concerned about the child's bleeding nose. The mother says "Doctor, Jane has been continuously bleeding for the last three hours. I have applied pressure but it doesn't stop. What should I do? Please do something!" You can sense that she is really worried about her child. How do you talk to her?

Label the emotion

- ➢ "Ms. Gordon, I hear that you are very worried about Jane's bleeding. Is that right?"

Understand the background

- ➢ "I understand that it is really hard to see her suffer like that."

Commend the patient

- ➢ "I appreciate that you called us for help at the right time. I recommend that you get Jane to the hospital immediately and we will be ready with our emergency team."
- ➢ "Do you want me to dispatch an ambulance for you?"

Keep it simple & support the patient

- ➢ "Please continue to apply pressure to her nose by pinching it and extend her head to face upwards."

Encourage the patient to elaborate Why-how-what approach

- ➢ Refer to D/D table to explain to the patient

Practice Question 19

Ms. Elle August, a 45 year old lady comes to your office complaining of sad mood and excessive sleepiness. She has recently been fired from work. Her question is "Doc, I am a single mom. How do I feed my children now? I have two girls. Who will take care of them?" And she starts crying.

How do you proceed?

- ✓ **Label the emotion**

- ✓ **Understand the background**

- ✓ **Commend the patient**

- ✓ **Keep it simple & support the patient**

- ✓ **Encourage the patient to elaborate Why-how-what approach**

Practice Question 20

A 24 year old gentleman, Mr. John Bond comes to the emergency room complaining of severe chest pain. He has a past medical history significant for sickle cell disease. He urges you to give him pain medication immediately but you request him to let you ask a few questions before choosing the right medicines. He responds by saying "It is all there in my Electronic Medical Records. I am telling you they give me Dilaudid all the time" What do you say next?

Label the emotion

> ➤ "Mr. Bond I can see that you are in severe pain."

Understand the background

> ➤ "I understand that these episodes can be very troublesome."

Commend the patient

> ➤ "Thank you for telling me about your sickle cell disease."

Keep it simple & support the patient

> ➤ "I will surely look into your electronic health records but before that please let me ask a few important questions."

Encourage the patient to elaborate Why-how-what approach

> ➤ "I assure you that it will be quick and that I will help you with your pain."

Practice Question 21

Ms. Hansen Koija, a 24 year old female comes to your office with multiple bruises on her neck and arms. Upon questioning she tells you that her dog bit her on the neck and that she is here for some injections or medications to help relieve the pain, and heal her bruises. On lifting her gown, you see that she has similar bite marks all over her abdomen. You suspect sexual abuse and ask her again, which makes her start crying. She says "Doc, I love my boyfriend but lately he has been acting strange. He beats me and uses me however he wants. I don't have anywhere else to go. What should I do?" How do you counsel her?

Label the emotion

> ➤ First offer her a tissue. Then patting on her shoulder gently say, "Ms. Koija I see that you are very troubled about the way your boyfriend has been behaving with you."

Understand the background

> ➤ Seek to understand for how long this has been going on and ask her about firearms at home. Ask her if she has any kids and whether they are safe or not.

Commend the patient

> ➤ "I admire your courage and honesty for sharing your difficulties with me. Do you have an exit plan (Food, Shelter, Clothes and Job)?"

Keep it simple & support the patient

> ➤ "I assure you that I am here to help. I would suggest that you call the social services for further assistance."

Encourage the patient to elaborate Why-how-what approach

> ➤ I want to dig deeper into the root cause of the problem and why he is doing that.
> ➤ F-Firearms
> ➤ I-illicit drugs
> ➤ R-Relationship outside the home
> ➤ E-Exit plan
> ➤ A-Alcohol, Tobacco

> ➤ R-Relationship inside the home
> ➤ M-Money
> ➤ S-Suicidal tendency and Sexual harassment
> ➤ Ms.Koija your safety is of utmost importance to us. In case you feel threatened, please do not hesitate to call us or the police.

Practice Question 22

A 68 year old male, Mr. Lee, has been diagnosed with atrial fibrillation recently and is on Coumadin prophylaxis. He comes to the ER with complaints of bleeding from the nose since this morning. As soon as you enter the room, he says "I won't take Coumadin anymore doctor, I know all this is happening to me because of Coumadin"

Label the emotion

- "Mr. Lee I see that you are very worried about the bleeding caused by Coumadin."

Understand the background

- "And it is very much possible that the bleeding is occurring because of Coumadin."
- "I would like to ask you a few questions to understand your concerns better."
- "When was the Coumadin started?"
- "How many episodes of bleeding have you had so far?"
- "Coumadin, diet and other drugs may interact with each other, therefore, I want to know everything about you."

Commend the patient

- "It was very nice of you that you came to me as soon as the adverse effects of Coumadin started bothering you."
- "I would recommend not to stop your medication cold turkey."

Keep it simple & support the patient

- "I assure you that I am here to help you out. I will perform a focused examination on you and then would like to do a few tests to confirm the cause of these recurrent bleeding episodes."
- "Then we will sit down together to make a plan of treatment which benefits both, your atrial fibrillation and your recurrent bleeding. Is that okay Mr. Lee?"

Encourage the patient to elaborate Why-how-what approach

- You should have the differential ready in the back of your mind.

Practice Question 23

A 56 year old gentleman comes to your office complaining of an inability to move the ring and little finger of his right hand. He works with an orchestra playing the piano. He is really concerned about his fingers and asks you "Doc, will I be able to play the piano again?" How do you proceed?

Label the emotion

Understand the background

Commend the patient

Keep it simple & support the patient

Encourage the patient to elaborate Why-how-what approach

Practice Question 24

Mrs. Ali is a hypertensive patient. She was prescribed a diuretic, hydrochlorothiazide for her blood pressure in a dose of 25 mg per day. Today, she comes to your office with complains of frequent urination, which interferes in her daily living. She refuses to take HCTZ anymore. How will you counsel her?

Label the emotion

> ➤ "Mrs Ali, I see that you are having troubles with this water pill, which you are taking for your high blood pressure."

Understand the background

> ➤ "I can imagine how inconvenient it would be for you with this medicine. Let me ask you a few more question regarding your problem and the medication so that I can help you better."

Commend the patient

> ➤ "Thank you for letting me know about the issue. I recommend that we run some tests to evaluate your symptoms."
> ➤ "I appreciate you being upfront and honest about the adverse effects of the medication."

Keep it simple & support the patient

> ➤ "I will review the dose and possibly change the medication after conducting a brief physical examination. Is that ok with you?"

Encourage the patient to elaborate Why-how-what approach

> ➤ "Don't worry; I will make sure that the new medicine doesn't cause this problem again."

Practice Question 25

Mr. John Sherman, a 65 year old gentleman comes to your clinic complaining of a swollen and painful left toe. He reports that his pain is 9/10 in severity, throbbing in nature and relieved by ibuprofen to some extent. He denies having any trauma or fever. He asks you "Do you think I have gout doctor?" What do you tell him?

Label the emotion

Understand the background

Commend the patient

Keep it simple & support the patient

Encourage the patient to elaborate Why-how-what approach

Practice Question 26

A 31 year old lady, Ms. Jules comes to you and says, "Doc, ever since I quit smoking, I have been gaining weight. Do you think it is because of the quitting tobacco?"

Label the emotion

> "Ms. Jules, I see that you are worried about your weight gain."

Understand the background

> "It is normal to regain some lost weight after quitting smoking because smoking makes you lose weight."

Commend the patient

> "I am happy that you are upfront with me about your thoughts about smoking."

Keep it simple & support the patient

> "But smoking would not be the appropriate thing to do. It can damage your lungs, heart, kidneys and many other organs in your body. It can cause many kinds of cancers. There are other ways to control weight, including dietary and lifestyle management."

Encourage the patient to elaborate Why-how-what approach

> "You have taken a really healthy decision by quitting smoking. I would want you to continue with it. I can refer you to weight management centers if you would like?"

Practice Question 27

Mr. Chen Lee, a 49 year old gentleman comes to your office for a routine health checkup. His past history is significant for HTN, DM and hypercholesterolemia. He reports having intermittent chest pain which resolves on its own in a few minutes. The pain is 5/10 in severity and dull aching in nature. He has smoked 1 PPD for the last 10 years. He requests a CT scan to rule out lung cancer. What do you tell him?

Label the emotion

Understand the background

Commend the patient

Keep it simple & support the patient

Encourage the patient to elaborate Why-how-what approach

Practice Question 28

You have a lady in your office today complaining of a sore throat. She works at a childcare center and she asks you, "Should I take a leave from work doctor, I am concerned about the children". What do you tell her?

Label the emotion

> ➢ "I can understand your concern and I am happy to hear that you care so much about the children. It is possible that you can transmit the infection."

Understand the background

Commend the patient

Keep it simple & support the patient

> ➢ "But let us first check what kind of infection it is. I would like to ask you a few questions and then briefly examine you."
> ➢ "Will that be ok with you?"

Encourage the patient to elaborate Why-how-what approach

> ➢ "I can assure you that I am here to help."

Practice Question 29

A 22 year old college going student comes to your office for a routine medical checkup and to get some health forms filled. He does not smoke, does not drink and has an overall healthy lifestyle. There is no significant family history. You suggest an annual flu vaccine to him, to which he replies "Doc, I don't want to take it. I have heard some people fall sick after that vaccine" How do you counsel him?

Label the emotion

Understand the background

Commend the patient

Keep it simple & support the patient

Encourage the patient to elaborate Why-how-what approach

Practice Question 30

A 27 year old Ms. Susan Lee, comes to your office complaining of bruises on her arms and legs. She seems to be anxious and is not giving you a proper history. You suspect a case of domestic abuse. How will you proceed?

Label the emotion

> "Ms. Lee, please be assured that whatever we discuss here is going to be strictly confidential and shall not be revealed to anyone else. I think that you might be victim of domestic abuse. I am here to help you and I understand that you are in a difficult situation right now. Please cooperate with me so that we can get to the bottom of this and then involved protection agencies for your care."

Understand the background

Commend the patient

Keep it simple & support the patient

Encourage the patient to elaborate Why-how-what approach

Practice Question 31

A 50 year old lady comes to your office for a breast cancer screening. She denies any symptoms but reports that her mother had died of breast cancer at the age of 65 years. She wants to get a mammogram to check for breast cancer. She asks you "Will it be covered by my insurance doctor?" How do you answer her question?

Label the emotion

Understand the background

Commend the patient

Keep it simple & support the patient

Encourage the patient to elaborate Why-how-what approach

Practice Question 32

An elderly gentleman is visiting you today. He complains of chronic fatigue and feeling low. He is not giving you a coherent history and upon repeated requests he breaks down and starts crying. He says "Doctor, my son doesn't love me. Our relations are pretty bad. I don't even know what is happening to my pension as he is the one who goes to the bank. I am really worried (sobbing)". How do you counsel this gentleman?

Label the emotion

- Offer him some tissues and a cup of water.
- "I understand that you are not at good terms with your son."

Understand the background

- "I suspect you may be a victim of elder abuse."

Commend the patient

- "I commend you for being so upfront with me."

Keep it simple & support the patient

- "Your safety is my most important concern right now. I can send in my social worker to discuss various shelter home options with you. She will also be able to help you with the aspects related to your pension."

Encourage the patient to elaborate Why-how-what approach

- "Please don't worry now. We are here to help you."

Practice Question 33

You have received a call from Mr. John Watson, father of three year old boy Robin Watson. He tells you that Robin has been having fever, runny nose and a productive cough for the past three days. Robin attends a day care center. You explain to him that it could be an infection and that the child should be brought to the hospital. John asks you "Do you think he got it from the day care center?" What do you tell him?

Label the emotion

Understand the background

Commend the patient

Keep it simple & support the patient

Encourage the patient to elaborate Why-how-what approach

Practice Question 34

Mr. John, a second year old college student sees you in your office. He complains of a cough and sore throat for the past four days. He also mentions that his girlfriend had the same condition a week ago. Now, he wants to play a soccer game with his college team tomorrow. What will you advice?

Label the emotion
- "John, I know that you are concerned about the game coming up."

Understand the background
- "But I think you might have a viral infection known as Infectious Mononucleosis which could have been transmitted from your girlfriend. This condition causes enlargement of an organ in your abdomen which puts it at risk for injury when you play contact sports."

Commend-Recommend-Commend
- "So I would advise you to wait for some test results to be back before engaging in any strenuous activity."

Keep it simple & support the patient
- Draw a line diagram for the patient about spleen and abdomen explaining the organs involved.

Start with "Y" - Encourage the patient to elaborate Why-how-what approach
- "The infection can be managed, so don't worry about it. I am here to help you."

Practice Question 35

A 78 year old male, Mr. Zachary Freeman comes to your office for follow up for his recently diagnosed prostate cancer. He reports that the previous doctor told him about numerous metastases in his spine. He is really concerned and asks you "How much time do you think I have doctor?" What should you tell this patient?

Label the emotion

> ➢ "Mr Freeman, I see that you are worried about your prostate cancer and the time you have."

Understand the background

> ➢ "I understand that your cancer has spread to the spine."

Commend the patient

> ➢ "I appreciate your concerns."

Keep it simple & support the patient

> ➢ Explain with line diagram about Batsons venous valveless plexus and spread of cancer.

Start with "Y" - Start Encourage the patient to elaborate Why-how-what approach

> ➢ "We have good treatment available for the spread of cancer, so you don't need to worry. We are here to help you."

Practice Question 36

Ms. Kelly, a 35 year old lady comes to your office complaining of coughing up blood since last night. She reports to have coughed up around 150 mL of blood already. She says "I think I am losing too much blood. Shouldn't you be giving me blood transfusion, doctor?" How do you respond?

Label the emotion

- ➢ "Ms. Kelly, I can see that you are worried about the blood loss and it can be scary to see blood in your sputum."
- ➢ ACT--> "Let me offer you some tissues."

Understand the background

- ➢ "You are absolutely right about blood transfusion after losing blood but we need to check your hemoglobin levels first."

Commend the patient

- ➢ "I appreciate you coming to our office with this concern."

Keep it simple & support the patient

- ➢ "Coughing up blood is an important symptom. Do not worry. We are here to help you."

Encourage the patient to elaborate Why-how-what approach

- ➢ "I would like to first get to the root cause of the problem by asking you some questions and performing a clinical examination."
- ➢ "Then we can plan our way forward."

Practice Question 37

Frank is your regular patient and he calls you up about his six year old daughter Susan. He tells you "Hey, I need a favor from you. We are all going for a vacation to Miami and Susan has this peculiar rash on her chest. Can you write a prescription for some lotion that would relive her of the rash?" How do you proceed with this call?

Label the emotion

Understand the background

Commend the patient

Keep it simple & support the patient

Encourage the patient to elaborate Why-how-what approach

Practice Question 38

Ms. Kelly, a 35 year old lady comes to your office complaining of coughing up blood since last night. She reports to have coughed up around 150 mL of blood already. She also gives a history of smoking around 1 pack a day for the last 10 years. Then she asks you "Doctor do you think this is cancer?" How do you counsel her?

Label the emotion

- "Ms. Kelly, I can understand your fears about lung cancer."

Understand the background

- "Smoking puts you at high risk for developing lung cancer among others."

Commend the patient

- "I appreciate your concern and knowledge about the problem. But there might be other causes also for this coughing up of blood. And I would like to conduct some investigations like a chest X-ray and blood tests to reach to a conclusion."

Keep it simple & support the patient

- "This is a very good question. Let me assure you that we are here to help you."

Encourage the patient to elaborate Why-how-what approach

- "I advise you to stop smoking immediately. I can help you with some of the options available to quit smoking. My social worker can give you a list of nearest rehabilitation centers if you would like that."

Practice Question 39

Ms. Kilson Nickolson, a 30 year old female comes to your office complaining of belly pain since this morning. She reports that the pain is 7/10 in severity, sharp, localized to the right side and not relieved with Tylenol. After taking her history, you request her for permission to examine. You begin by palpating her abdomen and as soon as you touch her belly she shouts out in pain saying "Stop it! You are hurting me doctor" How will you proceed now?

Label the emotion

Understand the background

Commend the patient

Keep it simple & support the patient

Encourage the patient to elaborate Why-how-what approach

Practice Question 40

A 40 year old construction worker Mr. Jason Cameron, comes to your office complaining of a 6/10 right knee pain since the past two days. He is concerned about his job. He asks "Doc, will I be able to still work at the construction site? I don't want to lose my job" How do you counsel him?

Label the emotion

- "Mr. Cameron I can understand that you worried about your work."

Understand the background

- "It is important that we first get to the root cause of this problem."

Commend the patient

- "I am happy that you expressed your concerns to me."

Keep it simple & support the patient

- "Let me please ask you a few questions and examine your knee before coming to a differential. Then I will order some investigations like X Ray and blood tests."

Encourage the patient to elaborate Why-how-what approach

- "Once we have a diagnosis, we can proceed with the management. Meanwhile I would advise you to not strain your knee."

Practice Question 41

A 67 year old lady, Ms. Pomella Schawenburg comes to your office complaining of dizziness and an unexpected fall today morning. She was standing and ironing her clothes when the fall happened. She denies any trauma or HEENT bleed. After the history and physical examination when you ask her to stand up and walk across the room to check her gait, she replies "Doc, I can't do it. I will fall down. Please don't make me do this" How do you counsel her?

Label the emotion

Understand the background

Commend the patient

Keep it simple & support the patient

Encourage the patient to elaborate Why-how-what approach

NOTES -

Section F

Counseling

Section F - Counseling

Closure: General Framework - ADICA

Make the patient comfortable:

After performing the physical examination, help the patient to sit as you need to maintain good eye contact when you are explaining things. Counseling a patient and having a conversation with them while they are lying down will be awkward for patient and the caregiver. It is important to not only listen attentively to the patient but also have a good eye contact in a patient-centered communication. To do this, patient and physician should be at the same level. Push back the leg rest extension of the bed. Drape them again, and make them comfortable. While doing this, keep talking to the patient:

- ✓ "Thank you Mr. Doe for cooperating with that. I believe I have gathered sufficient information. Now, I request you to kindly sit up so we can discuss further. Let me help you tie your gown again. Let me make you comfortable," and push back the leg rest.
- ✓ "Does this feel more comfortable, Mr. Doe?"

If patient is hurting and cannot sit, then please don't force the patient to sit. Patient comes first and their pain foremost.

Ask the patient:

- ✓ "Do you have any questions for me?"
- ✓ "Is there something you want to ask?"

The Closure Itself:

Closure in itself is a very important aspect of the patient encounter, not only in the Step 2 CS Examination, but also in the real life. Acquiring the skills of delivering a good closure requires practice and patience. The following methodology will help one learn to deliver a concise, yet comprehensive closure.

- ✓ **First and foremost**, there are no ideal closures! Every case, diagnosis, and every patient, (personal traits), will demand a unique closure. There is no way to pre-determine how to deliver the closure, or how much time will be spent on counseling the patient.
- ✓ **Do not confuse the patient with too much medical jargon.** The patient may be curious to know the disease he is suffering from, but this is not the right time to show extensive medical knowledge, or list the differential diagnosis! Names of common, and easily understood diseases, may be used, but don't overwhelm the patient. The job is to make their lives easier and simpler; lead them to the disease by using simpler phrases:
- ✓ Bacterial throat infection, (instead of Streptococcal Pharyngitis).
- ✓ If the patient has cholecystitis—
    - o Draw a simple line diagram of the liver and gallbladder while maintaining good eye contact.
    - o Explain to the patient, pointing towards the picture, "This is the liver and below it is the gallbladder. It stores bile juice for fat digestion. Swelling and infection of this organ is probably causing your symptoms."

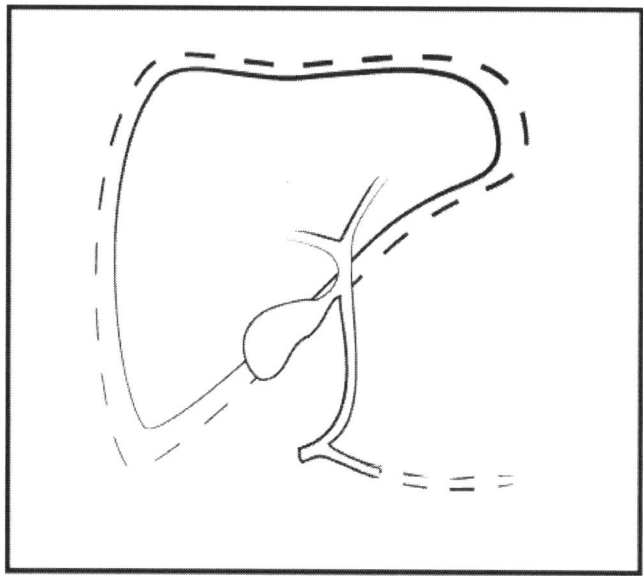

Fig.Chapter Closure

Do not assume that the patient will not understand medical terms. However, some patients may have already researched their symptoms and diseases, or visited other doctors. It should not come as a surprise if they ask, "Doc, am I suffering from chronic fatigue syndrome?" or "Doc, I read that Guillain Barre Syndrome can lead to weakness in the legs. Do you think I have Guillain Barre Syndrome?"

Use medical terms judiciously but without judging the patients!

Do not give false hope to the patient during the closure.

Now that the tricky aspects are evident, there can be a sigh of relief!
To make life easier as a student, (and Step two CS examiner), and also as a physician, here is a list of the basic elements that must be addressed in every closure. It is not difficult to deliver a great closure if one follows the basic skeleton, and addresses all the core components.

Skeletal Framework of the Closure:

Address the patient:

- ✓ Address the patient appropriately and use the correct salutation.

Disease:

- ✓ Talk a little about what **diseases** they MAY have.

Examine:

- ✓ Discuss with the patient, the **why, how and what** of all the **physical examinations** you are going to perform. Write in the patient note about the examination (breast exam, pelvic exam, rectal exam and corneal reflex) which you cannot perform in Step 2 CS exam.

Investigate:

- ✓ Discuss with the patient, the **why, how and what** of all the **investigations** (blood/radiological /special), you are going to perform to confirm the diagnosis.

Counsel:

- ✓ **Counsel** on various aspects of Dr.(Saw)³MD. See the chapters on counselling for the details. If there is no time, at least counsel on the lifestyle modifications which are essential for this patient, e.g. smoking cessation for a regular tobacco smoker.

Dr	✓ Doctor Follow-up
S	✓ Symptoms, Smoking, Salt restriction
A	✓ Activity, Alcohol
W	✓ Weight, Wine, Water restriction
M	✓ Medications and Side effects
D	✓ Diet and driving

Counsel More:

If there is time, talk about the extended Dr.(Saw)³MD.

T	✓ Tests to be done ✓ Transport for discharge and follow-up appointments ✓ Therapy
H	✓ Home Nursing ✓ Health insurance issues
R	✓ Resources for family ✓ Return to work ✓ Results pending
E	✓ Equipment: Walker, cane, glucometer, Oxygen etc.
E	✓ Expert in wound care, insulin injections, ostomy care

Draw:

Use the back side of the blue rough sheet for counselling. Draw, elaborate and write in bold letters to emphasize the point. (E.g. 'No alcohol' or 'Wine restriction' for a patient with suspected chronic liver disease or alcoholic liver disease.) Be gentle and polite, but firm.

Help:

Offer help and support to the patient with following suggestions:

- ✓ "We can get you enrolled in our hospital's obesity control program if you are interested."
- ✓ "I can ask our social worker to help you procure this equipment/medication that your insurance does not cover."
- ✓ "I strongly recommend that you quit smoking. There are various ways in which we can help you with that if you are interested."

Address the challenging question again:

Before finishing the closure, make sure to touch upon the challenging question again, if time permits. Give an elaborate explanation so as to score high on the Step 2 CS exam, as well as improve the patient experience when practicing medicine in the future.

Remember: **ADICA**: **A**ddress-**D**isease-**I**nvestigate-**C**ounsel-**A**ddress

After the closure:

Always finish the closure by asking the patient whether they have any questions.

- ✓ "Do you have any questions for me?"
- ✓ "Is there anything that you would like to discuss again?"

Thank the patient politely and leave the room after collecting all your belongings, (Blue sheets and clipboard, pen, stethoscope). Make sure to drape the patient, and make them comfortable before leaving.

Sample Closures:

Some sample closures are mentioned here. Also, sample closures are provided in each practice case. For e.g. If you are suspecting **Infectious Mononucleosis**-

- ✓ "Mr. Doe, after discussing your concerns and doing the physical examination, I believe that you are suffering from a viral infection which you may have acquired from your close contact. I believe it is a transient infection, however we will have to run some tests to ensure that we do not miss any serious disease. These tests include routine blood cell counts, seeing the cells under a microscope and the rapid test for the viral infection that I suspect. I would also like to take a throat swab and run tests on that.

- ✓ We will plan your follow up for this in near future. Meanwhile, I recommend that you do not take part in any activities involving contact sports, as there is a possible risk of trauma leading to rupture of the spleen in this condition.

- ✓ I would also like to make some routine recommendations which will help you achieve a healthy lifestyle. Tobacco smoking can lead to a number of diseases, I advise you to therefore quit smoking. We have a 'Quit-Tobacco' program in our hospital in which I can get you enrolled to help you quit, if you are interested.

- ✓ Also, I advise you to use condoms during sexual intercourse to protect yourself against STDs.

- ✓ Now, let us talk again about your concern about an HIV infection leading to your symptoms. Mr. Doe, it is too early for me to confirm or rule out an HIV infection. For that, I will have to run some blood tests which can not only test for any preexisting infection but also screen newly acquired infection. We will discuss the further steps to be taken after the results of these tests are back.
- ✓ Do you have any other questions for me, Mr. Doe?"

Now, let's discuss the components of this closure, according to the principles mentioned before:

Address the patient:

- ✓ "Mr. Doe, after discussing your concerns and doing the physical examination

Disease:

- ✓ I believe that you are suffering from a viral infection which you may have acquired from your close contact. I believe it is a transient infection

Investigate (and examine):

- ✓ However we will have to run some tests to ensure that we do not miss out any serious infection. These tests include routine blood cell counts, seeing the cells under a microscope and the rapid test for the viral infection that I suspect. I would also like to take a throat swab and run tests on that.

Counsel: Dr.(Saw)³MD: Follow up

- ✓ We will plan your follow up for this in near future.

Counsel: Dr.(Saw)³MD: Activities

- ✓ Meanwhile, I recommend that you do not take part in any activities involving contact sports as there is a possible risk of trauma leading to rupture of the spleen in this condition.

Counsel: Dr.(Saw)³MD: Smoking

- ✓ I would also like to make some routine recommendations which will help you achieve a healthy lifestyle. Tobacco smoking can lead to a number of diseases, I advise you to quit smoking.

Offer Help
- ✓ We have a 'Quit-Tobacco' program in our hospital in which I can get you enrolled to help you quit if you are interested.

Counsel More
- ✓ Also, I advise you to use condoms during sexual intercourse to protect yourself against STDs.

Address the challenging question again: (Do not give false hope to the patient)

- ✓ Now, let us talk again about your concern about an HIV infection leading to your symptoms. Mr. Doe, it is too early for me to confirm or rule out an HIV infection. For that, I will have to run some blood tests which can not only test for any pre-existing infection but also screen newly acquired infection. We will discuss the further steps to be taken after the results of these tests are back.

After the closure:

- ✓ Do you have any other questions for me, Mr. Doe?"

In our Vital Checklist Workshop, we use the following checklist to grade medical students when they are preparing for the exam. We are big proponents of immersion coaching and strongly believe in **"Perfect Practice Makes Perfect."**

Address the patient	✓
Diagnosis with diagram	✓
Investigations	✓
Counselling and Closure	✓
After the closure question	✓

VITAL CHECKLISTS

iCrush and Cope with Cancer

VCL	Areas	Ready Set iCrush	WIP	Ci	Pi
i	Infection.[1]	Do you have fever, chills, cough or redness in the area of medi-port?			
C	Chemo induced mental fogging.[2, 3]	Did you have any episodes of confusion?			
R	Renal or kidney failure (Labs).[4-6]	Do you have any kidney problems? Did you pass less amount of urine than usual?			
U	Urinary and bowel problems.[7-9]	Do you have leaky bladder or bowel?			
S	Skin.[10-12]	Do you notice any changes with your skin?			
H	Heart problems.[13, 14]	Do you have chest pain or shortness of breath?			
A	Appetite.[15]	Is there any change in your appetite?			
N	Nausea.[16]	Do you have any nausea or vomiting?			
D	Diarrhea.[17, 18]	Do you have diarrhea?			
C	Constipation.[19, 20]	Do you have constipation? When was your last bowel movement?			
O	Osteoporosis.[21, 22]	When did you get your DEXA scan and Vitamin D3 levels checked?			
P	Pain.[23]	Do you have pain? If yes, where is your pain? On a scale of 1 to 10, how bad is your pain?			
E	Erectile dysfunction.[24]	Do you have erectile dysfunction?			
W	Weight.[25]	Any changes in your weight?			
I	Insomnia.[26, 27]	Any changes in your sleep?			
T	Thyroid check-up.[28]	Do you have any heat or cold intolerance? Do you have any thyroid problems? Do you take synthyroid?			

H	Hair loss.[29, 30]	Have you noticed any hair loss?
C	Cognitive dysfunction.[31]	Do you have any difficulty remembering things?
A	Anxiety & depression.[32]	Do you feel depressed? Do you have anxiety? Since how long do you have these symptoms?
N	Neutropenia.[1]	What are the results of your blood tests? Do you have decreased white cell count?
C	Chemotherapy.[33]	What are the side effects of the chemotherapy?
E	Evaluate for response.[34]	Is the tumor responding to the chemotherapy?
R	Radiology-CT scans, X-rays, MRI.[35]	Did you get an X-Ray/ MRI/ CT scan done? What are the results of these tests?

Table: iCrush and Cope with Cancer
VCL- Vital Checklist; WIP-Work in Progress; Ci-Caregiver Initials; Pi-Patient Initials. This iCrush and Cope with Cancer Vital Checklist is designed using Kanban (Lean from Toyota Production System) and Theory of Constraints by Eliyahu Goldratt.
For commercial use, please contact us at hi@vitalchecklist.com; For non-commercial use, please contact Dr.Harpreet Singh MD, FACP via email drsingh@vitalchecklist.com; 2016 Copyrights and Trademarks reserved Harpreet Singh MD, FACP, Vital Checklist and (iCrush). If you are doing a research project using this checklist, please contact Dr. Harpreet Singh for permission. Email him at drsingh@icrush.org

1. Freifeld, A.G., et al., *Clinical practice guideline for the use of antimicrobial agents in neutropenic patients with cancer: 2010 update by the infectious diseases society of america.* Clin Infect Dis, 2011. **52**(4): p. e56-93.
2. Ito, Y., et al., *Cisplatin neurotoxicity presenting as reversible posterior leukoencephalopathy syndrome.* AJNR Am J Neuroradiol, 1998. **19**(3): p. 415-7.
3. Lyass, O., et al., *Cisplatin-induced non-convulsive encephalopathy.* Anticancer Drugs, 1998. **9**(1): p. 100-4.
4. Hayes, D.M., et al., *High dose cis-platinum diammine dichloride: amelioration of renal toxicity by mannitol diuresis.* Cancer, 1977. **39**(4): p. 1372-81.
5. Gonzales-Vitale, J.C., et al., *The renal pathology in clinical trials of cis-platinum (II) diamminedichloride.* Cancer, 1977. **39**(4): p. 1362-71.
6. Wittes, R.E., et al., *Combination chemothereapy with cis-diamminedichloroplatinum (II) and bleomycin in tumors of the head and neck.* Oncology, 1975. **32**(5-6): p. 202-7.
7. Teh, H.S., S.A. Fadilah, and C.F. Leong, *Transverse myelopathy following intrathecal administration of chemotherapy.* Singapore Med J, 2007. **48**(2): p. e46-9.
8. Cachia, D., et al., *Myelopathy following intrathecal chemotherapy in adults: a single institution experience.* J Neurooncol, 2015. **122**(2): p. 391-8.
9. Gagliano, R.G. and J.J. Costanzi, *Paraplegia following intrathecal methotrexate: report of a case and review of the literature.* Cancer, 1976. **37**(4): p. 1663-8.
10. Asnis, L.A. and A.A. Gaspari, *Cutaneous reactions to recombinant cytokine therapy.* J Am Acad Dermatol, 1995. **33**(3): p. 393-410; quiz 410-2.

11. Remlinger, K.A., *Cutaneous reactions to chemotherapy drugs: the art of consultation.* Arch Dermatol, 2003. **139**(1): p. 77-81.
12. Payne, A.S., W.D. James, and R.B. Weiss, *Dermatologic toxicity of chemotherapeutic agents.* Semin Oncol, 2006. **33**(1): p. 86-97.
13. Floyd, J.D., et al., *Cardiotoxicity of cancer therapy.* J Clin Oncol, 2005. **23**(30): p. 7685-96.
14. Monsuez, J.J., et al., *Cardiac side-effects of cancer chemotherapy.* Int J Cardiol, 2010. **144**(1): p. 3-15.
15. Davis, M.P. and D. Dickerson, *Cachexia and anorexia: cancer's covert killer.* Support Care Cancer, 2000. **8**(3): p. 180-7.
16. Hesketh, P.J., *Chemotherapy-induced nausea and vomiting.* N Engl J Med, 2008. **358**(23): p. 2482-94.
17. Saliba, F., et al., *Pathophysiology and therapy of irinotecan-induced delayed-onset diarrhea in patients with advanced colorectal cancer: a prospective assessment.* J Clin Oncol, 1998. **16**(8): p. 2745-51.
18. Hecht, J.R., *Gastrointestinal toxicity or irinotecan.* Oncology (Williston Park), 1998. **12**(8 Suppl 6): p. 72-8.
19. Anderson, H., et al., *VAD chemotherapy--toxicity and efficacy--in patients with multiple myeloma and other lymphoid malignancies.* Hematol Oncol, 1987. **5**(3): p. 213-22.
20. Holland, J.F., et al., *Vincristine treatment of advanced cancer: a cooperative study of 392 cases.* Cancer Res, 1973. **33**(6): p. 1258-64.
21. Pfeilschifter, J. and I.J. Diel, *Osteoporosis due to cancer treatment: pathogenesis and management.* J Clin Oncol, 2000. **18**(7): p. 1570-93.
22. Schwartz, A.M. and J.C. Leonidas, *Methotrexate osteopathy.* Skeletal Radiol, 1984. **11**(1): p. 13-6.
23. Portenoy, R.K., *Treatment of cancer pain.* Lancet, 2011. **377**(9784): p. 2236-47.
24. Nelson, C.J., et al., *Sexual bother following radical prostatectomyjsm.* J Sex Med, 2010. **7**(1 Pt 1): p. 129-35.
25. Martin, L., et al., *Diagnostic criteria for the classification of cancer-associated weight loss.* J Clin Oncol, 2015. **33**(1): p. 90-9.
26. Taylor, D.J., et al., *Comorbidity of chronic insomnia with medical problems.* Sleep, 2007. **30**(2): p. 213-8.
27. Howell, D., et al., *Sleep disturbance in adults with cancer: a systematic review of evidence for best practices in assessment and management for clinical practice.* Ann Oncol, 2014. **25**(4): p. 791-800.
28. Brabant, G., et al., *Hypothyroidism following childhood cancer therapy-an under diagnosed complication.* Int J Cancer, 2012. **130**(5): p. 1145-50.
29. Wu, C.Y., G.S. Chen, and C.C. Lan, *Erosive pustular dermatosis of the scalp after gefitinib and radiotherapy for brain metastases secondary to lung cancer.* Clin Exp Dermatol, 2008. **33**(1): p. 106-7.
30. Donovan, J.C., D.M. Ghazarian, and J.C. Shaw, *Scarring alopecia associated with use of the epidermal growth factor receptor inhibitor gefitinib.* Arch Dermatol, 2008. **144**(11): p. 1524-5.
31. Rubnitz, J.E., et al., *Transient encephalopathy following high-dose methotrexate treatment in childhood acute lymphoblastic leukemia.* Leukemia, 1998. **12**(8): p. 1176-81.
32. Holland, J.C., *Anxiety and cancer: the patient and the family.* J Clin Psychiatry, 1989. **50 Suppl**: p. 20-5.
33. Epstein, J.B., et al., *Oral complications of cancer and cancer therapy: from cancer treatment to survivorship.* CA Cancer J Clin, 2012. **62**(6): p. 400-22.
34. Gennari, A., et al., *Duration of chemotherapy for metastatic breast cancer: a systematic review and meta-analysis of randomized clinical trials.* J Clin Oncol, 2011. **29**(16): p. 2144-9.
35. Silvestri, G.A., et al., *Methods for staging non-small cell lung cancer: Diagnosis and management of lung cancer, 3rd ed: American College of Chest Physicians evidence-based clinical practice guidelines.* Chest, 2013. **143**(5 Suppl): p. e211S-50S.

Cytochrome P450 Inhibitors
PQRS In EKG or ECG are inhibitors

VCL	Areas	Ready Set iCrush	WIP	Ci	Pi
P	Paroxetine.[1]	Are you taking Paroxetine?			
Q	Quinolones, Quinidine.[2]	Are you taking Quinolones like Ciprofloxacin? Do you take Quinidine?			
R	Ritonavir.[3]	Do you take Ritonavir?			
S	Sertraline.[4]	Do you take Sertraline?			
In	Indinavir.[5]	Do you take Indinavir?			
E	Ethanol (acute intake).[6]	Did you take alcohol recently? How much alcohol did you drink?			
K	Ketoconazole or Itraconazole.[7]	Are you taking any anti-fungal drugs like Ketoconazole or Itraconazole?			
G	Grape Fruit Juice.[8]	Do you take grape juice?			
Or	Omeprazole.	Do you take anti-acid drugs like Omeprazole?			
E	Erythromycin.[9]	Do you take Erythromycin?			
C	Cimetidine, Cymbalta.[10]	Do you take Cimetidine? Do you take Cymbalta (Duloxetine)?			
G	Gemfibrozil.[11]	Do you take Gemfibrozil?			

The P.Q.R.S In EKG or ECG will inhibit P450 and thus warfarin will not be metabolized leading to an increase in INR.

Table: Cytochrome P450 Inhibitors
VCL- Vital Checklist; WIP-Work in Progress; Ci-Caregiver Initials; Pi-Patient Initials. This Cytochrome P450 Inhibitors Vital Checklist is designed using Kanban (Lean from Toyota Production System) and Theory of Constraints by Eliyahu Goldratt.
For commercial use, please contact us at hi@vitalchecklist.com; For non-commercial use, please contact Dr.Harpreet Singh MD, FACP via email drsingh@vitalchecklist.com; 2016 Copyrights and Trademarks reserved Harpreet Singh MD, FACP, Vital Checklist and (iCrush). If you are doing a research project using this checklist, please contact Dr. Harpreet Singh for permission. Email him at drsingh@icrush.org

1. Gu, L., et al., *Biotransformation of caffeine, paraxanthine, theobromine and theophylline by cDNA-expressed human CYP1A2 and CYP2E1*. Pharmacogenetics, 1992. **2**(2): p. 73-7.
2. Peterson, J.A. and S.E. Graham, *A close family resemblance: the importance of structure in understanding cytochromes P450*. Structure, 1998. **6**(9): p. 1079-85.
3. Smith, G., et al., *Molecular genetics of the human cytochrome P450 monooxygenase superfamily*. Xenobiotica, 1998. **28**(12): p. 1129-65.
4. Werck-Reichhart, D. and R. Feyereisen, *Cytochromes P450: a success story*. Genome Biol, 2000. **1**(6): p. Reviews3003.
5. Danielson, P.B., *The cytochrome P450 superfamily: biochemistry, evolution and drug metabolism in humans*. Curr Drug Metab, 2002. **3**(6): p. 561-97.
6. Watkins, P.B., *Drug metabolism by cytochromes P450 in the liver and small bowel*. Gastroenterol Clin North Am, 1992. **21**(3): p. 511-26.
7. Wrighton, S.A., M. VandenBranden, and B.J. Ring, *The human drug metabolizing cytochromes P450*. J Pharmacokinet Biopharm, 1996. **24**(5): p. 461-73.
8. Wilkinson, G.R., *Cytochrome P4503A (CYP3A) metabolism: prediction of in vivo activity in humans*. J Pharmacokinet Biopharm, 1996. **24**(5): p. 475-90.
9. Ketter, T.A., et al., *The emerging role of cytochrome P450 3A in psychopharmacology*. J Clin Psychopharmacol, 1995. **15**(6): p. 387-98.
10. Murray, M., *Mechanisms and significance of inhibitory drug interactions involving cytochrome P450 enzymes (review)*. Int J Mol Med, 1999. **3**(3): p. 227-38.
11. Nelson, D.R., et al., *The P450 superfamily: update on new sequences, gene mapping, accession numbers, early trivial names of enzymes, and nomenclature*. DNA Cell Biol, 1993. **12**(1): p. 1-51.

Cytochrome p450 Inducers/ Stimulators - PERCCS

VCL	Areas	Ready Set iCrush	WIP	Ci	Pi
P	Phenytoin.[1]	Do you take Phenytoin?			
E	Ethanol (chronic intake).[2]	Do you drink alcohol? How much do you take and since how long you have been drinking?			
R	Rifampin.[3]	Do you take Rifampin?			
C	Carbamazepine (Tegretol).	Do you take Carbamazepine (Tegretol)?			
C	(Carba and Barba) Barbiturates (Phenobarbital).	Do you take Phenobarbital or any other barbiturates?			
S	Steroids (Dexamethasone).	Do you take Dexamethasone or any other steroids?			

If you are getting PERK(c)s; You will stimulate the enzyme and warfarin will be metabolized sooner leading to a fall in INR.

Table: Cytochrome P450 Inducers/ Stimulators
VCL- Vital Checklist; WIP-Work in Progress; Ci-Caregiver Initials; Pi-Patient Initials. This Cytochrome P450 Inducers/ Stimulators Vital Checklist is designed using Kanban (Lean from Toyota Production System) and Theory of Constraints by Eliyahu Goldratt.
For commercial use, please contact us at hi@vitalchecklist.com; For non-commercial use, please contact Dr.Harpreet Singh MD, FACP via email drsingh@vitalchecklist.com; 2016 Copyrights and Trademarks reserved Harpreet Singh MD, FACP, Vital Checklist and (iCrush). If you are doing a research project using this checklist, please contact Dr. Harpreet Singh for permission. Email him at drsingh@icrush.org

1. Flockhart, D.A. and J.R. Oesterheld, *Cytochrome P450-mediated drug interactions.* Child Adolesc Psychiatr Clin N Am, 2000. **9**(1): p. 43-76.
2. Kalgutkar, A.S., R.S. Obach, and T.S. Maurer, *Mechanism-based inactivation of cytochrome P450 enzymes: chemical mechanisms, structure-activity relationships and relationship to clinical drug-drug interactions and idiosyncratic adverse drug reactions.* Curr Drug Metab, 2007. **8**(5): p. 407-47.
3. Stepan, A.F., et al., *Structural alert/reactive metabolite concept as applied in medicinal chemistry to mitigate the risk of idiosyncratic drug toxicity: a perspective based on the critical examination of trends in the top 200 drugs marketed in the United States.* Chem Res Toxicol, 2011. **24**(9): p. 1345-410.

Dementia symptoms - iCrush Senior Moments

VCL	Areas	Ready Set iCrush	WIP	Ci	Pi
i	Impaired recent short term memory.[1]	What did you had for breakfast this morning? Confirm the answer with family member or support at home.			
C	Challenges with event planning or problem solving/ managing finances/ driving around. Challenge with Check book. Challenge with controlling bowel and bladder functions.[2]	Who manages your bills? Do you have difficulty in remembering things? Do you often get lost when you are driving by yourself? Any changes in bladder and bowel habits? Have you lost control over your bowel and bladder?			
Rush	Rush and rash judgment and poor decisions.[3]	Has your family members noticed you make a rash decision?			
S	Speech problems.[4]	Do you have problems in communicating?			
E	Eyes- Visual hallucinations (Delirium or Lewy Body Dementia).[5]	Do you see things that others deny seeing?			
N	Nose-smell altered.[6]	Do you smell weird odors that others deny smelling?			
I	Impaired behavior & personality changes.[1]	Does your family members or support at home tell you about a change in your behavior or change in your personality?			

Or	Orientation to time, place, and person.[7]	What is your name? Where are you right now (which country/ state/ city/ building)? Which year/ month/ day is it today?
Mo	Motor incoordination.[8]	Did you notice any changes in your balance or increase in number of falls?
Me	Memory loss.[9]	Can you tell me your date of birth? When is your wedding anniversary? Confirm the answer with a family member or support at home.
N	Neglect activities of daily living.	Do you have difficulties in moving around your house/ taking shower/ getting dressed/ cooking for yourself/ feeding yourself?
T	Thoughts of depression.[10]	Do you feel depressed?
S	Stroke.[10]	Do you have a past h/o stroke or weakness or numbness in any parts of your body?

Table: Dementia Symptoms
VCL- Vital Checklist; WIP-Work in Progress; Ci-Caregiver Initials; Pi-Patient Initials. This Dementia Symptoms Vital Checklist is designed using Kanban (Lean from Toyota Production System) and Theory of Constraints by Eliyahu Goldratt.
For commercial use, please contact us at hi@vitalchecklist.com; For non-commercial use, please contact Dr.Harpreet Singh MD, FACP via email drsingh@vitalchecklist.com; 2016 Copyrights and Trademarks reserved Harpreet Singh MD, FACP, Vital Checklist and (iCrush). If you are doing a research project using this checklist, please contact Dr. Harpreet Singh for permission. Email him at drsingh@icrush.org

1. Pfeiffer, E., *A short portable mental status questionnaire for the assessment of organic brain deficit in elderly patients.* J Am Geriatr Soc, 1975. **23**(10): p. 433-41.
2. Tangalos, E.G., et al., *The Mini-Mental State Examination in general medical practice: clinical utility and acceptance.* Mayo Clin Proc, 1996. **71**(9): p. 829-37.
3. Grisso, T. and P.S. Appelbaum, *Comparison of standards for assessing patients' capacities to make treatment decisions.* Am J Psychiatry, 1995. **152**(7): p. 1033-7.
4. Anthony, J.C., et al., *Limits of the 'Mini-Mental State' as a screening test for dementia and delirium among hospital patients.* Psychol Med, 1982. **12**(2): p. 397-408.
5. Crum, R.M., et al., *Population-based norms for the Mini-Mental State Examination by age and educational level.* Jama, 1993. **269**(18): p. 2386-91.
6. Freidl, W., et al., *Mini mental state examination: influence of sociodemographic, environmental and behavioral factors and vascular risk factors.* J Clin Epidemiol, 1996. **49**(1): p. 73-8.

7. Folstein, M.F., S.E. Folstein, and P.R. McHugh, *"Mini-mental state". A practical method for grading the cognitive state of patients for the clinician.* J Psychiatr Res, 1975. **12**(3): p. 189-98.

8. Royall, D.R., J.A. Cordes, and M. Polk, *CLOX: an executive clock drawing task.* J Neurol Neurosurg Psychiatry, 1998. **64**(5): p. 588-94.

9. Borson, S., et al., *The mini-cog: a cognitive 'vital signs' measure for dementia screening in multi-lingual elderly.* Int J Geriatr Psychiatry, 2000. **15**(11): p. 1021-7.

10. Jorm, A.F., L. Fratiglioni, and B. Winblad, *Differential diagnosis in dementia. Principal components analysis of clinical data from a population survey.* Arch Neurol, 1993. **50**(1): p. 72-7.

Depression – DIGEST P CAPsule

VCL	Areas	Ready Set iCrush	WIP	Ci	Pi
D	Depression.[1]	Do you feel sad or depressed?			
I	Insomnia or hypersomnia.[2]	Did you notice any changes in your sleep?			
G	Guilt.[3]	Do you feel guilty about something in life?			
E	Energy loss.[4]	Do you feel loss of energy at all times?			
S	Suicidal ideation.[5]	Do you have any thoughts about hurting yourself? Did you ever plan about hurting yourself?			
T	Time more than 2 weeks (symptoms of depression for at least 2 weeks).[6]	Since how long do you feel depressed or sad?			
P	Pleasure loss.[7]	Do you think you have lost interest in all the activities that you used to love earlier?			
C	Concentration lapses[8]	Do you have difficulty in concentrating in your work?			
A	Appetite change or weight loss/gain[9]	Any changes in your appetite? Did you notice any changes in your weight?			
P	Psychotic symptoms, Somatic symptoms.[10]	Did you see or hear things that others denied? Did you feel that your limbs were heavy?			

Table: Depression
VCL- Vital Checklist; WIP-Work in Progress; Ci-Caregiver Initials; Pi-Patient Initials. This Depression Vital Checklist is designed using Kanban (Lean from Toyota Production System) and Theory of Constraints by Eliyahu Goldratt.
For commercial use, please contact us at hi@vitalchecklist.com; For non-commercial use, please contact Dr.Harpreet Singh MD, FACP via email drsingh@vitalchecklist.com; 2016 Copyrights and Trademarks reserved Harpreet Singh MD, FACP, Vital Checklist and (iCrush). If you are doing a research project using this checklist, please contact Dr. Harpreet Singh for permission. Email him at drsingh@icrush.org

1. Ansseau, M., et al., *High prevalence of mental disorders in primary care.* J Affect Disord, 2004. 78(1): p. 49-55.
2. McCullough, J.P., Jr., et al., *Comparison of DSM-III-R chronic major depression and major depression superimposed on dysthymia (double depression): validity of the distinction.* J Abnorm Psychol, 2000. 109(3): p. 419-27.
3. Yang, T. and D.L. Dunner, *Differential subtyping of depression.* Depress Anxiety, 2001. 13(1): p. 11-7.
4. Zimmerman, M., et al., *Diagnosing major depressive disorder X: can the utility of the DSM-IV symptom criteria be improved?* J Nerv Ment Dis, 2006. 194(12): p. 893-7.
5. Tidemalm, D., et al., *Risk of suicide after suicide attempt according to coexisting psychiatric disorder: Swedish cohort study with long term follow-up.* Bmj, 2008. 337: p. a2205.
6. Zimmerman, M., et al., *A simpler definition of major depressive disorder.* Psychol Med, 2010. 40(3): p. 451-7.
7. Andrews, G., et al., *Issues for DSM-V: simplifying DSM-IV to enhance utility: the case of major depressive disorder.* Am J Psychiatry, 2007. 164(12): p. 1784-5.
8. Zimmerman, M., et al., *Validity of a simpler definition of major depressive disorder.* Depress Anxiety, 2010. 27(10): p. 977-81.
9. Regier, D.A., et al., *DSM-5 field trials in the United States and Canada, Part II: test-retest reliability of selected categorical diagnoses.* Am J Psychiatry, 2013. 170(1): p. 59-70.
10. Tylee, A. and P. Gandhi, *The importance of somatic symptoms in depression in primary care.* Prim Care Companion J Clin Psychiatry, 2005. 7(4): p. 167-76.

Hypothyroidism - LESS THYROID

VCL	Areas	Ready Set iCrush	WIP	Ci	Pi
L	Lower lung function- decreased respiratory capacity. Lower heart function- decreased cardiac output and contractility. Libido is decreased in men.[1-5]	Do you have any cough/ chest pain/ shortness of breath? Do you have any light-headedness/ black-outs/ swelling of feet? Is there a decrease in libido?			
E	Energy loss. Eye Swelling.[6]	Do you feel loss of energy at all times? Did you notice a swelling around your eyes?			
S	Skin is dry and thin. Sweating is decreased.[7]	Did you notice any dryness of your skin?			

S	Sensory loss. Carpal tunnel syndrome + Other neurological findings.[8]	Do you have any tingling/ numbness/ weakness in any parts of your body?
T	Temperature- cold intolerance. Tired and fatigued.	Have you ever noticed that you feel cold when others in the room are comfortable? Do you feel tired and fatigued at all times?
H	Hypertension.[9, 10]	Were you diagnosed to have high blood pressure at the same time when these symptoms (tired & fatigue) started?
Y	"Y" are you Dull (Memory loss), Down (Menorrhagia), Depressed (Depression).[11]	Have you become forgetful recently? Do you have increased bleeding during your menstrual cycles? Do you feel sad or depressed?
R	Reproductive issues.[12]	Are you having problems with conceiving? Do have irregular menstrual cycles with heavy bleeding?
O	Obesity.[13]	Did you notice any unintentional weight gain, without any changes in your diet?
I	Insomnia (sleep apnea, as patients may have enlarged gland, tongue) Or Increased sleepiness.[14]	Did you notice any changes in your sleep? Do you snore while sleeping?
D	Digestive system- Constipation.[15, 16]	Do you have constipation?

Table: Hypothyroidism
VCL- Vital Checklist; WIP-Work in Progress; Ci-Caregiver Initials; Pi-Patient Initials. This Hypothyroidism Vital Checklist is designed using Kanban (Lean from Toyota Production System) and Theory of Constraints by Eliyahu Goldratt.
For commercial use, please contact us at hi@vitalchecklist.com; For non-commercial use, please contact Dr.Harpreet Singh MD, FACP via email drsingh@vitalchecklist.com; 2016 Copyrights and Trademarks reserved Harpreet Singh MD, FACP, Vital Checklist and (iCrush). If you are doing a research project using this checklist, please contact Dr. Harpreet Singh for permission. Email him at drsingh@icrush.org

1. Laroche, C.M., et al., *Hypothyroidism presenting with respiratory muscle weakness.* Am Rev Respir Dis, 1988. **138**(2): p. 472-4.
2. Zhou, K.R., *[X-ray diagnosis of the downward displacement of the tricuspid valve (author's transl)].* Zhonghua Fang She Xue Za Zhi, 1979. **13**(2): p. 69-71.
3. Siafakas, N.M., et al., *Respiratory muscle strength in hypothyroidism.* Chest, 1992. **102**(1): p. 189-94.
4. Ladenson, P.W., P.D. Goldenheim, and E.C. Ridgway, *Prediction and reversal of blunted ventilatory responsiveness in patients with hypothyroidism.* Am J Med, 1988. **84**(5): p. 877-83.
5. Klein, I. and K. Ojamaa, *Thyroid hormone and the cardiovascular system: from theory to practice.* J Clin Endocrinol Metab, 1994. **78**(5): p. 1026-7.
6. Smith, T.J., R.S. Bahn, and C.A. Gorman, *Connective tissue, glycosaminoglycans, and diseases of the thyroid.* Endocr Rev, 1989. **10**(3): p. 366-91.
7. Heymann, W.R., *Cutaneous manifestations of thyroid disease.* J Am Acad Dermatol, 1992. **26**(6): p. 885-902.
8. Duyff, R.F., et al., *Neuromuscular findings in thyroid dysfunction: a prospective clinical and electrodiagnostic study.* J Neurol Neurosurg Psychiatry, 2000. **68**(6): p. 750-5.
9. Klein, I. and S. Danzi, *Thyroid disease and the heart.* Circulation, 2007. **116**(15): p. 1725-35.
10. Fommei, E. and G. Iervasi, *The role of thyroid hormone in blood pressure homeostasis: evidence from short-term hypothyroidism in humans.* J Clin Endocrinol Metab, 2002. **87**(5): p. 1996-2000.
11. Osterweil, D., et al., *Cognitive function in non-demented older adults with hypothyroidism.* J Am Geriatr Soc, 1992. **40**(4): p. 325-35.
12. Krassas, G.E., et al., *Disturbances of menstruation in hypothyroidism.* Clin Endocrinol (Oxf), 1999. **50**(5): p. 655-9.
13. Diekman, T., et al., *Prevalence and correction of hypothyroidism in a large cohort of patients referred for dyslipidemia.* Arch Intern Med, 1995. **155**(14): p. 1490-5.
14. Haupt, M. and A. Kurz, *Reversibility of dementia in hypothyroidism.* J Neurol, 1993. **240**(6): p. 333-5.
15. Shafer, R.B., R.A. Prentiss, and J.H. Bond, *Gastrointestinal transit in thyroid disease.* Gastroenterology, 1984. **86**(5 Pt 1): p. 852-5.
16. Lauritano, E.C., et al., *Association between hypothyroidism and small intestinal bacterial overgrowth.* J Clin Endocrinol Metab, 2007. **92**(11): p. 4180-4.

Questions to ask about secretions or discharge from the body - ABCDEF

VCL	Areas	Ready Set iCrush	WIP	Ci	Pi
A	Amount.[1]	What is the amount of your discharge?			
B	Blood/ No blood.[2]	Does your discharge has blood? What is the color of discharge- bright red/ coffee colored? Is it blood tinged or whole blood?			
C	Color, Consistency.[3]	What is the color of your discharge? What is the consistency of your discharge?			

D	Duration.[4]	Since how long are you having this discharge?
E	Episodes.[5]	How often do you have this discharge?
F	Foul odor, Fever.[6]	Does it have any foul smell? Did you have any fevers with it?

Table: Questions to ask about discharge or Secretions From the body
VCL- Vital Checklist; WIP-Work in Progress; Ci-Caregiver Initials; Pi-Patient Initials. This Questions to ask about discharge or Secretions From the body Vital Checklist is designed using Kanban (Lean from Toyota Production System) and Theory of Constraints by Eliyahu Goldratt.
For commercial use, please contact us at hi@vitalchecklist.com; For non-commercial use, please contact Dr.Harpreet Singh MD, FACP via email drsingh@vitalchecklist.com; 2016 Copyrights and Trademarks reserved Harpreet Singh MD, FACP, Vital Checklist and (iCrush). If you are doing a research project using this checklist, please contact Dr. Harpreet Singh for permission. Email him at drsingh@icrush.org

1. Hussain, A.N., C. Policarpio, and M.T. Vincent, *Evaluating nipple discharge.* Obstet Gynecol Surv, 2006. **61**(4): p. 278-83.
2. Isaacs, J.H., *Other nipple discharge.* Clin Obstet Gynecol, 1994. **37**(4): p. 898-902.
3. Murad, T.M., G. Contesso, and H. Mouriesse, *Nipple discharge from the breast.* Ann Surg, 1982. **195**(3): p. 259-64.
4. Jardines, L., *Management of nipple discharge.* Am Surg, 1996. **62**(2): p. 119-22.
5. King, T.A., et al., *A simple approach to nipple discharge.* Am Surg, 2000. **66**(10): p. 960-5; discussion 965-6.
6. Dixon, J.M., et al., *Periductal mastitis and duct ectasia: different conditions with different aetiologies.* Br J Surg, 1996. **83**(6): p. 820-2.

iCRUSH STROKE

Do you any of these risk factors? You have more chances of stroke if you have any?					
VCL	**Areas**	**Ready Set iCrush**	**WIP**	**Ci**	**Pi**
i	Irregular heartbeat.[1]	Did you ever experience irregular heart beat?			
C	Cholesterol problems.[2]	Do you have high cholesterol?			
R	Recreational Drugs and alcohol.[3]	Do you use recreational drugs or alcohol?			
U	Uncontrolled diabetes mellitus.[4]	Do you have diabetes? In what range your blood sugar levels? What was your last HbA1c?			

S	Smoking or tobacco in any form.[5]	Do you smoke? Do you chew tobacco?
H	Hypertension (high BP)/ Heart disease.[6]	Do you have high blood pressure? Do you have a heart disease?
	Did you experience any of the following symptoms of stroke?	
S	Sudden onset severe headache, Slurred speech.[7]	Did you ever have a sudden onset severe headache? Do you notice a change in your speech?
T	Topple over (Dizziness). Trouble walking (imbalance).[8]	Do you have dizziness or did you ever black-out? Do you ten to lose balance while walking?
R	Raise your arms. Raise your legs.[9]	Do you have weakness in your arms or legs?
O	Orientation to time, place, and person. Change in behavior.[10]	What is your name? Where are you now (country/state/city/building)? What is the year/ month/ day/ time of the day? Did any family members notice any change of behavior in you?
K	(K) Confusion. (K) Coordination.[11]	Ask family members or home support for any confusion and difficulties with balance?
E	Examine for vision changes, facial droop.[12, 13]	Do you having blurring of vision or changes in vision? Did you notice any facial droop or numbness of face?

Table: (iCrush) Stroke
VCL- Vital Checklist; WIP-Work in Progress; Ci-Caregiver Initials; Pi-Patient Initials. This (iCrush) Stroke Vital Checklist is designed using Kanban (Lean from Toyota Production System) and Theory of Constraints by Eliyahu Goldratt.
For commercial use, please contact us at hi@vitalchecklist.com; For non-commercial use, please contact Dr.Harpreet Singh MD, FACP via email drsingh@vitalchecklist.com; 2016 Copyrights and Trademarks reserved Harpreet Singh MD, FACP, Vital Checklist and (iCrush). If you are doing a research project using this checklist, please contact Dr. Harpreet Singh for permission. Email him at drsingh@icrush.org

1. Caplan, L.R., *Brain embolism, revisited.* Neurology, 1993. **43**(7): p. 1281-7.
2. Yaghi, S. and M.S. Elkind, *Lipids and Cerebrovascular Disease: Research and Practice.* Stroke, 2015. **46**(11): p. 3322-8.
3. Hankey, G.J., *Potential new risk factors for ischemic stroke: what is their potential?* Stroke, 2006. **37**(8): p. 2181-8.
4. Luitse, M.J., et al., *Diabetes, hyperglycaemia, and acute ischaemic stroke.* Lancet Neurol, 2012. **11**(3): p. 261-71.

5. Kurth, T., et al., *Smoking and risk of hemorrhagic stroke in women*. Stroke, 2003. **34**(12): p. 2792-5.
6. Lewington, S., et al., *Age-specific relevance of usual blood pressure to vascular mortality: a meta-analysis of individual data for one million adults in 61 prospective studies*. Lancet, 2002. **360**(9349): p. 1903-13.
7. Gorelick, P.B., et al., *Headache in acute cerebrovascular disease*. Neurology, 1986. **36**(11): p. 1445-50.
8. Hemphill, J.C., 3rd, et al., *Guidelines for the Management of Spontaneous Intracerebral Hemorrhage: A Guideline for Healthcare Professionals From the American Heart Association/American Stroke Association*. Stroke, 2015. **46**(7): p. 2032-60.
9. Kothari, R., et al., *Early stroke recognition: developing an out-of-hospital NIH Stroke Scale*. Acad Emerg Med, 1997. **4**(10): p. 986-90.
10. Connolly, E.S., Jr., et al., *Guidelines for the management of aneurysmal subarachnoid hemorrhage: a guideline for healthcare professionals from the American Heart Association/american Stroke Association*. Stroke, 2012. **43**(6): p. 1711-37.
11. Goldstein, L.B. and D.L. Simel, *Is this patient having a stroke?* Jama, 2005. **293**(19): p. 2391-402.
12. Adams, H.P., Jr., et al., *Baseline NIH Stroke Scale score strongly predicts outcome after stroke: A report of the Trial of Org 10172 in Acute Stroke Treatment (TOAST)*. Neurology, 1999. **53**(1): p. 126-31.
13. *Generalized efficacy of t-PA for acute stroke. Subgroup analysis of the NINDS t-PA Stroke Trial*. Stroke, 1997. **28**(11): p. 2119-25.

Smoking Cessation Counselling - DrSPADE

VCL	Areas	Ready Set iCrush	WIP	Ci	Pi
Dr.	Doctor or Caregiver.	Doctor or caregiver will assess trigger, routine, and risks.			
S	Survey the routine and triggers.[1]	Survey if patient smokes and document it.			
P	Point out.	Point out the risks of Smoking			
A	Assess.	Assess the willingness to quit within 30 days.			
D	Drugs, Device.[2]	Discuss medications and devices that can help with quitting smoking			
E	Evaluate.	Evaluate and follow up the patient			

Table: Smoking Cessation Counselling
VCL- Vital Checklist; WIP-Work in Progress; Ci-Caregiver Initials; Pi-Patient Initials. This Smoking Cessation Counselling Vital Checklist is designed using Kanban (Lean from Toyota Production System) and Theory of Constraints by Eliyahu Goldratt.
For commercial use, please contact us at hi@vitalchecklist.com; For non-commercial use, please contact Dr.Harpreet Singh MD, FACP via email drsingh@vitalchecklist.com; 2016 Copyrights and Trademarks reserved Harpreet Singh MD, FACP, Vital Checklist and (iCrush). If you are doing a research project using this checklist, please contact Dr. Harpreet Singh for permission. Email him at drsingh@icrush.org

1. Kenfield, S.A., et al., *Smoking and smoking cessation in relation to mortality in women*. Jama, 2008. **299**(17): p. 2037-47.
2. Rigotti, N.A., *Clinical practice. Treatment of tobacco use and dependence*. N Engl J Med, 2002. **346**(7): p. 506-12.

Smoking - LET'S CRUSH (Smoking) OKAY

VCL	Areas	Ready Set iCrush	WIP	Ci	Pi
L	Lungs: Risk of having: COPD Asthma Lung Cancer.[1-4]	Do you have productive cough/ shortness of breath/ blood in phlegm/ weight loss? Do you have COPD/ Asthma/ lung cancer?			
E	Endocrine: Risk of Diabetes.[5]	Do you have Diabetes? Do you have increased frequency of urination/ increased appetite/ increased thirst?			
T	Teeth & Oral Cavity: Risk of having: Gingivitis, Periodontitis, Tongue cancer, Cancer of floor of mouth Buccal cancer.[6]	Do you have any pain or swelling or bleeding in your gums? Do you have any whitish or red colored patch in your mouth? Do you have any non-healing ulcer on your tongue or in mouth? Do you have any tongue cancer or cancer of mouth?			
S	Skin.[7]	Do you have nicotine stains on your fingers or nails?			
C	Cholesterol, Clots, Cancer (Colon/ Esophageal/ Bladder/ Cervix).[8-10]	Do you have high cholesterol? Did you ever had blood clots? Do you have anemia or blood in stools? Do you have difficulty in swallowing? Do you have any blood in urine? Do you have foul smelling cervical discharge? Do you have any cancer of colon/ bladder/ esophagus/ cervix?			
R	Reproductive organs.[11]	Do you have erectile dysfunction? Did you ever had complications during pregnancy like Abruptio placenta, Preterm premature rupture of membranes, Still birth, Low birth weight?			

U	Ulcer: Peptic ulcer disease.[12-15]	Do you have peptic ulcer disease?
S	Stroke, Sleep apnea, Snoring.[16-20]	Did you ever had stroke? Do you snore during sleep? Do you have an interrupted sleep at night? Do you feel sleepy even after you wake up in the morning?
H	Hypertension, Hear attack, Heart failure.[21]	Do you have high blood pressure? Do you have a heart disease? Do you have shortness of breath, swelling of feet?
O	Osteoporosis.[22-24]	Did you get a bone scan done?
K	Kidney Cancer.[14]	Did you ever have abdominal pain, blood in urine and palpable mass in the flanks? Do you have kidney cancer?
A	Artery: Risk of Peripheral artery disease.[25]	Do you have any pain in your legs on walking which becomes better with rest?
Y	Yearly expense: Approx. 8$ per pack	Are you aware of the yearly expense of smoking?

Table: Lets Crush (Smoking) Okay
VCL- Vital Checklist; WIP-Work in Progress; Ci-Caregiver Initials; Pi-Patient Initials. This Lets Crush (Smoking) Okay Vital Checklist is designed using Kanban (Lean from Toyota Production System) and Theory of Constraints by Eliyahu Goldratt.
For commercial use, please contact us at hi@vitalchecklist.com; For non-commercial use, please contact Dr.Harpreet Singh MD, FACP via email drsingh@vitalchecklist.com; 2016 Copyrights and Trademarks reserved Harpreet Singh MD, FACP, Vital Checklist and (iCrush). If you are doing a research project using this checklist, please contact Dr. Harpreet Singh for permission. Email him at drsingh@icrush.org

1. *Smoking-attributable mortality, years of potential life lost, and productivity losses--United States, 2000-2004.* MMWR Morb Mortal Wkly Rep, 2008. **57**(45): p. 1226-8.
2. Doll, R. and A.B. Hill, *Smoking and carcinoma of the lung; preliminary report.* Br Med J, 1950. **2**(4682): p. 739-48.
3. Wynder, E.L. and E.A. Graham, *Etiologic factors in bronchiogenic carcinoma with special reference to industrial exposures; report of eight hundred fifty-seven proved cases.* AMA Arch Ind Hyg Occup Med, 1951. **4**(3): p. 221-35.
4. Willemse, B.W., et al., *The impact of smoking cessation on respiratory symptoms, lung function, airway hyperresponsiveness and inflammation.* Eur Respir J, 2004. **23**(3): p. 464-76.
5. Willi, C., et al., *Active smoking and the risk of type 2 diabetes: a systematic review and meta-analysis.* Jama, 2007. **298**(22): p. 2654-64.

6. Zee, K.Y., *Smoking and periodontal disease.* Aust Dent J, 2009. **54 Suppl 1**: p. S44-50.
7. Rigotti, N.A., *Clinical practice. Treatment of tobacco use and dependence.* N Engl J Med, 2002. **346**(7): p. 506-12.
8. Wyss, A., et al., *Cigarette, cigar, and pipe smoking and the risk of head and neck cancers: pooled analysis in the International Head and Neck Cancer Epidemiology Consortium.* Am J Epidemiol, 2013. **178**(5): p. 679-90.
9. Blot, W.J., et al., *Smoking and drinking in relation to oral and pharyngeal cancer.* Cancer Res, 1988. **48**(11): p. 3282-7.
10. Spitz, M.R., *Epidemiology and risk factors for head and neck cancer.* Semin Oncol, 1994. **21**(3): p. 281-8.
11. Dillner, J., et al., *Etiology of squamous cell carcinoma of the penis.* Scand J Urol Nephrol Suppl, 2000(205): p. 189-93.
12. Ladeiras-Lopes, R., et al., *Smoking and gastric cancer: systematic review and meta-analysis of cohort studies.* Cancer Causes Control, 2008. **19**(7): p. 689-701.
13. Lynch, S.M., et al., *Cigarette smoking and pancreatic cancer: a pooled analysis from the pancreatic cancer cohort consortium.* Am J Epidemiol, 2009. **170**(4): p. 403-13.
14. Cumberbatch, M.G., et al., *The Role of Tobacco Smoke in Bladder and Kidney Carcinogenesis: A Comparison of Exposures and Meta-analysis of Incidence and Mortality Risks.* Eur Urol, 2016. **70**(3): p. 458-66.
15. Parasher, G. and G.L. Eastwood, *Smoking and peptic ulcer in the Helicobacter pylori era.* Eur J Gastroenterol Hepatol, 2000. **12**(8): p. 843-53.
16. Anthonisen, N.R., et al., *The effects of a smoking cessation intervention on 14.5-year mortality: a randomized clinical trial.* Ann Intern Med, 2005. **142**(4): p. 233-9.
17. Vollset, S.E., A. Tverdal, and H.K. Gjessing, *Smoking and deaths between 40 and 70 years of age in women and men.* Ann Intern Med, 2006. **144**(6): p. 381-9.
18. Kenfield, S.A., et al., *Smoking and smoking cessation in relation to mortality in women.* Jama, 2008. **299**(17): p. 2037-47.
19. Ikeda, F., et al., *Smoking cessation improves mortality in Japanese men: the Hisayama study.* Tob Control, 2012. **21**(4): p. 416-21.
20. Cao, Y., et al., *Cigarette smoking cessation and total and cause-specific mortality: a 22-year follow-up study among US male physicians.* Arch Intern Med, 2011. **171**(21): p. 1956-9.
21. Ezzati, M., et al., *Role of smoking in global and regional cardiovascular mortality.* Circulation, 2005. **112**(4): p. 489-97.
22. Kanis, J.A., et al., *Smoking and fracture risk: a meta-analysis.* Osteoporos Int, 2005. **16**(2): p. 155-62.
23. Cornuz, J., et al., *Smoking, smoking cessation, and risk of hip fracture in women.* Am J Med, 1999. **106**(3): p. 311-4.
24. Oncken, C., et al., *Impact of smoking cessation on bone mineral density in postmenopausal women.* J Womens Health (Larchmt), 2006. **15**(10): p. 1141-50.
25. Conte, M.S., et al., *Society for Vascular Surgery practice guidelines for atherosclerotic occlusive disease of the lower extremities: management of asymptomatic disease and claudication.* J Vasc Surg, 2015. **61**(3 Suppl): p. 2s-41s.

Complications of Diabetes and follow up - iCRUSH DIABETES

VCL	Areas	Ready Set iCrush	WIP	Ci	Pi
i	Infection of the feet or other skin issues.[1, 2]	Do you pay regular visits to your foot doctor?			
C	Cholesterol(checked every 3-6 months if uncontrolled).[3]	Do you go for regular follow-ups to your Primary Care Physician and get your blood tests done?			
R	Record of low and high blood sugars.[4]	Do you check your blood glucose levels regularly at home and maintain a log book with the readings of low and high levels?			
U	Urine protein and kidney function.[5]	Do you go for regular follow-ups to your Primary Care Physician and get your blood and urine tests done?			
S	Sleep apnea.[6]	Do you snore while you sleep? Do you feel that you did not have a good sleep at night? Do you feel sleepy and fatigued during the day?			
H	Heart disease.[7, 8]	Do you have a heart disease?			
D	Depression.[9]	Do you feel sad or depressed?			
I	Impotence.[10]	Do you have an erectile dysfunction?			
A	A1C.[11, 12]	Did you have your A1C checked regularly?			
B	Blood pressure.[13]	Do you have high blood pressure?			
E	Eye: Diabetic retinopathy.[14, 15]	Do you go for regular eye exams to the eye doctor?			
T	Tingling/ numbness in limbs: Diabetic Neuropathy.[16]	Diabetic neuropathy, peripheral circulation and loss of sensation			
E	Ear check-up (Peripheral neuropathy).[17]	Do you have any changes in your hearing or problems with your balance?			
S	Stomach problems (Gastroparesis, constipation).[18-20]	Do you experience early satiety, nausea, bloating sensation after meals? Do you have constipation?			

Counselling: Case or Disease Based

A Picture Speaks a Thousand Words

Why-How-What of 2D pictures in patient counseling.

The Why of the problem

Health literacy is the degree to which individuals have the capacity to obtain, process, and understand basic health information and services needed to make appropriate health decisions.

Healthcare providers often encounter scenarios where there is a need to explain the normal anatomy, pathological processes, signs and symptoms or the mechanism of action of a medication to the patient/s and their caregivers. In such situations, doctors often resort to using printed pictures, charts, posters, anatomical models etc. However, during the 15 minutes patient encounter in the clinic, time may be too short to even gather the necessary tools for proper counseling of the patient, especially on a busy day, with other patients waiting. Even if we have these tools, research done by National Adult Literacy Survey (NALS) has shown

- ✓ 66% of U.S. adults age 60 and over have inadequate or marginal literacy skills.
- ✓ 50% of welfare recipients read below fifth grade level.
- ✓ 50% of Hispanic Americans and 40% of African Americans have reading problems.
- ✓ Inadequate literacy was an independent risk factor for hospital admission among 3,260 elderly managed care enrollees.
- ✓ Health literacy problems were independently associated with worse glycemic control among 408 English and Spanish speaking patients with diabetes.

Not to mention, that in the 15 minute Step 2 CS patient encounter when having to demonstrate a high level of interpersonal skills and effectively counsel the standardized patient, these types of tools are not be provided.

To properly activate and educate the patient, we need to discuss things with head, heart and hands and be focused on the patient 100% time.

I always tell my students: "Don't be a pamphlet doctor!"
~Dr. Harpreet Singh

How will you solve it?

The following will be provided:

- ✓ A pen
- ✓ The backside of the blue scrap sheet (which will be referred to as the 'Patient Education Sheet')
- ✓ A picture speaks a thousand words - Draw picture!

As per John Medina's book *Brain Rules*, vision trumps all other senses and recognition improves with the pictures. He also explains in his book immediate recall improves. Indeed, **'Seeing is believing'** and human beings tend to remember things experienced with all the senses more than things that are just heard. To add touch-points to the counselling make use of 2D pictures.

What does a caregiver or medical student need to do?

Vital Checklist Workshop can help students create, and garner, the skills to draw simple, elegant and descriptive 2D pictures during the exam. It is certain that these can be used effectively in a real clinical practice as well; these pictures are time-tested by the Vital Checklist team.
Let's get set to ace the Step 2 CS Exam!

General Counselling:

General counselling, as the term suggests, incorporates the generalized coaching that should be provided to all patients, regardless of the specific case at hand. It will cover most of the aspects of healthcare follow-up, urgent care needs, medications and lifestyle modifications.

To make it easier, an easy to remember & hard to forget Vital Checklist-Dr. Saw M.D. is elaborated here.

Dr.Saw MD	
Dr	Doctor Follow up Name_____, Date_____, Time_____, Place_____
Symptoms	
Activity	
Weight	
Medications and its side effects	
Diet and Driving	

Ci- Caregiver initials; Pi Patient initials
© 2016 Harpreet Singh MD, FACP | Vital Checklist | (iCrush)

Now, let's delve into some details.

Doctor Follow-up

The patient should first be advised as to when to visit again. He should be given a date he prefers, or advised to call up to the office to set up an appointment.

- ✓ Q: "I would like you to come back after a week for a check-up."
- ✓ Q: "Please contact my secretary to schedule your next appointment with me."
- ✓ Q: "I would like to see you again in a few weeks, please call the office and schedule a time at your convenience within two weeks."

Symptoms

- ✓ Tell the patient about the specific symptoms or signs that they should watch out for and keep track of. Explain in what cases they should contact emergency services.
- ✓ Leave a business card with them, so that if the symptoms worsen they can call.
- ✓ "I would like you to watch out for breathlessness and call me if you have problems breathing again."
- ✓ "I want you to give me a call if you having breathing problems when you go to sleep."
- ✓ "If you notice any blood or red color in your urine, please call 911 immediately."
- ✓ "If you have a chest pain again, then please take a baby aspirin and call 911 immediately."

Try and think of other warning symptoms the patient should make note of.

Don't come out of the patient's room before 15 minutes is up. Use every minute to interact with the standardized patient. Educate the standardized patient. The more you communicate in the exam; the better is the chance of passing the exams.

	Patient Activation Card *Ready→ Set→ Ask & Act* **Warning Symptoms→ (iCrush) S.T.R.O.K.E™**
I	✓ I/V site and infections ✓ Inspection of incisions→ clean; dry; intact ✓ Intestinal symptoms→ appetite, abdominal pain, weight gain/loss, diarrhea, vomiting, nausea
C	✓ Chest pain or chest pressure→ call 9-1-1 ✓ Irregular heartbeat (palpitations); dizziness
R	✓ Records of high temp, blood pressure, blood sugar ✓ Records of vital signs ✓ Fever or chills
U	✓ Urinary symptoms ✓ Bloody, frequent u.r.i.n.e. (circle one) ±pain ✓ Urgency, retention, incontinence, night time urine, excessive urine
S	✓ Shortness of breath- sports→walking uphill→mild elevation→ activities of daily living (adl)→ talking ✓ Surgical wounds
H	✓ Hurt; are you hurting somewhere? pain scale is important
	If you see somebody with symptoms of S.T.R.O.K.E; Call 9-1-1. <u>Time lost is brain lost</u>. If clot busting drug T.P.A (tissue plasminogen activator) is given in timely fashion, there is increased chance of recovery and decrease chance of long term disability
S	✓ Severe and sudden headache ✓ Slurred/strange speech
T	✓ Topple over (dizziness) ✓ Trouble walking (losing balance)
R	✓ Raise your arms ✓ Raise your legs
O	✓ Orientation to time, place and person. also ask situation ✓ Behavior
K	✓ (K) confusion ✓ (K) coordination
E	✓ Examine eyes for problems in seeing ✓ Examine face for facial droop & numbness ✓ Emotional→ sad, angry, nervous, happy
	How to teach warning symptoms to patients? **(iCrush)S.T.R.O.K.E™** ©Harpreet Singh MD FACP 2015;

Activity

Describe the activities the patient shouldn't do.

- ✓ "Please don't do aggressive activity and you must rest often when you have to do heavy exercise."
- ✓ "Please don't lift any heavy weights at home."
- ✓ "Please don't drive after taking these medications."
- ✓ "Please don't indulge in heavy work-outs."

Weight

Always ask the patient to monitor his/her weight. This is very important to do in certain cultures, and can help pick up on lifestyle diseases at an early stage.

- ✓ "Please monitor your weight regularly". Patient might ask "But why doctor, I am not fat." Politely respond by saying "It is just my protocol. I tell everyone to monitor their weight." Advise them to keep a journal or a log book.

Different Clinical Scenarios
1. There may be a clinical scenario with obesity.
2. There may be a clinical scenario with metabolic syndrome.
3. There may be a clinical scenario where the patient has cholesterol problems, diabetic problems, or hypertension.

- ✓ Whenever there is a patient that is overweight or obese, always counsel about obesity, diabetes mellitus, hypertension, and hyperlipidemia. Always ask the patient to monitor weight and log into a journal. This will help to connect to metabolic syndrome.

Medications

- ✓ If the patient is getting a prescription, then give complete advice about the medication.
- ✓ "Please take your medications as prescribed and let me know if you have any side-effects from them"
- ✓ "I have prescribed you some medications. I would like you to take them as directed and let me know of any side-effects immediately."

Diet

If there is opportunity to give advice about dietary modification, it is always a bonus point.

- ✓ "I want you to avoid fatty foods."
- ✓ "I want you to eat lots of fruits and vegetables."
- ✓ "I want you to drink at least 4 glasses of water every day."

Driving

Certain medications, like narcotics, warrant an advisory against driving.

- ✓ "Some of the drugs that you require might make you a bit drowsy and I would strongly recommend that you avoid driving yourself while on these medications."
- ✓ "It is important that you have an assigned driver with you because these drugs might make you drowsy."

Now let's add more to it. Remember Dr. (Saw)² MD.

Dr.Saw² MD	
Dr	Doctor Follow up Name_____, Date_____, Time_____, Place_____
Symptoms	
Activity	
Weight	
Smoking Cessation	
Alcohol Restriction	
Wine Restriction	
Medications and its side effects	
Diet and Driving	

Additional points:

Smoking cessation

It is very important to coach a patient to QUIT smoking if he does smoke, and to appreciate and encourage the patient who has already quit smoking.

- ✓ "Mr. Doe, I recommend that you quit smoking immediately. If you agree, I can help you with various options to quit the habit."

- ✓ "We have various options and programs to help you quit smoking, if you would like I will send my social worker to help you with it."
- ✓ "I really appreciate that you have stopped smoking and I would like you to continue with your decision. I am there to help you if needed."

Challenging Question
"Doctor, If I quit smoking can I chew tobacco instead? Tobacco helps to reduce my stress."
✓ Clinical Scenario- Tobacco Cessation Counseling ✓ Use Dr. Spade methodology.

Alcohol restriction

Always ask the patient to restrict his alcohol intake if he is consuming more than the safe limit, especially if he has heart, liver, or kidney failure.

- ✓ "Mr. Doe, I seriously recommend that you decrease the amount of alcohol you consume and I am there to help you with the process if you decide to do it"
- ✓ "Alcohol can result in liver failure as well as many other things, and I would like you to watch your consumption and lower it. I am there to help you if needed."

Wine restriction

Some patients might say NO to alcohol consumption, but on further probing might admit to consuming wine. Coach them to restrict wine consumption, if it is more than the safe limit.

- ✓ "I want you to keep a watch on your wine consumption and lower it."
- ✓ "I can help you with lowering your wine consumption if you want. It would really help you to do so"

Challenging Question
Improve HDL and Wine use

Remember Dr. (Saw)³MD!	
Dr	Doctor Follow-up
S	✓ Symptoms ✓ Smoking cessation ✓ Salt restriction
A	✓ Aggressive activity, alcohol restriction
W	✓ Weight ✓ Wine restriction ✓ Water restriction
T	✓ Tests to be done ✓ Transport for discharge and follow-up appointments ✓ Therapy
H	✓ Home nursing ✓ Health insurance issues
R	✓ Resources for family ✓ Results pending ✓ Return to work
E	✓ Equipment: walker, cane, glucometer, oxygen etc.
E	✓ Expert in wound care, insulin injections, ostomy care
M	✓ Medications
D	✓ Diet and driving

Some additional points:

Sodium restriction

This is specifically useful for patients with a heart, liver or kidney problem. Ask the patient to restrict their salt consumption to below 2000mg/day.

- ✓ "I would like you to restrict your total sodium intake to a maximum of 2000 milligrams per day. This will help manage your condition."

Water restriction

This is also useful for patients with a heart, liver or kidney problem. Ask the patient to restrict their water intake to below 2000 mL/day.

- ✓ "I would like you to restrict your total fluid intake to a maximum of 2000 mL per day. This will help manage your condition."

Tests to be done

Tell the patient what investigations should be ordered.

- ✓ "I would like to draw blood, as well as get an ultrasound of your abdomen to come to a final diagnosis."
- ✓ "A blood draw and a CT scan would be highly useful for me to reach a conclusion about your problem."

Challenging Question
How will you explain the CT scan, ultrasound or other radiological studies to the patients?

Transport

Discuss their concerns about transportation to and from the hospital, and offer the help of a social worker.

- ✓ "I understand that you have some concerns regarding your transportation to the follow-up visits. Please don't worry, I will send in my social worker to help you with this issue."

Home nursing

Discuss the requirement of a health nurse at the patient's home if he does not already have good social support.

- ✓ "I can understand that you are concerned about your care at home, but I am here to help, and I will send in my social worker to discuss the various home nursing options with you."

Health insurance

Many times, the patient will refuse your investigations or treatment, citing a lack of finances and health insurance. It is your duty to help him by offering to send in the social worker.

- ✓ "I am sorry to hear about your situation but I strongly recommend that you go ahead with the investigations. I will send in my social worker to help you with the financial issues."
- ✓ "I will send in my social worker to answer your questions about health insurance"

Resources for family

Offer information about help groups and reading material to the patient and his family.

- ✓ "My social worker can help you with information regarding various help groups and reading material about your condition. I can send her in if you want."

Results pending

"We will discuss about the pending results in near future. Please make a note of these tests."

Return to work

If the patient asks about his capability to return to work, then advise accordingly.

- ✓ "I think you should rest for a week before returning to work."
- ✓ "It is not the best time to return to work, I sincerely recommend a rest for a minimum of three days."

Equipment

Discuss the availability of walkers, canes and oxygen equipment with the patient.

- ✓ "You will be requiring a walker to assist you in walking for a few days. I will send in my social worker to discuss the various options available."
- ✓ "My social worker will help arrange oxygen equipment for your use at home."

Expert care

Discuss the need of an expert to manage wounds, ostomies and injections if required by the clinical scenario.

- ✓ "You will need daily wound dressings and I will send in my social worker to help you find an expert who can come to your home and do it."
- ✓ "You will need help in administering insulin injections at home and my social worker can help you with the various options in this regard."

How to Improve Health Literacy?

Billions of dollars are spent on billboards and marketing so that patients can be enticed to the healthcare facilities. I believe that if we need strong word of mouth marketing, our front-end health caregivers should have tools and should spend time to improve health literacy. Patient Experience begins with the Patient Education. Trust develops when a doctor sits and explains the disease process in an elaborate manner.

Handing out pamphlets will not improve any health literacy. These pamphlets are usually stored in the drawers, shredded when they reach home, or left in the car trunk. To improve patient education, patient should understand the numbers have oral literacy and print literacy. This can only happen if we try involving more senses of the patients. Memory increases when the number of sensory organs has increased—vision, auditory, reading, writing and kinesthetic. Patient need to be immersed in the learning of their disease process and that can only happen if we can draw pictures, explain with help of metaphors and analogies. To improve the memory, patients should be able to trace back what their doctors told. This can happen if they have chunked Vital Checklist and this can be remembered by easy repetition. Once they have explained the patients in the layman language, it's easy to leave a mark on the patient and improve patient satisfaction. In USMLE Step 2 CS exam, you have pen, paper and your communication skills to improve health literacy of the standardized patients. Don't rush through this part and spend adequate time. Many students will complete the clinical scenarios in 12-13 minutes and you must use this opportunity to talk, discuss and draw a picture to explain the clinical conditions.

Use this phrase to continue the discussion.

Though I am done with the clinical scenario and I have explained everything, but I do have a few more minutes before I am called. Do you want to discuss anything else?

Don't ask close-ended question, "Can I explain anything else with a picture?"

Just do it! Just explain with the help of picture. Obviously, you should be well versed with the anatomy and physiology to explain the disease process. These will help to showcase your communication skills and help you pass the exam in the first attempt.

U Listen, W.R.I.T.E., Draw & Memorize with Vital Checklist		
U	Understanding numeracy	Numeracy (using and understanding numbers)[1, 2]
Listen	Listen and speak	Oral literacy [1]
W	Write[3, 4]	Write (Print literacy)[1]
R	Read[3]	Read (Print literacy)[1]
I	Integrate[5]	Integrating the multiple sensory pathways increase retention[3]
T	Touchpoint tools[3, 6, 7]	Hands-on training and immersion coaching[8]
E	Explain with metaphors and analogies	May enhance physicians' ability to communicate thus improving better patient perception[9, 10]
Draw	Draw—2-D-line diagrams	Picture superiority effect[11-13]
Memorize	Memory	Short-term memory→long-term memory[5]
With		
Chunked	Chunking	Probability of recall is greater when the "chunking" strategy[14]
Vital	The checklist manifesto [15]	Safe surgery checklist saved lives[17]
Checklist	Central line checklist[16]	Checklist reduced infections [16]

Copyright 2016: Harpreet Singh MD, FACP, Vital Checklist and/or iCrush
For permission please contact: drsingh@vitalchecklist.com

References:
[1] I. o. M. U. C. o. H. Literacy, L. Nielsen-Bohlman, A. M. Panzer, and D. A. Kindig, "What Is Health Literacy?," 2004 2004.
[2] B. D. Weiss, M. Z. Mays, W. Martz, K. M. Castro, D. A. DeWalt, M. P. Pignone, *et al.*, "Quick Assessment of Literacy in Primary Care: The Newest Vital Sign," *The Annals of Family Medicine,* vol. 3, pp. 514-522, 2005.
[3] N. Fleming and C. Mills, ""Not Another Inventory, Rather a Catalyst for Reflection"," *To Improve the Academy,* vol. 11, p. 18, 1-1-1992 1992.
[4] K. Klein and A. Boals, "Expressive writing can increase working memory capacity.," *Journal of Experimental Psychology: General,* vol. 130, p. 520, Sep 2001 2001.
[5] J. Medina, *Brain rules : 12 principles for surviving and thriving at work, home, and school,* 1st ed. Seattle, WA: Pear Press, 2008.

[6] D. Conant and M. Norgaard, *TouchPoints: Creating Powerful Leadership Connections in the Smallest of Moments*: Jossey-Bass, 2011.

[7] D. Conant, N. affiliation, M. Norgaard, and N. affiliation, "TouchPoints: The power of leading in the moment," *Leader to Leader,* vol. 2012, pp. 44-49, 2016.

[8] A. Robbins. (2015, 13th December). *The Training Effect | Personal Development | Tony Robbins.* Available: https://www.tonyrobbins.com/coaching/training-effect/

[9] D. Casarett, A. Pickard, J. M. Fishman, S. C. Alexander, R. M. Arnold, K. I. Pollak, *et al.*, "Can Metaphors and Analogies Improve Communication with Seriously Ill Patients?," in *J Palliat Med.* vol. 13, ed, 2010, pp. 255-60.

[10] H. Osborne, *Health literacy from A to Z : practical ways to communicate your health message*, 2nd ed. Burlington, MA: Jones & Bartlett Learning, 2013.

[11] A. Paivio, J. M. Clark, N. Digdon, and T. Bons, "Referential processing: reciprocity and correlates of naming and imaging," *Mem Cognit,* vol. 17, pp. 163-74, Mar 1989.

[12] P. S. Houts, C. C. Doak, L. G. Doak, and M. J. Loscalzo, "The role of pictures in improving health communication: a review of research on attention, comprehension, recall, and adherence," *Patient Educ Couns,* vol. 61, pp. 173-90, May 2006.

[13] B. A. Ally, C. A. Gold, and A. E. Budson, "The picture superiority effect in patients with Alzheimer's disease and mild cognitive impairment," *Neuropsychologia,* vol. 47, pp. 595-8, Jan 2009.

[14] G. A. MILLER, "The magical number seven plus or minus two: some limits on our capacity for processing information," *Psychol Rev,* vol. 63, pp. 81-97, Mar 1956.

[15] A. Gawande, *The checklist manifesto : how to get things right*, 1st ed. New York: Metropolitan Books, 2010.

[16] P. Pronovost, D. Needham, S. Berenholtz, D. Sinopoli, H. Chu, S. Cosgrove, *et al.*, "An intervention to decrease catheter-related bloodstream infections in the ICU," *N Engl J Med,* vol. 355, pp. 2725-32, Dec 2006.

[17] A. B. Haynes, T. G. Weiser, W. R. Berry, S. R. Lipsitz, A. H. Breizat, E. P. Dellinger, *et al.*, "A surgical safety checklist to reduce morbidity and mortality in a global population," *N Engl J Med,* vol. 360, pp. 491-9, Jan 2009.

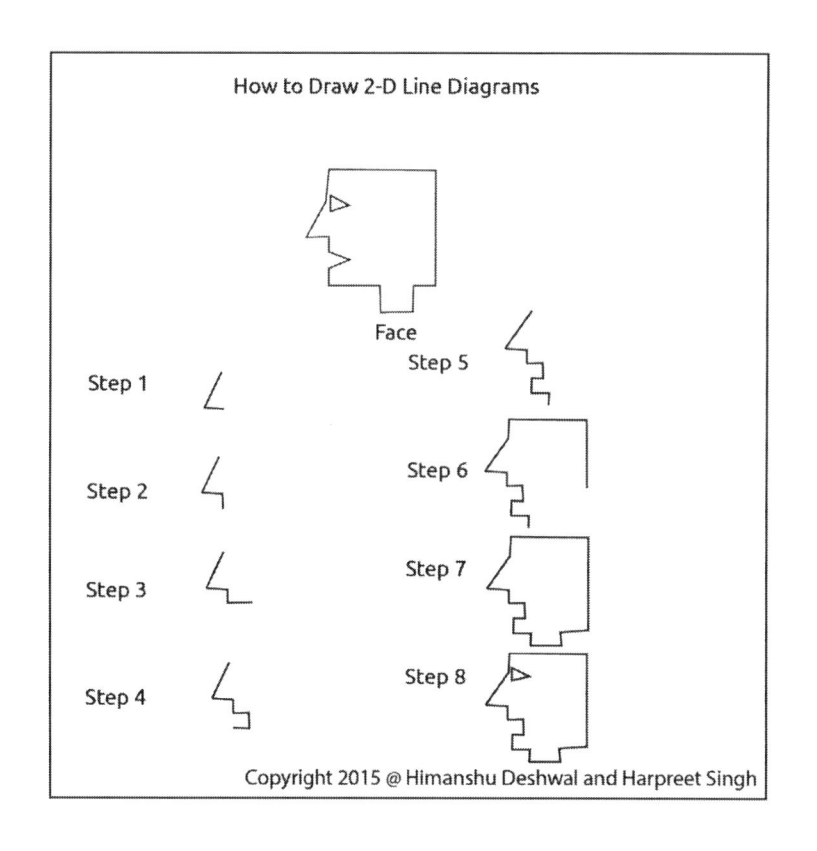

How to Draw 2-D Line Diagrams

Face

Step 1

Step 2

Step 3

Step 4

Step 5

Step 6

Step 7

Step 8

Copyright 2015 @ Himanshu Deshwal and Harpreet Singh

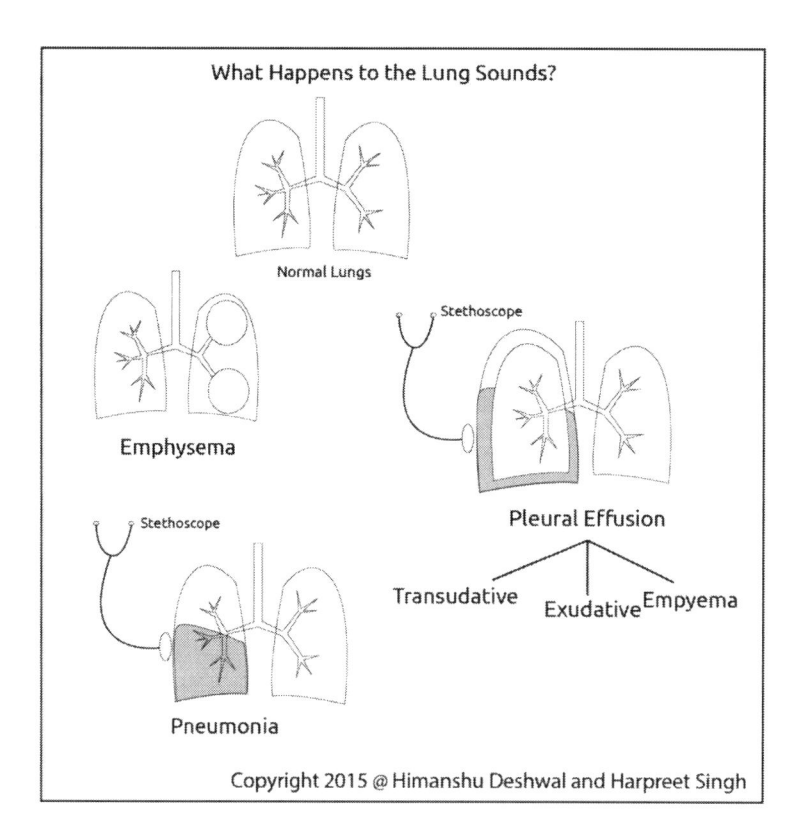

What Happens to the Lung Sounds?

Normal Lungs

Emphysema

Stethoscope

Pleural Effusion

Transudative   Exudative   Empyema

Stethoscope

Pneumonia

Copyright 2015 @ Himanshu Deshwal and Harpreet Singh

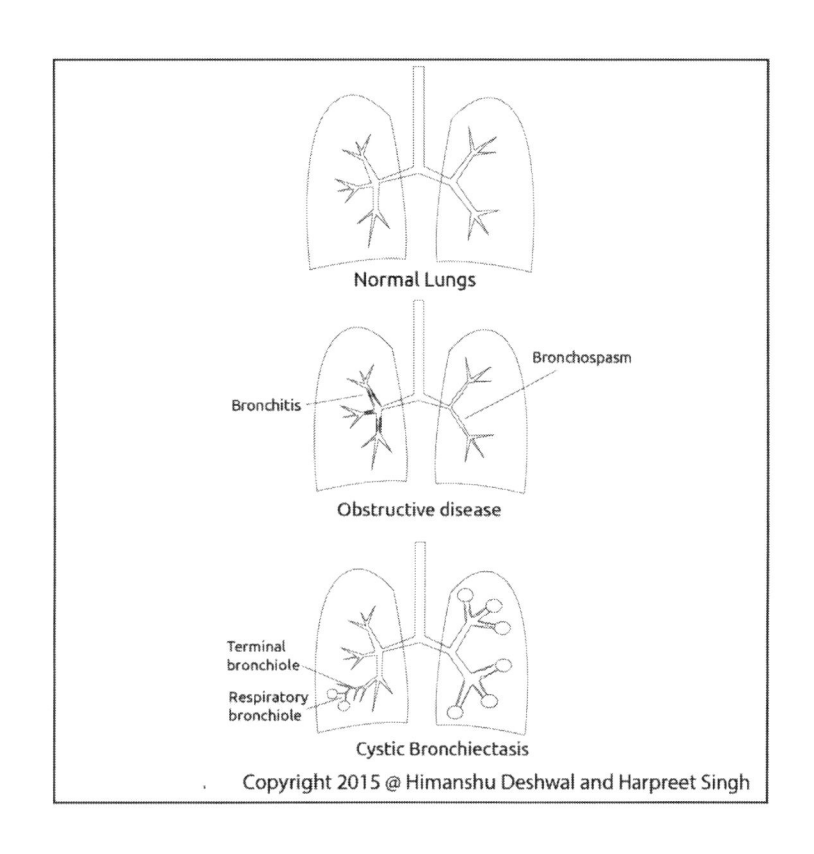

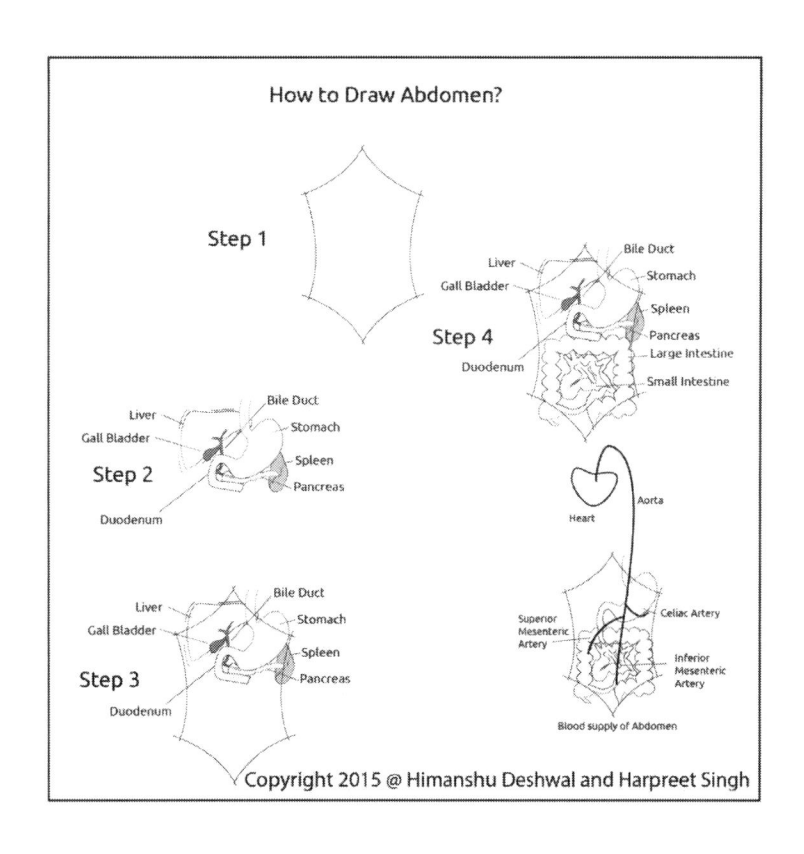

278

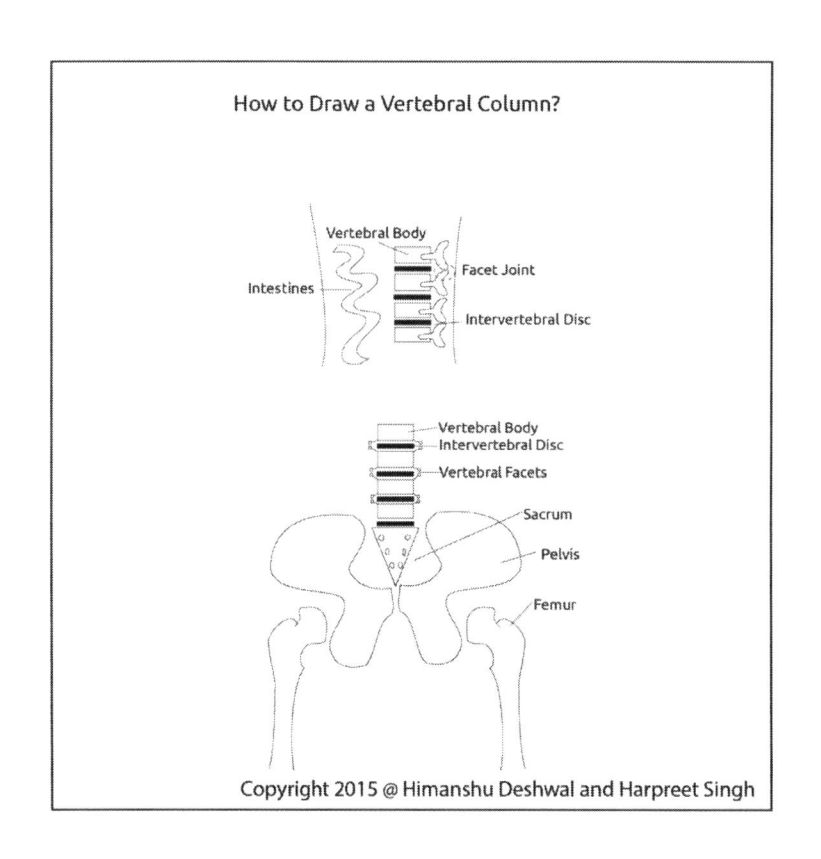

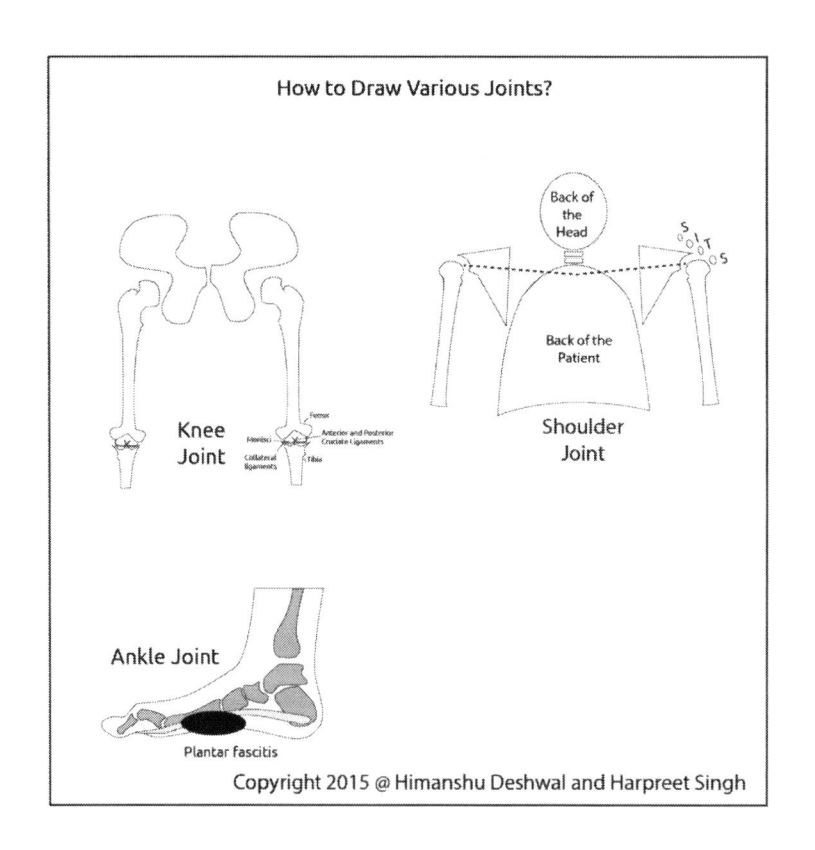

How to Explain Complaints of Upper Respiratory Tract?

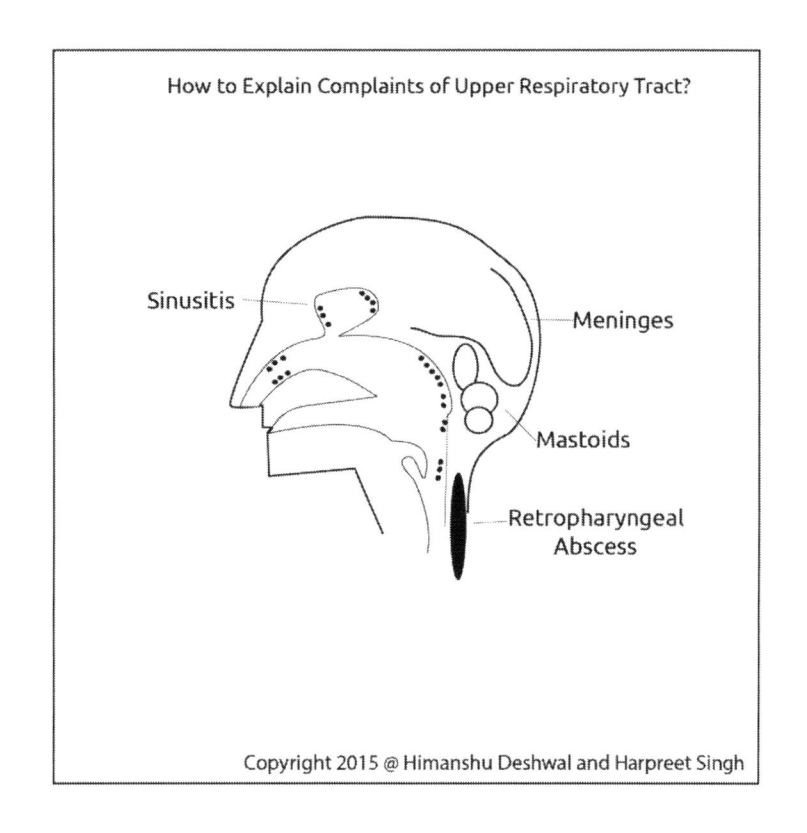

- Sinusitis
- Meninges
- Mastoids
- Retropharyngeal Abscess

Copyright 2015 @ Himanshu Deshwal and Harpreet Singh

How to Explain Causes of Renal Failure?

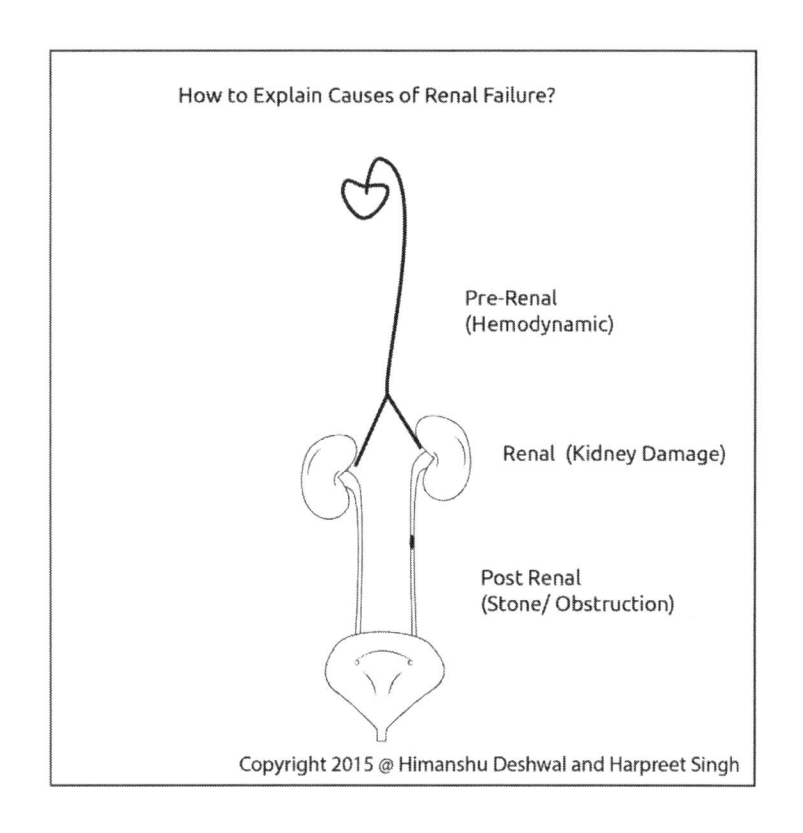

- Pre-Renal (Hemodynamic)
- Renal (Kidney Damage)
- Post Renal (Stone/ Obstruction)

Copyright 2015 @ Himanshu Deshwal and Harpreet Singh

How to Explain the Function of Sildenafil?

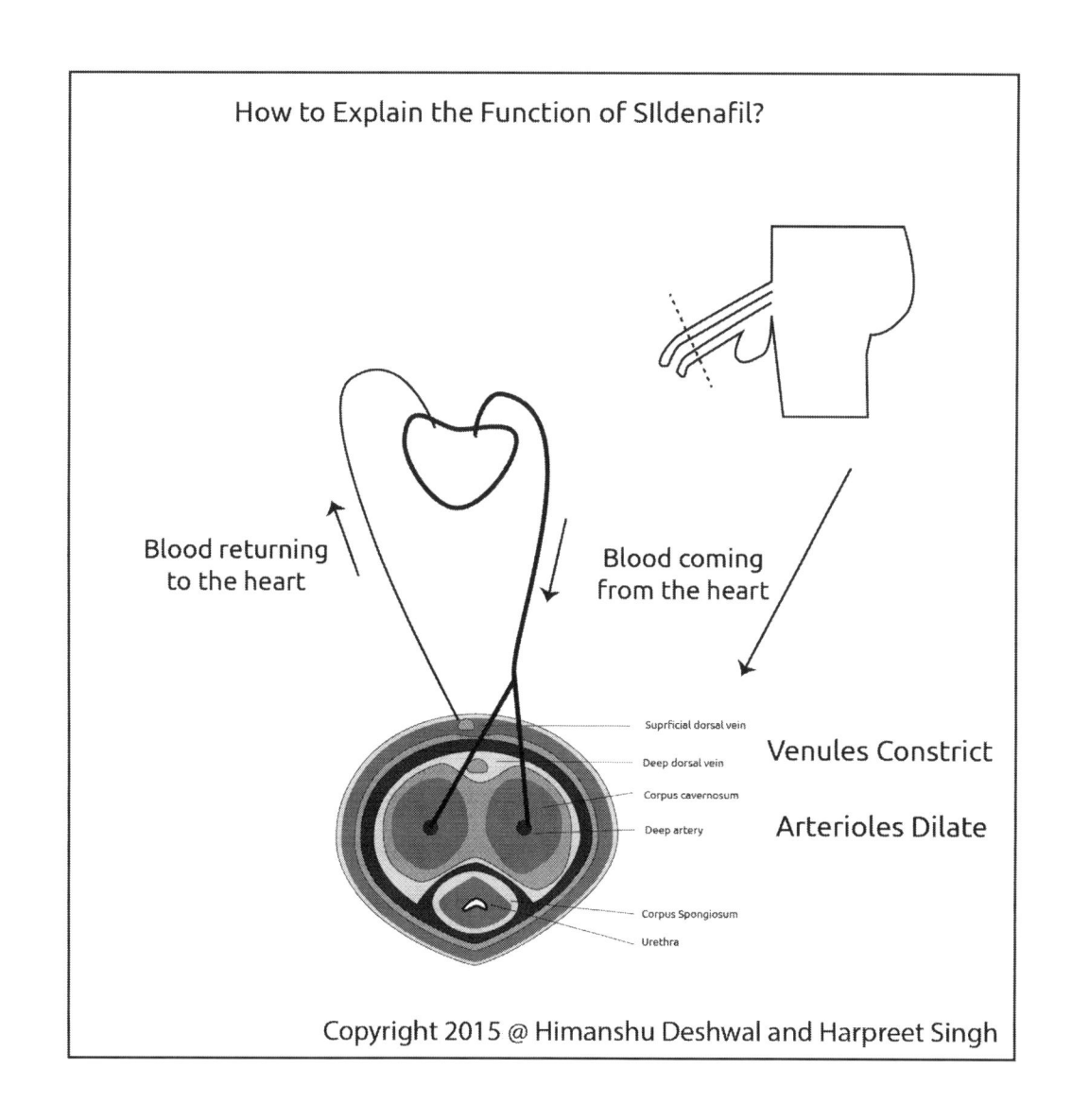

Blood returning to the heart

Blood coming from the heart

- Superficial dorsal vein
- Deep dorsal vein
- Corpus cavernosum
- Deep artery
- Corpus Spongiosum
- Urethra

Venules Constrict

Arterioles Dilate

Copyright 2015 @ Himanshu Deshwal and Harpreet Singh

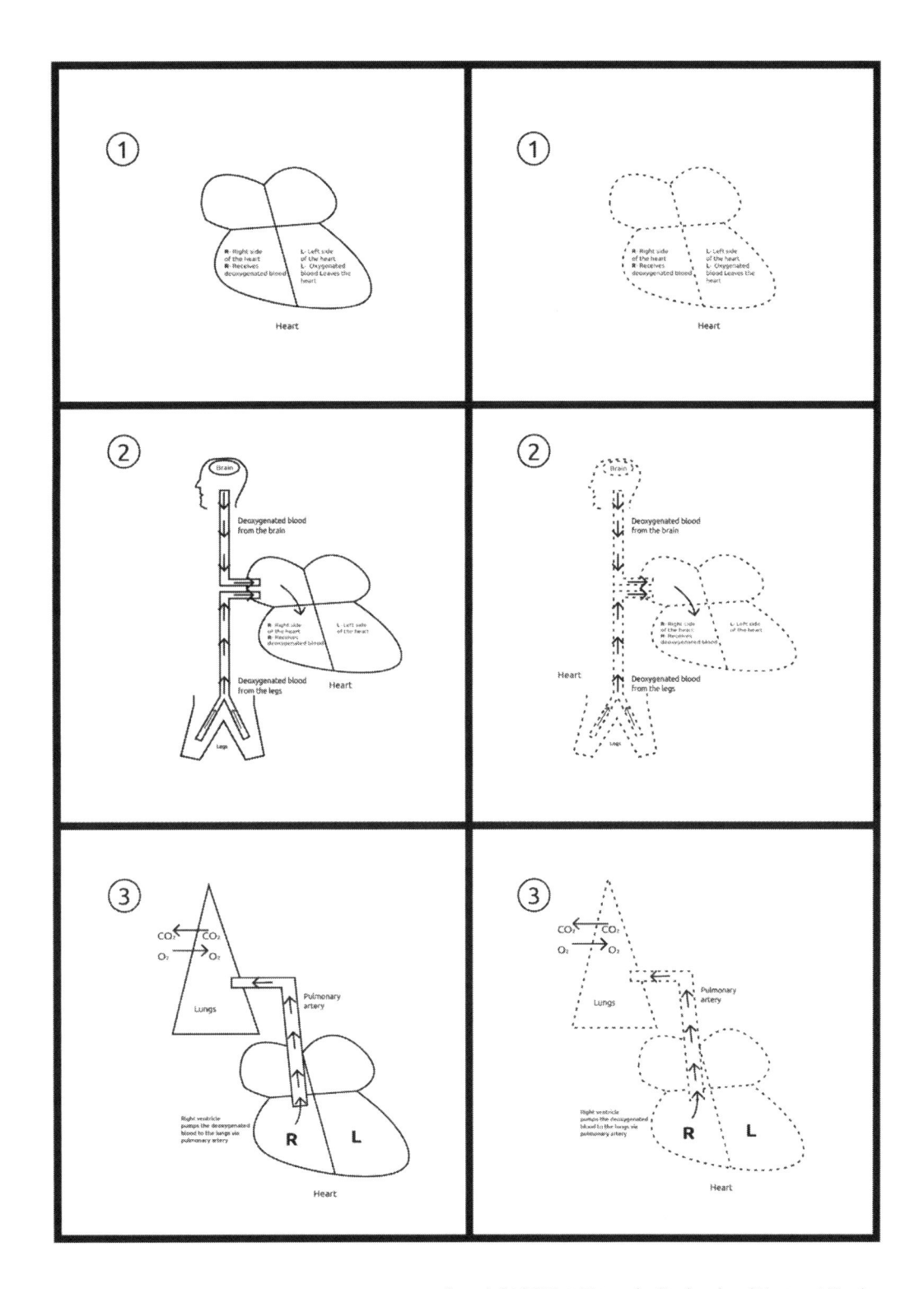

Copyright 2015 @ Himanshu Deshwal and Harpreet Singh

⑦

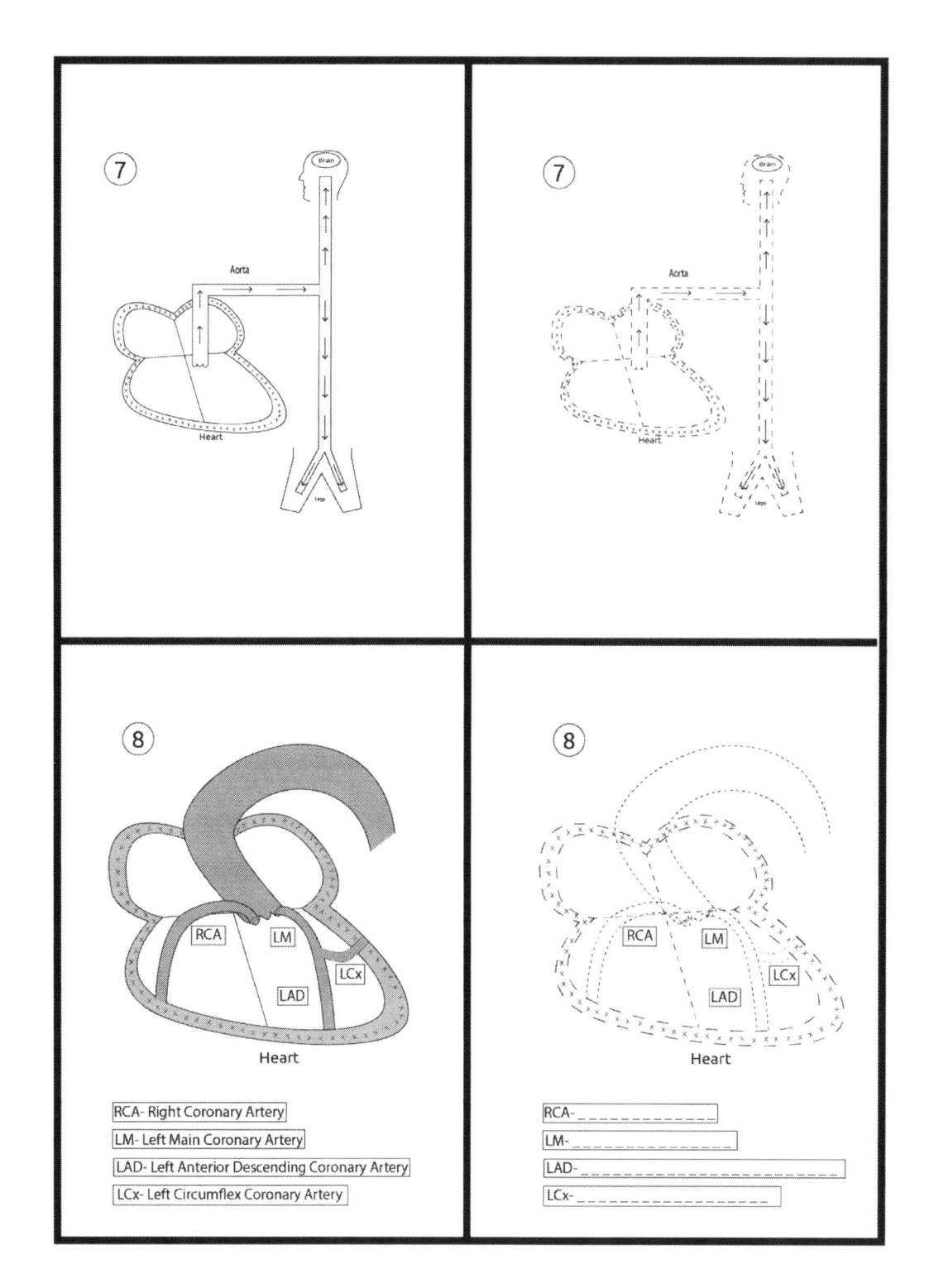

Aorta
Brain
Heart
Legs

⑦

Aorta
Brain
Heart
Legs

⑧

RCA | LM
LAD | LCx

Heart

RCA- Right Coronary Artery
LM- Left Main Coronary Artery
LAD- Left Anterior Descending Coronary Artery
LCx- Left Circumflex Coronary Artery

⑧

RCA | LM
LAD | LCx

Heart

RCA- _____
LM- _____
LAD- _____
LCx- _____

Copyright 2015 @ Himanshu Deshwal and Harpreet Singh

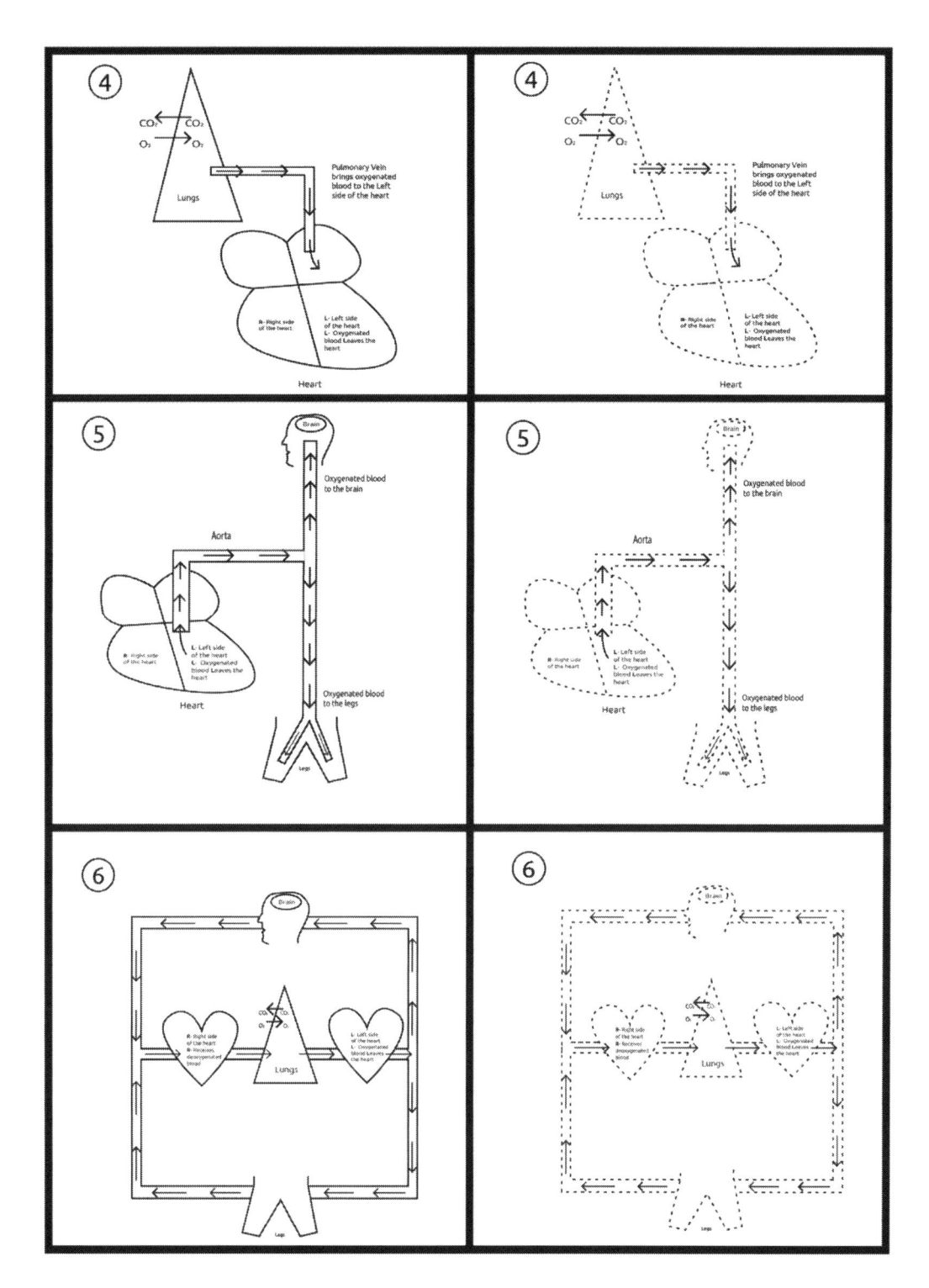

Copyright 2015 @ Himanshu Deshwal and Harpreet Singh

283

Let's discuss this topic with an example. In this we will elaborate Bell's palsy and meningitis using pictures and Vital Checklist.

(U→ Listen→ W.R.I.T.E →Draw → Memorize with Vital Checklist)

Bell's Palsy

The term Bell's palsy relates to late Sir Charles Bell, who first described the anatomy and function of the facial nerve. It was initially described in relation with traumatic facial nerve paralysis, but has now become more generalized over the years to involve an "acute facial paralysis of unknown origin"

Facial paralysis is a clinical syndrome of various causes and a thorough clinical examination and assessment is required to reach to a diagnosis.

Anatomy

The course of the facial nerve can be very easily explained if we divide it into three segments- the first segment is the origin, the facial nerve originates at the ponto-medullary junction and traverses to enter the cranial bone from the internal auditory meatus.

The second segment is the nerve's journey through the bone via the facial canal. An important point to remember is that the narrowest part is the labyrinthine segment, which is the most common site of nerve entrapment.

The third segment is the exit of the nerve out of the stylo-mastoid foramen and giving out peripheral branches through the parotid gland.

Function

The facial nerve as the name suggests is the main nerve supplying muscles of facial expression and carries a substantial amount of sensations from the face.

It is also involved in taste sensations from anterior 2/3 of the tongue via the chorda tympani branch.

It acts as the efferent arc of the corneal reflex as well.

Differential diagnosis Of Bell's palsy

Here are the differential diagnoses that should be kept in mind while evaluating a case of Bell's palsy.

Let us use our standard mnemonic "Vital Signs" to find an easy way to encompass all DD's of Bell's palsy.

	Etiology	CAUSES
V	**V**ascular	- Herpes Simplex is one of the causes that can be associated with Bell's palsy. The evidence is not conclusive but it has been widely accepted due to association of the virus with demyelination and inflammation.
- Reactivation of inactive herpes zoster virus is the second most common viral association with Bell's palsy.
- HIV Infection
I	**I**nflammation	- Stroke is one of the most important life threatening conditions that should be ruled out in case of facial palsy.
T	**T**rauma	- Trauma to the facial nerve secondary to a base of skull fracture.
A	**A**utoimmune	- Diabetes has been known to cause this disease by microvascular damage leading to diabetic mono and poly neuropathy.
- The nerve degenerates secondary to blockage of small vessels supplying the nerve due to hypercoagulability disorders.
L	**L**abs	- Rickettsial disease: This can affect virtually any cranial nerve but facial nerve is by far the most commonly affected, in as many as 8 percent of all cases of Lyme's disease. It is one of the most important causes of bilateral facial paralysis.
S	**S**ocial & Drugs	- Any disease process affecting the extracellular space or causing edema can lead to Bell's palsy. Examples include pregnancy and hypothyroid myxedema.
I	**I**nfection	- Other infections apart from herpes zoster and simplex – including EBV, Coxsackie, Rubella, Mumps and adenovirus.
G	**G**enetic	- There is convincing evidence to suggest that there might be a genetic predisposition to the disease.
N	**N**eurological/**N**eoplasm	- Tumors of the temporal bone, internal acoustic canal or cerebellopontine angle.
- Parotid tumors and surgical treatment of the tumors has been shown to cause paralysis of the facial nerve secondary to iatrogenic damage.
S	**S**ystemic	- Neurosarcoidosis is an important cause of bilateral bell's palsy.

Clinical Features of Bell's Palsy

We would like to explain the clinical features of Bell's palsy using a picture that will depict the symptoms and signs to elicit.

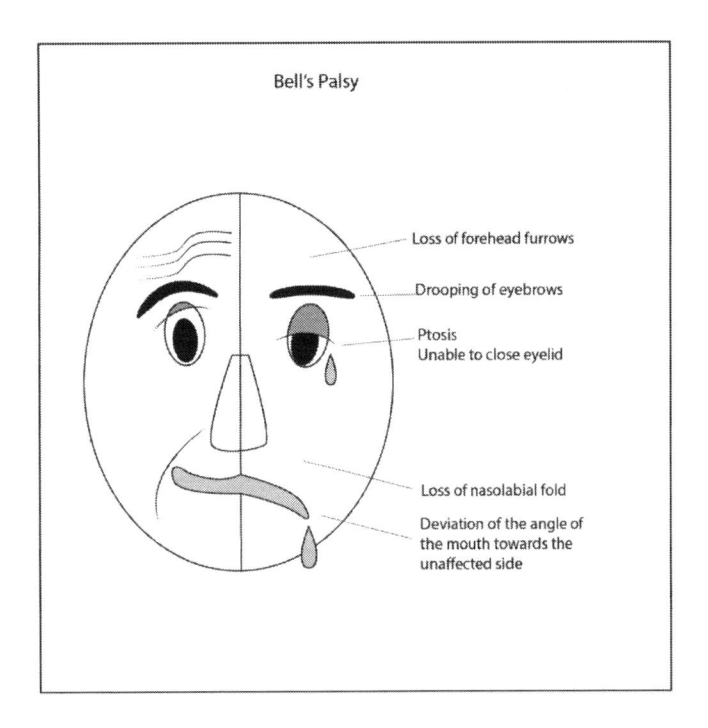

Sensation, decreased tearing and hyperacusis - these features indicate a high lesion in the facial canal and have very limited clinical relevance.

UMN and LMN lesions of the Facial Nerve

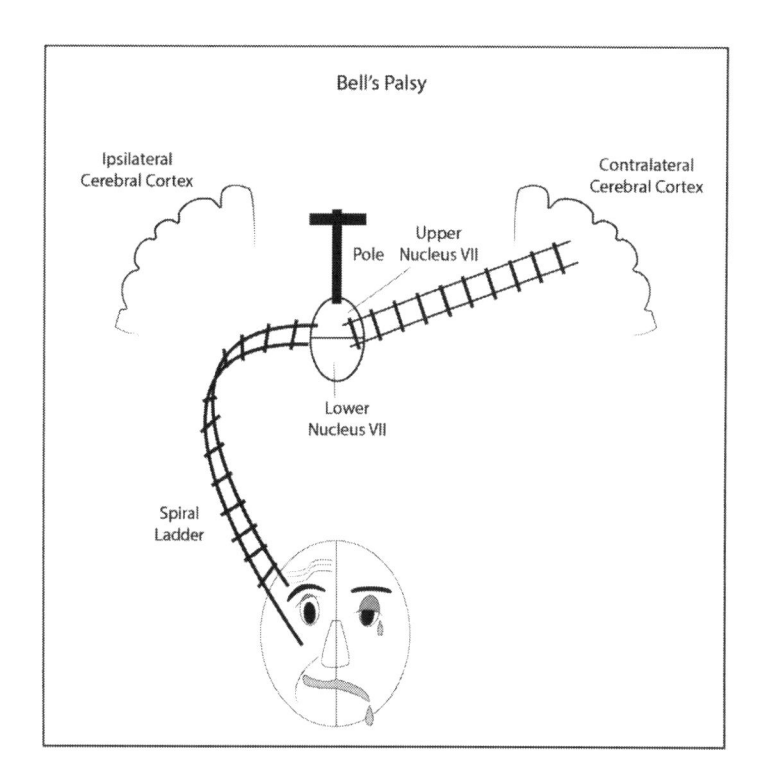

It is vital to know the difference between an UMN lesions of the brain and LMN lesions of the facial nerve.

Let us try to differentiate the lesions using our "Monkey and the Bell" technique

There are three monkeys in our brain whose main aim in life is to deliver bells to the face!

These monkeys are on a pole, on a spiral ladder and on a straight ladder.

The pole depicts connection between the upper nucleus and the ipsilateral side of the brain cortex- Pay heed to the fact that only the upper nucleus is connected to the pole.. The straight ladder depicts the connection between the contralateral cortex and the upper and the lower nucleus of the facial nerve. The spiral ladder depicts the tortuous course of the LMN facial nerve.

- ✓ If there is a break in the spiral ladder (Facial Nerve itself- LMN) no bell can ever reach the face and this leads to full facial paralysis.

- ✓ If there is a break in the straight ladder – Stroke in contralateral cortex- the monkey on the straight ladder cannot deliver the bells to the monkey on the spiral ladder. Seeing this the monkey on the pole comes and gives a bell to the upper nucleus- notice that the upper nucleus only innervates the upper part of face.

- ✓ Hence in an UMN lesion the upper part of facial musculature- forehead and eyebrows are functioning due to innervation of upper nucleus from ipsilateral cortex.

History and Physical Examination

We suggest that you take a comprehensive history using DOCTOR AID @ PM. The aim of gathering the history should be to reach to a prospective diagnosis.

The knowledge of differential diagnoses will let you take a relevant negative history to rule out a pathological process causing the symptoms.

Now do a focused clinical examination of the neurological system, followed by an examination of the facial nerve. We suggest that you start from top to bottom of the face.

- ✓ Ask the patient to raise his eyebrows- or to furrow his forehead.
- ✓ Ask the patient to close his eyes- you may ask him to close his eyes tightly.
- ✓ Ask the patient to blow his cheeks and try to whistle.
- ✓ Ask the patient to smile while observing for asymmetry.
- ✓ Ask the patient to clench his neck muscles and observe for movements in the platysma.
- ✓ Make sure you do a brief ear examination and document that no vesicles were seen to rule out herpes zoster.

Document that taste and lacrimation was not tested due to limitations in examination scenario.

Diagnosis of Bell's Palsy

The diagnosis of Bell's palsy is mainly clinical and imaging and diagnostic tests are mainly directed to rule out potential surgical causes of facial palsy that can be promptly treated.

Diagnostic Criterion for Bell's Palsy

- ✓ Acute onset of diffuse facial nerve involvement showing up as palsy of facial muscles with or without taste and lacrimation involvement.
- ✓ The symptoms progress to maximal over 2-3 weeks and then gradually subside or get better over the next 6 months.

Electro diagnostic tests like the electromyography and nerve conduction study can be done to evaluate the prognosis and the potential for recovery.

Contrast Enhanced CT scan and Gadolinium contrast MRI can be used to rule out a space-occupying lesion causing paralysis. These studies should include brain parotic gland and temporal bone.

Other tests-

- ✓ Serological testing for Lyme's disease (ELISA)- especially if patient gives history of travel to endemic areas like New Mexico and history of tick bite.
- ✓ Test for HIV if history of high risk sexual behavior.
- ✓ Blood glucose, HbA1c and Serum lipid profile as a precautionary measure.

Treatment of Bell's Palsy

Early commencement of glucocorticoid therapy remains the mainstay of treatment for idiopathic facial nerve paralysis. The drug of choice is prednisolone.

Several clinical trials have demonstrated no added benefit of giving antiviral therapy.

Supportive care includes eye drops and eye patches, psychological counseling and multivitamin supplements.

Now practice a case of Bell's palsy with your study partner using the case scenario below.

Notes for the Standardized Patient/Study Partner:

History:

You are a 46-year-old man who noticed some drooling of saliva from the corner of your mouth. You have been struggling to keep your left eye open as well. You have presented to the clinic in absolute panic.

Act very agitated and keep asking the doctor " Do I have a stroke Doctor?"

- ✓ You noticed that the left side of your face looks very different to the right side which appears almost normal.
- ✓ You have insulin dependent diabetes and are on thyroid replacement for hypothyroidism.

(You can say no to other symptoms and build the rest of the details not mentioned here based on your judgment.)

Examination: Pretend no discomfort on any maneuver.

- ✓ When asked to close eyes- shut only the right side forcefully.
- ✓ When asked to blow your cheeks – pretend to have a weakness and fail to do that.
- ✓ When asked to smile, try a crooked smile which deviates to the right

Challenging Question:

"Doc, Am I having a Stroke? Is there something wrong with my brain?"

Meningitis

Meningitis is one of the most common infections of the Central Nervous System and one of the 10 most common causes of deaths due to an infection. Every year around 1.2 million cases of bacterial meningitis are reported worldwide.

The USMLE will test you on some CNS cases and Meningitis will fall into the differential of almost all of the cases. Thus a clear understanding of the clinical features and diagnostic tests involved will come in handy during the exam and in real life patient encounters as well!

Causative Agents

Now the causative agents usually give a good insight into the processes involved in causing meningitis. We suggest an easy way of remembering the causes, which will point towards 2 of the most common clinical features of meningitis as well- " Not So Loud- I Cant See". This mnemonic sheds light on the - photophobia and phonophobia.

Causative Organisms in Meningitis			
Mnemonic	Organism	Predisposing Conditions	Special Clinical Features If Any
"Not"	Nisseria Meningitidis	Living in Closed Quarters, Like a Hostel- Usually Teenage-Early twenties Age Group	Can Cause Skin petechiae and palpable purpura. Can lead to Arthritis as well.
"So"	Streptococcus Pneumoniae	Anything that breaches the barrier to brain- Cribiform Fracture, Basilar Skull Fracture, Cochlear Implant	
"Loud"	Listeria Monocytogenes	Cell mediated Immunity is Deficient- Transplant, Steroids, Alcoholism, Malignancy.	Tendency to have focal neurological deficit and seizures early in the course of disease.
"I"	Hemophilus Influenzae	Humoral Immunity is Deficient	In individuals with no documented vaccination status.
"Cant"	Coagulase Negative Staphylococcus	Surgery and Foreign Body.	
"See"	Staphylococcus Aureus	Surgery, Endocarditis, Ventricle Drains, Cellulitis.	

Clinical Features

We would like to divide the clinical features to the Classical Triad and special features linked to particular organisms.

The classical triad of meningitis is

Classical Triad Of Meningitis	
Symptoms	Details
Fever	Almost 95 % Patients have high fevers >38 degrees Celsius.
Nuchal Rigidity	Almost 80-90% complain of signs of meningeal irritation.
Change in Mental Status	This includes confusion or lethargy.

Other clinical features include headache that may be generalized. Focal seizures, and neurological deficit may also be a presenting sign.

History and Physical Examination

We suggest that you use our time-tested method of taking history of the symptoms- DOCTOR AID @ PM

For the clinical examination we suggest that you make sure that you follow the following very important points that could cost you dearly if omitted!

Pitfalls of the Meningitis case!	
Situation	Your Reaction
Patient is lying on the bed and does not get up to greet you as you enter.	Do not ask him to get up- the SP's are trained actors and never do anything without a reason. They may be pointing you towards a diagnosis.
The lights in the room are very dim.	Do not switch on the lights. Ask the patient if the lights are bothering him and offer to dim them if he ever complains of a headache.
You are suspecting migraine or meningitis.	Never shine a light in the patients eyes, they might have photophobia and you will lose marks for being inconsiderate towards the patient.
The patient is complaining of pain on bending the neck	It may be a sign of meningeal irritation but do not keep repeating the exam. As a rule if a manoeuvre is painful make it a point to do it only once.

Do a focused physical examination. The Kernig's sign and the Brudzinki's sign are important and should be attempted unless the patient has already mentioned that bending the neck hurts him.

- ✓ Kernig's Sign- the patient is unable to extend the knee when the hip is flexed. An easy way to remember this is the fact that "K" is common between Knee and Kernig.

- ✓ Brudzinki's Sign- Bending the neck reflexively leads to bending of the hips. "B" is common between Bending and Brudzinki.

The concept behind these findings is the fact that there is meningeal irritation. The spinal cord and the terminal nerves are wrapped inside the meninges. The meninges are acting as snug blankets around these CNS structures. When the meninges are inflamed and body movement causes the nerves/spinal cord to move a minuscule bit, there is excruciating pain. The counter mechanisms like bending the hip in Brudzinki's sign applies counter traction on the cord and stops it from moving. Imagine this as 2 equally strong wrestlers pulling on a rope and it ends up not moving at all.

Laboratory Tests

The importance of getting an early lumbar puncture is emphasized by our Vital Checklist "LP Can Save The Brain"

Lab Tests for Meningitis		
Vital Checklist	Lab Test	Importance
"LP"	Lumbar Puncture	✓ CSF White cell count- 1000-5000/ microL ✓ RBC suggest a traumatic tap and the WBC count should be adjusted in this case ✓ Gram stain of the sample can point towards the etiology ✓ Various Rapid Tests are available to rule out different organisms ✓ PCR for microbe proteins can be performed. ✓ High opening pressure values suggest bacterial causes as well.
"Can"	CT Scan	Indication for delaying a LP and doing a CT first are ✓ Features of raised ICP- papilledema, Focal neuro deficit ✓ Immunocompromised- HIV ✓ H/O CNS disease ✓ Abnormal level of consciousness.
"Save"	Serum Electrolytes	Full range of electrolytes- to rule out a metabolic acidosis or hyponatremia
"The"	TLC	Total leucocyte count becomes very important and solidifies the diagnosis.
"Brain"	Blood Cultures	Two sets of blood cultures should be obtained prior to induction of antibiotics to get a full drug sensitivity and susceptibility.

Management of Meningitis

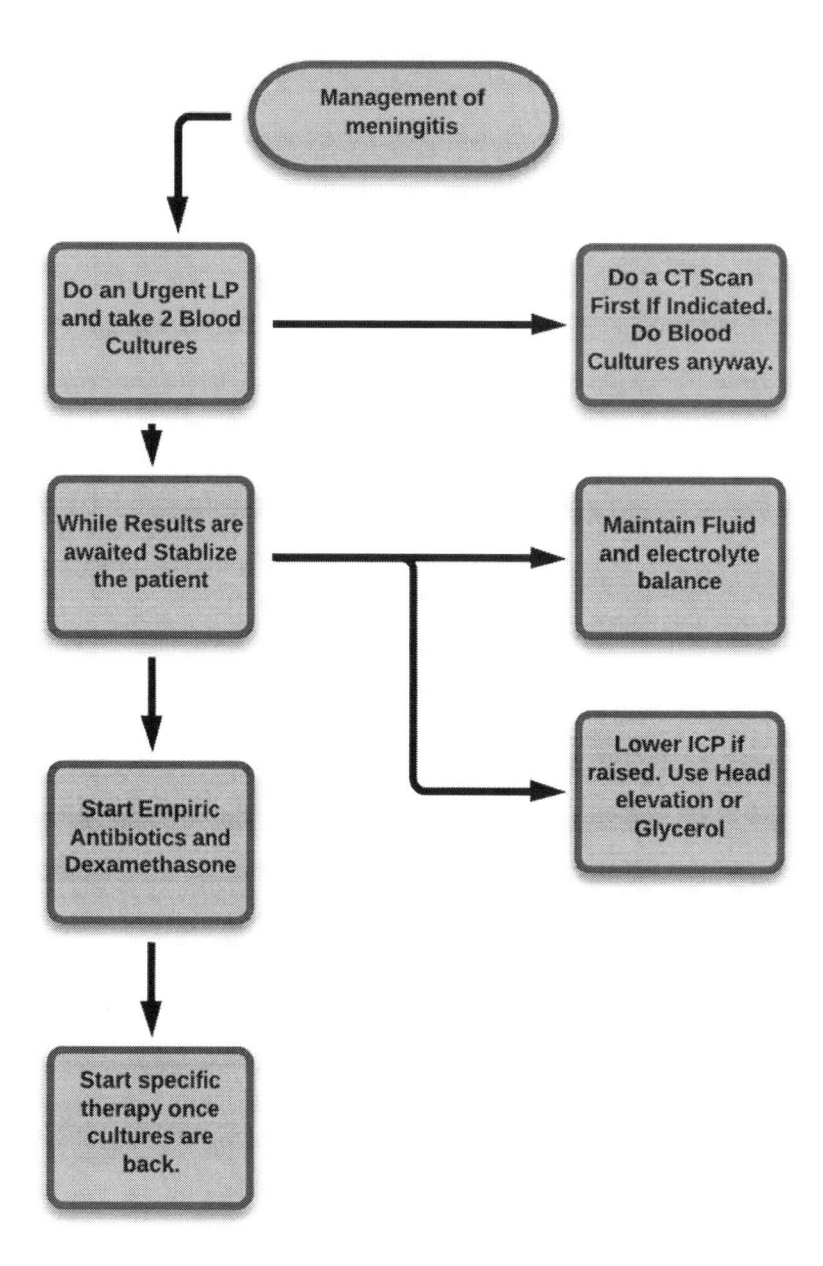

```
                    ┌─────────────────┐
                    │  Management of  │
                    │    meningitis   │
                    └─────────────────┘
                            │
                            ▼
        ┌──────────────────┐      ┌──────────────────┐
        │  Do an Urgent LP │─────▶│   Do a CT Scan   │
        │  and take 2 Blood│      │ First If Indicated.│
        │     Cultures     │      │    Do Blood      │
        └──────────────────┘      │ Cultures anyway. │
                │                 └──────────────────┘
                ▼
        ┌──────────────────┐      ┌──────────────────┐
        │ While Results are│─────▶│  Maintain Fluid  │
        │ awaited Stablize │      │  and electrolyte │
        │   the patient    │      │     balance      │
        └──────────────────┘      └──────────────────┘
                │
                │                 ┌──────────────────┐
                │                 │   Lower ICP if   │
                │────────────────▶│ raised. Use Head │
                ▼                 │   elevation or   │
        ┌──────────────────┐      │     Glycerol     │
        │   Start Empiric  │      └──────────────────┘
        │  Antibiotics and │
        │   Dexamethasone  │
        └──────────────────┘
                │
                ▼
        ┌──────────────────┐
        │  Start specific  │
        │  therapy once    │
        │   cultures are   │
        │      back.       │
        └──────────────────┘
```

The following flowchart should be used to describe management of suspected meningitis

An example of empiric therapy is Ceftriaxone + Vancomycin + Ampicillin (if patient is >50 years of age). This is a good regimen for individuals with no known immunodeficiency.

In patients with impaired cell mediated immunity, switch Ceftriaxone with Cefepime and give the other 2 drugs in the above regime with it.
In Hospital acquired meningitis, delete the ampicillin, give just the cefepime and vancomycin.

Practice Case

Now practice this case with your study partner

Notes for the Standardized Patient/Study Partner:

History:

You are a 37 year old female. You are presenting to the clinic with acute headache. You are feeling very ill, and you have a problem with loud sounds and bright lights.

Keep lying on the bed when the examinee enters. Do not move or offer your hand as a greeting.

Pretend to be agitated if the examinee switches on/brightens the light.

Medications: Tylenol and OCP

You do not have any vomiting, seizures, previous history of seizures, brain tumour.

(You can say no to other symptoms and build the rest of the details not mentioned here based on your judgment.)

Examination:

You have excruciating pain on bending your neck, and if the examinee flexes your hips, promptly bend your knees.

Challenging Questions:

"Doctor- I don't want to get a lumbar puncture! Do I need It?"

For the examinee:

DOORWAY INFORMATION:

Opening Scenario

Mrs. Anne Jones, a 37-year-old female, comes to the clinic complaining of an excruciating headache.

Vital Signs
BP: 144/86 mmHg
Temp: 102.3°F
RR: 22/minute
HR: 120/minute, regular

Examinee Tasks
1. Take a focused history.
2. Perform a focused physical exam (do not perform rectal, genitourinary, or female breast exam).
3. Explain your clinical impression and workup plan to the patient.
4. Write the patient note after leaving the room.

Now, start your stopwatch and begin the practice. Make sure you practice management of front side of blue rough sheet. Write "Patient Education Sheet" on top of the back side of the Blue rough sheet and use it during this encounter to your advantage.

After the patient encounter, practice typing your patient notes. If you do not have access to a computer immediately, then practice on the patient note sheet provided here.

Later, you can review and compare your DDx with that written by the Vital Checklist Team for this case.

Section G

Differential Diagnosis

Section G – Differential Diagnosis

Narrowing the Diagnosis

After you have taken a thorough history, sometimes you are still not sure of the diagnosis. You need to ask associated symptoms, but because of time constraints, you don't know where to start. If you don't remember the associated symptoms of all the disease processes, then you must ask review of symptoms using GHALEN and GHULAM approach as explained below.

Review of Symptoms

Skin- Remember skin is the largest organ. Ask for moles, skin cancer and scars.
Be RESPECTFUL (Signs of Inflammation)
R- Redness; ES-Excessive Swelling; P-Pain; EC-Excessive Calor; (T); FUL- Functional Loss

G	General Examination		G	Glands
H	Heart (Cardiovascular)		H	HEENT/ Hematology
A	Abdomen		U	Urogenital-Bowel and Bladder
L	Lungs		L	Lumbosacral
E	Extremities		A	Anal bleeding, Buttocks/Prostate
N	Neurological		M	Musculoskeletal-Muscles and Joints

Psychiatric-SAD
S-Sad (Depression)
A-Anxiety
D-Day time somnolence ❼ Fatigue ❼ Do you know the D/D

© 2016 Harpreet Singh MD, FACP | Vital Checklist| (iCrush)

Table: Review of Symptoms—An easy to remember and hard to forget Vital Checklist for Review of Symptoms

This GAHLEN/GHULAM approach will help you to narrow the differential diagnosis. All medical students are different and learn in a different manner. Many health caregivers learn with the aid of checklist, some with pictures, and a few learn without acronyms. We have done due diligence to show the variety of ways to narrow the differential diagnosis. This will also prevent cognitive tunneling, and you will not freeze in front of the patient during the stressful encounter.

In real practice the more associated symptoms you have, the narrower the diagnosis is and you can tailor the investigations and tests to that specific assessment. You will save healthcare dollars and your ICD-10 documentation will improve.

Some students have told us that they don't have any time to ask many questions and therefore it is important to ask relevant associated symptoms and learn these tables.

Differential Diagnosis

On the basis of ASSOCIATED SYMPTOMS

Nervous System

ASSOCIATED SYMPTOMS	DIFFERENTIAL DIAGNOSIS

Headache

ASSOCIATED SYMPTOMS	DIFFERENTIAL DIAGNOSIS
Blurring of vision	✓ Glaucoma, Giant Cell Arteritis, Migraine
Double vision	✓ SAH, Sinus venous thrombosis
Hearing Loss	✓ TMJ dysfunction, Acoustic neuroma
Tearing of eyes and rhinorrhea	✓ Cluster headache
"Worst headache of my life"	✓ Subarachnoid hemorrhage
Worse on intake of cheese, wine, chocolate or OCPs	✓ Migraine
Abnormal vision/ smell preceding headache (Aura)	✓ Migraine
Early morning headache	✓ Space Occupying lesion (Brain tumor), Raised ICP (Pseudotumor cerebri), COPD (CO_2 retention)
After the weekend/holiday (more in the afternoon)	✓ Tension type headache
Tingling and numbness in upper limbs	✓ Cervical arthritis/ spondylosis

ASSOCIATED SYMPTOMS   **DIFFERENTIAL DIAGNOSIS**

Loss of consciousness

Associated Symptoms	Differential Diagnosis
Warmth, sweating and light-headedness	✓ Vasovagal syncope, Situational syncope
LOC during cough, urination, defecation or laughter	✓ Situational syncope
LOC with jerky movements	✓ Seizures, Convulsive syncope
Loss of bowel or bladder control	✓ Seizures
Post-ictal weakness/confusion	✓ Seizures
Focal neurological deficit	✓ Stroke, TIA, Intracerebral hemorrhage

Dizziness

Associated Symptoms	Differential Diagnosis
Vertigo (spinning sensation)	✓ Inner ear pathology or central pathology
Tinnitus and hearing loss	✓ Inner ear pathology, CN VIII pathology
Worsens on lying down or rolling over in bed	✓ Benign paroxysmal positional vertigo (BPPV)
Ear fullness	✓ Meniere's disease
Sweating and LOC	✓ Vasovagal syncope, cardiac arrhythmia
Lightheadedness	✓ Cardiac arrhythmia, orthostatic hypotension
Drugs	✓ Diuretics, antihypertensive drugs
Blurring of vision/painful vision	✓ Multiple sclerosis

ASSOCIATED SYMPTOMS		DIFFERENTIAL DIAGNOSIS

Tingling and Numbness

Glove and stocking pattern	✓	Peripheral neuropathy/metabolic (diabetes mellitus)
Associated dizziness, bloating/abdominal fullness, erectile dysfunction, orthostatic hypotension	✓	Autonomic neuropathy, Diabetes mellitus
Single limb numbness and tingling	✓	Radiculopathy, multiple sclerosis
Hypopigmented rash with tingling and dumbness	✓	Leprosy
Back pain	✓	Lumbar stenosis, lumbar disc herniation, multiple myeloma
Perioral tingling	✓	Hypocalcemia, panic attack

Muscle weakness

More in the evening	✓	Myasthenia gravis
Improves by evening	✓	Lambert Eaton Syndrome
Ascending muscle paralysis	✓	Guillain-Barré Syndrome (GBS)
Descending muscle paralysis	✓	Botulism
Remitting and relapsing type	✓	Multiple sclerosis, Transverse myelitis
Hemiparesis	✓	Stroke/TIA
Restlessness with inactivity	✓	Restless leg syndrome
Muscle weakness with loss of temperature and pain sensation in the upper limbs	✓	Syringomyelia
Loss of bowel and bladder control with muscle weakness	✓	Cauda equina syndrome, GBS
Traumatic nerve injury	✓	Brown Sequard syndrome

ASSOCIATED SYMPTOMS	DIFFERENTIAL DIAGNOSIS

Tremors

Intentional tremors	✓ Essential tremors, Cerebellar tremor
Resting tremors	✓ Parkinsonism
Jaundice	✓ Alcoholic liver disease, Liver failure (Hepatic encephalopathy)
Caffeine intake	✓ Caffeine induced tremors
Shortness of breath/cough	✓ COPD, CO_2 narcosis
Abnormal gait	✓ Cerebellar disorders, Parkinson disease

Seizures

Loss of Consciousness	✓ Complex partial seizure, Generalized Tonic Clonic Seizures
No LOC	✓ Partial seizure
High fever in children (Age < 5 years)	✓ Febrile seizure
Neck rigidity with fever	✓ Meningitis, Encephalitis
H/o Alcoholism/ benzodiazepine abuse	✓ Withdrawal seizure
Illicit drug abuse	✓ Cocaine induced
Blank stare	✓ Absence seizure
Pre-seizure aura (visual/auditory/foul smell/focal neurological symptoms	✓ Encephalitis
No Postictal weakness or loss of bowel and bladder control	✓ Convulsive syncope

| ASSOCIATED SYMPTOMS | | DIFFERENTIAL DIAGNOSIS |

Confusion

Associated Symptoms		Differential Diagnosis
Vomiting and diarrhea	✓	Metabolic cause of delirium, chronic renal disease
Elderly patient	✓	Drug induced, diabetic complication, electrolyte imbalance
Muscle weakness/focal neurological signs	✓	Stroke, TIA
Post-ictal weakness	✓	Seizures
Memory loss	✓	Dementia

Memory Loss

Associated Symptoms		Differential Diagnosis
Acute onset memory loss with confusion and violent behaviour	✓	Drug induced, metabolic, infections
Rapid onset (weeks to months) with myoclonus	✓	Creutzfeldt-Jakob disease
Stepwise worsening	✓	Vascular dementia, multiple strokes, heart disease
Parkinson-like features	✓	Lewy-body dementia
Dementia, Diarrhea and Dermatitis	✓	Pellagra Vitamin B3 Deficiency
Associated change in behaviour, psychosis	✓	Pick's disease (fronto-temporal dementia)
Loss of orientation to time, place, person and situation and anosognosia	✓	Alzheimer disease
Pseudo dementia (patient complains of forgetfulness) plus depressive symptoms (DIGEST P CAPSULE)	✓	Major Depression
h/o Head injury	✓	Retrograde (old memories)/ anterograde (new memories) amnesia

ASSOCIATED SYMPTOMS **DIFFERENTIAL DIAGNOSIS**

Loss of Vision

Painful Loss of vision	✓	Glaucoma, Uveitis, keratitis, optic neuritis (Multiple sclerosis)
Painless Loss of vision	✓	Complete retinal vein occlusion (CRVO), Complete retinal artery occlusion (CRAO), Vitreous haemorrhage, retinal detachment
Tunnel vision, blurring of vision	✓	Glaucoma, MS
Photophobia (unilateral/bilateral)	✓	Uveitis, Keratitis
Eye swelling	✓	Orbital cellulitis

Hearing Loss

Ear pain and discharge	✓	Chronic Suppurative Otitis media (CSOM)/Acute Suppurative Otitis media (ASOM), Malignant otitis externa
Vertigo and tinnitus	✓	Meniere's disease, labyrinthitis, Sensory neural hearing loss (SNHL)
Ear fullness	✓	Meniere's disease
Headache/ Jaw pain	✓	TMJ dysfunction
Alcohol/NSAIDS/Loop diuretics/ Aminoglycosides/ Chemotherapy	✓	SNHL
Hearing loss to particular frequencies	✓	Presbycusis (Age related)
h/o Noise pollution, ear trauma, war/ factories	✓	Traumatic hearing loss

Cardiovascular System

ASSOCIATED SYMPTOMS   **DIFFERENTIAL DIAGNOSIS**

Chest pain

Associated Symptoms		Differential Diagnosis
Shortness of breath	✓	Myocardial Infarction (MI), Pulmonary Embolism (PE), Acute CHF, Acute exacerbation of COPD
Dizziness/Syncope	✓	Aortic stenosis, Arrhythmia, Aortic dissection
Excessive sweating	✓	MI, arrhythmia
Palpitation	✓	MI, arrhythmia, mitral or aortic regurgitation
Hemoptysis	✓	Acute PE, Mitral stenosis
Tearing pain radiating to the back	✓	Aortic dissection
Chest pain worsens on inspiration	✓	Pleuritis, pericarditis
Chest pain on pushing at costochondral junction	✓	Musculoskeletal pain (costochondritis)
Chest pain improves on bending forward	✓	Pericarditis
Fever	✓	Infective endocarditis (Other stigmata like Osler's node, Roth's spot, Janeway lesions, hematuria may also be present).
h/o Sudden deaths in family	✓	Hypertrophic Obstructive Cardiomyopathy (HOCM)

ASSOCIATED SYMPTOMS   DIFFERENTIAL DIAGNOSIS

Palpitation

Regular palpitation	✓	Panic attacks, excessive caffeine intake and hyperdynamic states like severe anemia, hyperthyroidism, wet beri beri, mitral/aortic regurgitation
Irregular palpitation	✓	Cardiac arrhythmia, HOCM, Atrial fibrillation, Atrial flutter
Dizziness/Syncope	✓	Arrhythmia
Chest pain	✓	MI, COPD
Shortness of breath	✓	Arrhythmia, MI
Tremors/weight loss/sweating	✓	Hyperthyroidism, panic attack
h/o blood loss, malnutrition	✓	Anemia
h/o drug intake	✓	Cocaine use, excessive caffeine intake
Post-palpitational diuresis	✓	Arrhythmia leading to left ventricular dysfunction and raised atrial pressures causing it to release natriuretic peptide. This leads to excretion of water and sodium.

Respiratory System

ASSOCIATED SYMPTOMS   DIFFERENTIAL DIAGNOSIS

Shortness of breath

Associated Symptoms		Differential Diagnosis
Orthopnea /Paroxysmal Nocturnal dyspnea (PND)	✓	Cardiac cause of shortness of breath (Left ventricular failure, cardiogenic pulmonary edema)
Chest pain	✓	Veno-Thromboembolism (VTE), COPD, MI, Acute MR, pleuritis
Leg pain	✓	VTE
Wheezing	✓	Asthma, COPD, exercise induced asthma, heart failure
Sneezing, Post-nasal drip, rhinorrhea, nasal stuffiness	✓	URI, Allergic rhinitis, flu, sinusitis
Cough	✓	Bronchitis, Asthma, COPD, Heart failure, Sinusitis
Fever	✓	Pneumonia, Bronchitis
Weight loss	✓	Tuberculosis, Lung cancer, COPD
Phlegm	✓	Chronic bronchitis (teaspoonful), Bronchiectasis (cupful), heart failure (Pink frothy), Aspergillosis (black colored)
Hemoptysis	✓	Tuberculosis, cancer, Aspergillosis, Pulmonary embolism, Mitral stenosis, AV fistula

ASSOCIATED SYMPTOMS   **DIFFERENTIAL DIAGNOSIS**

Sore throat

Associated Symptoms		Differential Diagnosis
Fever, myalgia, cough, nasal stuffiness	✓	Flu
Skin rash, joint ache, hematuria	✓	Streptococcal pharyngitis
Ulcers in the throat	✓	Coxsackie virus infection/Herpangia
Loss of appetite	✓	Infectious mononucleosis, Acute HIV
Dysphagia, change in voice, fever	✓	Retropharyngeal abscess
Acid reflux, cough, halitosis	✓	GERD, Zenker's diverticulum

Snoring

Associated Symptoms		Differential Diagnosis
Weight gain, cold intolerance, dry skin or constipation	✓	Hypothyroidism
Excessive daytime symptoms	✓	Obstructive Sleep apnea (OSA)
Excessive daytime symptoms, change in voice and dysphagia	✓	Central sleep apnea/bulbar palsy
h/o Recurrent tonsillitis	✓	Adenoid/tonsillar hypertrophy
Shortness of breath	✓	Secondary pulmonary hypertension due to Chronic OSA

Gastrointestinal System

ASSOCIATED SYMPTOMS	DIFFERENTIAL DIAGNOSIS

Abdominal pain

Associated Symptoms	Differential Diagnosis
Nausea/vomiting	✓ Pancreatitis, Gastroenteritis, Acute appendicitis, Acute bowel obstruction.
Hematemesis	✓ Peptic Ulcer, Esophageal Varices
Diarrhea	✓ Gastroenteritis, Carcinoid Syndrome, Lactose Intolerance
Bloody Diarrhea	✓ Intussusception, Acute mesenteric ischemia, Shigella/Yersinia/Campylobacter/Salmonella/ Hemorrhagic E.coli infection
Weight loss	✓ Malabsorption, GI Malignancy, Mesenteric Ischemia, Gastric Ulcer, Pancreatitis.
Increases with food intake, increases with fatty food	✓ Gallstones, Pancreatitis, Gastric Ulcer, Mesenteric ischemia.
Decreases with food intake	✓ Duodenal Ulcer
Radiates to the back	✓ Pancreatitis, Duodenal Ulcer, Abdominal Aortic Aneurysm, Hodgkin's Lymphoma, Pyelonephritis, Renal Cell carcinoma
Loud Bowel Sounds	✓ Small Bowel Disease, Partial obstruction, Enteric Fever, Malabsorption
Bleeding PV, Menstrual Problems	✓ Ectopic Pregnancy, PID, Endometriosis
Painful Defection	✓ Rectal disorder, Proctalgia fugax

ASSOCIATED SYMPTOMS	DIFFERENTIAL DIAGNOSIS

Dysphagia

Eating solids and liquids	✓ Achalasia
Eating solids>liquids	✓ Mechanical obstruction: Esophageal Cancer, Schatzki ring , Plummer-Vinson Syndrome
GERD	✓ Zenker's Diverticulum, Schatzki ring, Scleroderma, CREST syndrome, Barret's Esophagus
Weight loss	✓ ALS, Esophageal Cancer
Change of voice	✓ Zenker's Diverticulum, Schatzki Ring
Brainstem Lesions	✓ CSA, ALS

Weight Loss

h/o laxative abuse, diet pills, excessive exercising, restricted eating habits	✓ Anorexia Nervosa
Night sweats	✓ TB, Cancer
Palpitations, sweating, cold/heat intolerance	✓ Hyperthyroidism
Flushing, Hypertension, palpitations	✓ Pheochromocytoma
Polyuria, polydipsia	✓ DM
Abdominal Pain	✓ Malabsorption, GI Malignancy, Mesenteric Ischemia, Gastric Ulcer, Pancreatitis

ASSOCIATED SYMPTOMS & DIFFERENTIAL DIAGNOSIS

Vomiting

Associated Symptoms	Differential Diagnosis
H/o nausea	✓ Gastroenteritis, Pregnancy, Chemotherapy, Intestinal Obstruction
No H/o nausea	✓ Increased Intra-cranial pressure
Abdominal pain	✓ Gastroenteritis, Intestinal Obstruction, Malabsorption, GI malignancy, Pancreatitis, Appendicitis, Cholecystitis.
Weight loss	✓ Gastric Ulcer, Mesenteric Ischemia, Obstruction, GI Malignancy
Dysphagia	✓ Zenker's Diverticulum, Esophageal obstruction (Achalasia, Malignancy, Schatzki Ring, PVS)
Diarrhea	✓ Gastroenteritis, Malabsorption

Diarrhea

Associated Symptoms	Differential Diagnosis
Fever, Bloody diarrhea	✓ Bacterial Enteritis (Campylobacter species, EHEC, Salmonella, Shigella, Entamoeba histolytica)
H/o recent antibiotic use	✓ Clostridium difficile infection
H/o Diarrhea alternating with constipation	✓ IBS
Malabsorption, rash, arthritis	✓ Celiac disease, IBD
H/o travel to an endemic area	✓ Enterotoxigenic E. Coli, Giardiasis
H/o mucus with blood, vomiting	✓ C.difficile infection,
Crampy abdominal pain	✓ Campylobacter infection
H/o step-ladder fever, chills, weakness	✓ Salmonella infection
Flushing, wheezing	✓ VIPoma, Carcinoid syndrome
Laxative abuse, weight loss	✓ Anorexia nervosa

ASSOCIATED SYMPTOMS	DIFFERENTIAL DIAGNOSIS

Jaundice

Associated Symptoms	Differential Diagnosis
Itching	✓ Gallstones, Pancreatic Cancer
H/o travel to an endemic area	✓ Hepatitis A, Hepatitis E
Pregnancy	✓ Intrahepatic Cholestasis of Pregnancy
H/o drugs	✓ OCPs, Amiodarone, Methyldopa, Halothane, Isoniazid, Chlorpromazine, Anabolic steroids
H/o hair loss, alcohol, sleep disturbances, testicular atrophy, spider nevi	✓ Liver cirrhosis, Liver Failure, Hepatic Carcinoma
Non-specific symptoms	✓ Auto-immune Hepatitis

Bloody Vomiting

Associated Symptoms	Differential Diagnosis
Nausea, black stools, feeling of fullness after meals	✓ Gastritis
Abdominal pain, light headedness, melena	✓ Esophageal varices
Loss of appetite, epistaxis, jaundice, weight loss, ascites, edema	✓ Cirrhosis
Abdominal pain, retching, fatigue, weight loss	✓ GI Cancer (stomach/esophageal)
Abdominal pain, bloating, decrease in pain after meals	✓ Duodenal Ulcer
Abdominal pain, weight loss, appetite changes, chest pain	✓ Peptic Ulcer
Abdominal pain, easy bruising, jaundice, weight loss	✓ Liver cancer
Dysphagia, sore throat, hoarseness of voice, abdominal pain, heartburn	✓ Esophagitis

ASSOCIATED SYMPTOMS   **DIFFERENTIAL DIAGNOSIS**

Bloody Stools

Black colored stools (Melena)	✓	GE varices, Mallory-Weiss syndrome, Gastritis, Bleeding gastric ulcer, Trauma
Mucus and abdominal pain	✓	C.difficile infection
Malabsorption, bloody diarrhea, arthritis, uveitis, skin rash, weight loss	✓	IBD
Severe abdominal pain	✓	Mesenteric ischemia
Painful defecation with streaks of blood on stool	✓	Anal fissure
Painless fresh blood	✓	Diverticulosis, hemorrhoids, IBD, Intestinal infection

Fatigue with Pallor

Blood Loss	✓	Anemia, GI bleed (Upper/Lower)
Weight gain	✓	Hypothyroidism, muscle weakness, chronic fatigue syndrome, Depression
Weakness	✓	Anemia, fibromyalgia, Hep C/Hep B

Endocrine System

| ASSOCIATED SYMPTOMS | DIFFERENTIAL DIAGNOSIS |

Polyuria

Increased hunger, increased thirst, weight loss, visual changes	✓ Diabetes Mellitus
Headaches	✓ Pituitary tumor
Head injury	✓ Diabetes Insipidus
H/o drugs intake	✓ Diuretics, Demeclocycline, caffeine, water pills, ethanol, lithium
Excessive water ingestion	✓ Primary polydipsia
Increased frequency, painful urination	✓ UTI
H/o hesitancy	✓ BPH

Weight gain

Excessive eating, inactivity	✓ Overeating, immobility
Heat/cold intolerance, weakness, rough/dry skin, constipation, decreased libido	✓ Hypothyroidism
H/o sadness, stress, sleep disturbances, loss of interest, suicidal thoughts	✓ Depression
Moonface, fat around neck(buffalo's hump), purple/pink striae around abdomen	✓ Cushing's syndrome
Headache, lethargy, diplopia, blurred vision	✓ Insulinoma
Menstrual changes, hirsutism, infertility, acne	✓ PCOS
Missed periods, morning sickness	✓ Pregnancy

ASSOCIATED SYMPTOMS   DIFFERENTIAL DIAGNOSIS

Neck Mass

Associated Symptoms	Differential Diagnosis
Heat/cold intolerance, weight gain, dry skin	✓ Hypothyroidism
Weight loss, palpitations, exophthalmos, tremors	✓ Hyperthyroidism, Grave's Disease
Weight loss	✓ Cancer, Lymphoma, HIV, TB
Chronic cough, lymphadenopathy, weight loss	✓ TB
Draining sinuses, mass moves with swallowing	✓ Thyroglossal cyst, branchial cyst
Difficulty breathing/eating	✓ Retrosternal thyroid
H/o hoarseness of voice, weight loss	✓ Cancer
Difficulty in neck movement, abnormal neck movement	✓ Torticollis (TIP: Always do an X-Ray to rule out TB)
Halitosis, h/o undigested food on pillow in the morning	✓ Zenker's diverticulum

Musculoskeletal System

| ASSOCIATED SYMPTOMS | DIFFERENTIAL DIAGNOSIS |

Knee Pain

Associated Symptoms	Differential Diagnosis
Pain in the evening, crepitus, bony enlargement	✓ Osteoarthritis
H/o early morning stiffness lasting >1 hr, stiffness in PIP and MCP joints	✓ Rheumatoid arthritis
Worsened on going down the stairs	✓ Meniscal injury
Redness of joint, chills and fever, recent h/o flu, GI infection	✓ Septic arthritis
H/o accident/fall, Swelling, immobility/difficulty in movement	✓ Trauma, Fracture, dislocation
Playing sports like football and basketball	✓ Jumper's knee - Tendonitis
H/o kneeling for long time, sweeping floors while sitting	✓ Bursitis

Ankle pain

Associated Symptoms	Differential Diagnosis
Early morning pain on standing up, after resting	✓ Plantar fasciitis
H/o accident, trauma, fall, twisting, swelling, bruising	✓ Sprain, Calcaneal fracture
Old age, morning stiffness, crepitus, bony enlargement	✓ Osteoarthritis
Medial side pain	✓ Bony spur
Increases on squeezing calves	✓ Achilles tendon rupture
H/o fever, swelling, injury, long standing, excessive movement	✓ Tenosinovitis

ASSOCIATED SYMPTOMS		DIFFERENTIAL DIAGNOSIS

Elbow pain

Associated Symptoms		Differential Diagnosis
H/o fall, swelling, bruising, difficulty moving	✓	Injury, trauma, dislocation, fracture, olecranon bursitis (pain at tip of elbow)
Fever, swelling, inflammation post abrasion	✓	Cellulitis
Worsened with shaking hands, opening jars, door knobs, playing golf/tennis	✓	Tennis elbow (lateral), Golfer's elbow (medial) - synovitis

Shoulder pain

Associated Symptoms		Differential Diagnosis
Stiffness, swelling, difficulty moving	✓	Frozen shoulder, Arthritis (osteo and rheumatoid)
H/o fall, swelling, immobility	✓	Trauma, fracture, dislocation
Pain on lifting arm above head, on combing hair, reaching behind the back	✓	Rotator cuff injury
Headache, jaw pain, scalp tenderness, Giant Cell Arteritis	✓	Polymyalgia Rheumatica
Neck pain, stiffness, dizziness	✓	Whiplash injury
Fever, redness, swelling	✓	Septic arthritis
Numbness and tingling on medial side of arm and forearm	✓	Thoracic outlet syndrome

ASSOCIATED SYMPTOMS		DIFFERENTIAL DIAGNOSIS

Back pain

Excessive exercising, accident, fall	✓	Trauma, muscle sprain
Fever, tenderness	✓	TB
Decreases with cycling, bending forward	✓	Spinal stenosis
Bowel and bladder incontinence	✓	Cauda Equina Syndrome
Increases with extending the back	✓	Disc herniation
BPH, old age, urgency, frequency	✓	Prostate cancer mets to spine
Swelling, fever	✓	Abscess

Urology and Reproductive System

ASSOCIATED SYMPTOMS   DIFFERENTIAL DIAGNOSIS

Bloody Urine

Associated Symptoms	Differential Diagnosis
Urgency, frequency, burning	✓ UTI, stones, BPH
Fever	✓ Pyelonephritis, cystitis
Flank pain	✓ Pyelonephritis, stones
Difficulty urination	✓ BPH, Cystitis
Fever, sore throat, microscopic hematuria	✓ Glomerulonephritis, IgA nephropathy, Strep infection, Diabetic, Viral
Weight loss, smoking	✓ Transitional cell carcinoma, Kidney cancer, prostate cancer
Hemoglobinuria	✓ Sickle cell anemia, Alport syndrome
H/o blow/injury	✓ Accident, injury to kidney, contact sports
H/o drug intake	✓ Cyclophosphamide, Penicillin, Rifampin, Heparin, Aspirin
Myoglobinuria	✓ Excessive exercise, Trauma, Burns
Consumption of beetroot	✓ Diet related
Rashes, bruises	✓ HUS, ITP, HSP

Burning Urination

Associated Symptoms	Differential Diagnosis
Urgency, vaginal discharge	✓ STD (Chlamydia, gonorrhea), Bacterial infection of Urinary tract, Cystitis
Hematuria	✓ Bladder Cancer, UTI, Stones
Dysuria, frequency, urgency	✓ UTI, Stones, Cystitis
Dysuria, old age, incomplete voiding	✓ BPH

ASSOCIATED SYMPTOMS   **DIFFERENTIAL DIAGNOSIS**

Incontinence

Associated Symptoms		Differential Diagnosis
Flank pain	✓	Stone, UTI
Lower abdominal pain, urgency, frequency	✓	Cystitis, UTI
Amenorrhea	✓	Pregnancy
Old age	✓	Normal phenomenon due to muscle weakness, menopause, BPH
Hemiplegia	✓	Stroke
Bradykinesia, tremors, rigidity	✓	Parkinson's disease
Headache	✓	Brain tumor
H/o accident, back pain	✓	Spinal injury
Weight loss, urgency, frequency, dysuria	✓	Prostate Carcinoma
Polyuria, polydipsia	✓	Diabetes
Low back pain, feeling of fullness in lower abdomen, dysuria	✓	Uterine Prolapse
Diet	✓	Alcohol, caffeine, spicy food, corn syrup, carbonated drinks

ASSOCIATED SYMPTOMS   DIFFERENTIAL DIAGNOSIS

Lower Abdominal Pain

Associated Symptoms	Differential Diagnosis
Infrequent bowel movements, hard stools, bloating	✓ Constipation
Nausea, vomiting, fever	✓ Gastroenteritis, appendicitis, diverticulitis
2 weeks after LMP	✓ Ovulation pain
Irregular periods/spotty, nausea, vomiting	✓ Ovarian cyst
Dysuria, frequency, urgency, hematuria	✓ Kidney infection, kidney stones
Missed periods, spotting	✓ Ectopic pregnancy
Coinciding with menses	✓ Dysmenorrhea, endometriosis

Pregnancy

Associated Symptoms	Differential Diagnosis
Increased nausea, vomiting	✓ Hyperemesis Gravidarum, morning sickness
Spotting	✓ Miscarriage (threatened abortion/complete abortion)
Passage of vesicular mass per vagina	✓ Gestational Trophoblastic Neoplasia, Molar pregnancy
Spotting, severe abdominal pain	✓ Ectopic pregnancy
H/o multiple miscarriages	✓ APLA syndrome, other autoimmune diseases
High blood sugar	✓ GDM
High BP	✓ Hypertension, Gestational Hypertension

ASSOCIATED SYMPTOMS	DIFFERENTIAL DIAGNOSIS

Inability to conceive

Headache, milky discharge from nipples, vision changes	✓ Pituitary tumor (prolactinoma)
Weight gain, fatigue, cold/heat intolerance, amenorrhea	✓ Hypothyroidism
H/o long duration of drugs intake	✓ OCPs, Norplant
No h/o menses	✓ Genetic diseases (Turner's syndrome), imperforate hymen, Androgen insensitivity syndrome, 5-alpha reductase deficiency
Irregular menses, hirsutism, weight gain, acne	✓ PCOS
Abdominal pain, h/o chlamydia/gonorrhea infection	✓ PID

Erectile Dysfunction

Smoking	✓ PVD, Leriche's syndrome
Polydypsia, polyuria, polyphagia	✓ DM
Increased BP	✓ CVS, HTN, stroke
Tremors, bradykinesia, rigidity	✓ Parkinson's disease
Headaches, nipple discharge	✓ Pituitary tumor (prolactinoma)
Difficulty in getting an erection, painful erection	✓ Peyronie's disease, Penile fracture, cavernous fibrosis
H/o Drug intake	✓ Anabolic steroids (hypogonadism), antihypertensives, antipsychotics, antidepressants.
Neurological disease	✓ Spinal cord lesions, brain stem lesions, MS

| ASSOCIATED SYMPTOMS | DIFFERENTIAL DIAGNOSIS |

Vaginal Bleeding

H/o previous amenorrhea, abdominal pain	✓ Miscarriage, ectopic pregnancy
H/o LMP 2 weeks ago	✓ mid-cycle ovulation bleeding
H/o irregular menses, hirsutism, acne, weight gain	✓ PCOS
H/o bleeding after intercourse, douching	✓ PID
Excessive bleeding during menses	✓ Uterine fibroids
H/o uterine prolapse or polyp	✓ Carcinoma cervix, uterine, vagina
Post-menopausal	✓ Vaginal atrophy, cancer, polyps, endometrial hyperplasia, post-menopausal hormonal therapy

Pain during sex (Dyspareunia)

Old age	✓ Vaginal atrophy
H/o surgery, trauma	✓ Child birth, pelvic surgery, sexual abuse
H/o spasm	✓ Vaginismus
Amenorrhea	✓ Imperforate hymen, vaginal agenesis
Dysmenorrhea	✓ Endometriosis, uterine fibroids
Stress, depression, anxiety	✓ Psychological factors
H/o skin diseases	✓ Eczema
H/o drugs	✓ Antidepressants, anti-hypertensive drugs, antihistamines, OCPs

Psychiatry

ASSOCIATED SYMPTOMS   DIFFERENTIAL DIAGNOSIS

Depressed mood

ASSOCIATED SYMPTOMS	DIFFERENTIAL DIAGNOSIS
Dry skin, constipation	✓ Hypothyroidism
Changes in sleep, appetite, weight, death/suicidal ideation	✓ Major Depressive disorder
Depressed mood <2 months after the death of a loved one	✓ Normal Bereavement
Depressed mood with irritability, anxiety, appetite changes, breast tenderness, joint swelling/bloating weight gain	✓ PMS
Depressed mood with alternating mood to mania characterized by grandiosity, flight of ideas and increased activity	✓ Bipolar disorder
Mood swings from mild depression to emotional highs for more than 2 years	✓ Cyclothymia
Depressed mood for at least 2 years in adults and 1 year in adolescents and children, poor appetite and concentration, feeling of helplessness Transient euthymic episodes of up to 2 months during the course if dysthymia	✓ Dysthymia

ASSOCIATED SYMPTOMS	DIFFERENTIAL DIAGNOSIS
Hallucinations	

Anxiety, suspiciousness, social withdrawal, ongoing unusual thoughts and beliefs	✓ Psychosis
Behavioral symptoms like flattened affect, catatonia, violent behaviour, positive or negative symptoms	✓ Schizophrenia
Excessive alcohol intake, anxiety, agitation, irritability, delirium, delusions, nightmares, restlessness	✓ Delirium tremens
Throbbing, pulsating headaches with nausea, vomiting, extreme sensitivity to light	✓ Migraines
Fluctuations in cognition, attention, alertness, behavioral and mood symptoms, impaired thinking	✓ Lewy Body Dementia
Increased appetite, difficulty solving problems, decreased coordination and concentration, insomnia, irritability, anxiety	✓ Marijuana abuse
Excessive daytime drowsiness, sudden loss of muscle tone, sleep paralysis	✓ Narcolepsy
Jerky movements, tingling, dizziness, loss of consciousness, biting the tongue, loss of bladder and bowel control	✓ Seizure disorder

ASSOCIATED SYMPTOMS		DIFFERENTIAL DIAGNOSIS

Insomnia

Associated Symptoms		Differential Diagnosis
Snoring with excessive day time sleepiness	✓	Sleep apnea
Sleep paralysis, hypnagogic and hypnopompic hallucinations (Gogic-Go to bed) (Pomp and show when you get up or waking up)	✓	Narcolepsy
H/o Alcohol/Drug abuse, depressed mood, withdrawal symptoms	✓	Substance abuse
Fatigue, dehydration/malaise, headache, indigestion, lack of concentration, irritability, muscle pain, recent travel from different time zone	✓	Jet Lag
Exophthalmos, palpitations, weight loss, excessive sweating, heat intolerance	✓	Hyperthyroidism
Irresistible urge to move the legs, leg cramps, restlessness, uncomfortable tingling and burning	✓	Restless leg syndrome
Excessive day time sleepiness, unintended dozing, impaired mental acuity, irritability, reduced performance and accident proneness	✓	Shift work sleep disorder

ASSOCIATED SYMPTOMS   DIFFERENTIAL DIAGNOSIS

Anxiety

Associated Symptoms	Differential Diagnosis
Restlessness, fatigue, concentration problems, irritability, muscle tension, sleep disturbances	✓ Generalized Anxiety Disorder (GAD)
Fear triggered by specific stimulus or situation (e.g. heights, fire or insects etc.)	✓ Specific phobias
Intense fear and avoidance of negative public scrutiny, public embarrassment, humiliation /social interaction	✓ Social phobias/Anxiety
Trembling, shaking, confusion, dizziness, nausea/difficulty breathing, chest tightness, feeling of impending doom.	✓ Panic disorder
Obsessive thoughts followed by certain behaviors to relieve anxiety (Obsessions and Compulsions) Patients knows it is not right and has trouble dealing with it. (Ego dystonic)	✓ Obsessive Compulsive Disorder (OCD)
Following certain behaviors because the person feels that is the right way or the only way to do it. (Obsessions and Compulsions) Patients feels that he is absolutely normal (Ego syntonic). Usually complaints are from other people who get annoyed by their behaviors	✓ Obsessive Compulsive Personality Disorder (OCPD)
Flashbacks, nightmares, sleep disturbances, aggression, agitation, anger, general discontent, guilt, hopelessness. H/o of trauma, sexual assault or obnoxious insult in the past.	✓ Post-Traumatic Stress Disorder ✓ (PTSD)

Pediatrics

ASSOCIATED SYMPTOMS   **DIFFERENTIAL DIAGNOSIS**

Dehydration

Associated Symptoms	Differential Diagnosis
Nausea, vomiting	✓ Gastroenteritis, Intussusception, Meckel's Diverticulum
Diarrhea	✓ Gastroenteritis (Viral/bacterial), Celiac disease (Malabsorption), Inflammatory Bowel disease, IBS
Polyuria, polydipsia, weight loss	✓ DM/DI, DKA
Excessive sweating in hot weather	✓ Hyperthermia/electrolyte disturbances

Wheezing

Associated Symptoms	Differential Diagnosis
SOB, chest tightness, cough, getting worsened by particular season/allergies	✓ Asthma
Hives, itching, feeling of warmth, weak rapid pulse, nausea, vomiting, diarrhea, dizziness/fainting	✓ Anaphylaxis
Runny and stuffy nose, cough, slight fever, difficulty breathing	✓ Bronchiolitis, cold (allergies)
Fever, chills, cough, chest pain, SOB, fatigue, nausea, vomiting, diarrhea	✓ Pneumonia
Congested/runny nose, dry cough, low grade fever, sore throat, mild headache. In severe cases, it can lead to a lower respiratory tract illness, cyanosis, severe cough and difficult breathing	✓ RSV or Bronchiolitis or Pneumonia
Atypical crying/irritability, apnea, failure to thrive (poor appetite), sore throat, recurrent pneumonitis	✓ Pediatric GERD

ASSOCIATED SYMPTOMS **DIFFERENTIAL DIAGNOSIS**

Seizures

Associated Symptoms		Differential Diagnosis
High fever	✓	Febrile seizures
Jerky movements of the body with incontinence of urine and stools	✓	Generalized Tonic Clonic Seizures
Blank staring	✓	Absence seizures
Headache, neck stiffness, fever	✓	Meningitis
Diarrhea	✓	Electrolyte disturbances

Enuresis

Associated Symptoms		Differential Diagnosis
Excessive thirst, urination, dehydration, high blood sugar	✓	DM, DI
Burning micturition	✓	UTI
Incontinence with recurrent UTIs	✓	Vesicoureteral reflux
Nerve damage	✓	Spina-bifida
Unfamiliar social situations, angry parents, overwhelming family events such as the birth of a brother/sister	✓	Anxiety

ASSOCIATED SYMPTOMS	**DIFFERENTIAL DIAGNOSIS**

Fever

Cough, SOB, Chest pain	✓ Pneumonia
Headache, neck stiffness, nausea, vomiting, chills	✓ Meningitis, brain abscess
Runny nose, sore throat, malaise, rash	✓ Viral infections
Diarrhea, poor appetite, dehydration	✓ Viral/bacterial gastroenteritis
Stridor, sore throat, difficult and painful swallowing, drooling and anxiety	✓ Epiglottitis
Bone pain, nausea, vomiting	✓ Osteomyelitis
Burning micturition, polyuria, bloody urine	✓ UTI, Renal stones
Joint pain	✓ Septic arthritis, JRA

Section H

Approach to Investigations

Section H - Approach to Investigations

Investigations are done for screening a disease, diagnosing a disease, confirming a diagnosis and monitoring treatment response.

Remembering the Hippocrates dictum: Do No Harm, therefore follow three golden rules when ordering investigations.

1. *DO NO HARM TO PATIENTS' HEALTH*
2. *DO NO HARM TO PATIENTS' WEALTH*
3. *DO NO HARM TO PATIENTS' PEACE OF MIND*

What investigations to do?
How will the test be done?
Why are you ordering this investigation.

S.N	WHAT	WHY	HOW
1.	**CBC (Complete blood counts)**	To check for haemoglobin that carries oxygen. Low haemoglobin signifies anemia. To check the level of different cells in the blood. WBC—Infections Platelet – Bleeding disorders	Usually by inserting a needle into the vein of the arm and withdrawing blood, collecting it in a blood vial and sending to lab for the test.
2.	**Iron studies**	Iron level Iron saturation TIBC Ferritin Anemic patient or hemochromatosis	Usually by inserting a needle into the vein of the arm and withdrawing blood, collecting it in a blood vial and sending to lab for the test.
3.	**Liver function test**	To see whether liver is functioning Liver cell damage Any obstruction in the bile duct	Usually by inserting a needle into the vein of the arm and withdrawing blood, collecting it in a blood vial and sending to lab for the test.
4.	**Kidney function test**	To see the kidney is damaged due to the poor perfusion from the heart or it is an intrinsic damage to the kidney	Usually by inserting a needle into the vein of the arm and withdrawing blood, collecting it in a blood vial and sending to lab for the test.
5.	**Thyroid function test**	This test is used to see thyroid hormonal levels, it is important for diagnosis and management of thyroid diseases: To see if the thyroid is under functioning or over functioning. To evaluate if the thyroid is being attacked by autoantibodies	Usually by inserting a needle into the vein of the arm and withdrawing blood, collecting it in a blood vial and sending to lab for the test. Fasting state
6.	**Lipid profile**	This test is done to assess the good and bad cholesterol, levels of fat molecules in blood	Same as above in fasting state

7.	**MRI**	This test uses radio waves in the magnetic fields to create an image of our internal body organs. Our body is composed of 70% H_2O. When human body is placed in the magnetic field, all water molecules line up and they emit small minuscule of energy which is transmitted as radio waves and captured by the computer. The images are displayed as thin slices.	In this test patient is made to lie in a hollow tube machine in which pictures are taken. These machines produce sound which can be disturbing sometimes. *use caution in patients with claustrophobia
8.	**X-ray**	In this test X-ray beam enters the body and different parts of body absorb X-rays and image is recorded on a plate depending on tissue density that helps in diagnosing diseases.	In this test patient can be in standing or lying or in sitting position. It involves radiation exposure and is non-invasive and takes little time
9.	**CT scan (Computed Tomography)**	In this test X-rays enters the body at different angles and the image is produced is in form of cross sections and provide 3D view of the internal structure of the body.	In this test the patient is made to lie on a narrow table which slides into a scanner and then using X-rays pictures in form of thin slices are taken of the body organs to see for bleeding, abnormal growths etc. It is superior to X rays as it provides more details about the abnormal structure and better location.
10.	**PET scan (Positron Emission Tomography)**	In this test, radioactive tracers are injected into the body.	In this test the patient is asked to lie on a narrow table which slides into a CT/MRI scanner and a radioactive tracer is injected through the vein which is taken up by various tissues of the body and then the function of the tissue can be evaluated based on images produces.

11.	**USG (Ultrasoundgraphy)**	In this test high frequency sound waves are used to produce images of the internal body organs.	In this test a transducer is kept on the patients' body surface which sends sound waves into the body tissue and these waves bounce off the structures in the body tissues which are then reflected back to the transducer which coverts these signals into images. It involves no radiation exposure.
12.	**ECG/EKG (Electrocardiogram)**	In this test the movement of electrical current through the heart and heart muscle during the heartbeat is traced on a paper and it helps detect any abnormality in the heart's rate, conduction pathways and rhythm.	In a standard 12 lead ECG the electrodes (round sensors that stick to skin) are placed on the patient's skin over the chest, arms and legs. These electrodes are connected to a machine which measures the electrical activity of the heart and produces an amplified tracing on a paper.
13.	**EEG (Electroenchephalography)**	In this procedure the brain's electrical activity is recorded as wave patterns using electrodes and helps detect any abnormal electrical activity especially in seizure and helps distinguish the origin of seizure in part of brain.	In this procedure the electrodes (round sensors that stick to skin) are placed on the patient's skin over the scalp and connected by wires to a machine which produce a tracing of small changes in voltage detected by electrodes.
14.	**Autoimmune panel (ANA, Anti-Ro, La, Anti-TPO)**	In these tests levels of auto antibodies are checked in the blood; these are cells of the immune system which have malfunctioned and these cells attack the body's own cells as if they are foreign to the body.	Same as for CBC

15.	**EMG (Electromyogram)**	In this test the electrical activities of the muscle is detected at rest and while the muscle is in contraction. It helps to detect problems of the muscle at the level of muscle or nerve supply to the muscle or spinal root level.	In this test small needles are inserted into the muscle to record its electrical activity and specific patterns (tracings) are produced in specific disorders of muscle and nerves.
16.	**Nerve conduction test**	In this test we measure the speed at which motor or sensory nerves conduct impulses. This test helps to distinguish disorder at the level of peripheral nerve or neuro muscularjunction.	In this test several electrodes are placed on the surface of skin or several small needles inserted along the pathway of nerves and the speed of nerve conduction is calculated.
17.	**Contrast enhanced CT/MRI**	In this test a dye is used to illuminate the organ of interest and also the abnormalities e.g abscesses become well defined and are easier to see than in plain	Dye is injected into the vein of arm which is taken up by tissue of interest in few minutes and then a CT or MRI is done which called as contrast enhanced MRI/CT.
18.	**Basic metabolic panel**	In this test we measure the levels of electrolyte e.g. sodium, potassium , calcium in the body which helps us to know body function at the cellular level as these levels are tightly maintained for normal tissue function.	Usually by inserting a needle into the vein of the arm and withdrawing blood, collecting it in a blood vial and sending to lab for the test.
19.	**HbA1c**	In this test we measure the average glucose concentration attached to the haemoglobin molecule across the life span of RBC that is approximately 120 days.	Usually by inserting a needle into the vein of the arm and withdrawing blood, collecting it in a blood vial and sending to lab for the test.
20.	**Coagulation studies**	In this test we measure the markers responsible for maintaining blood clotting mechanism and thickness of the blood	Usually by inserting a needle into the vein of the arm and withdrawing blood, collecting it in a blood vial and sending to lab for the test.

21.	**Stool tests**	In this test stool sample is examined under microscope for cysts and ova of parasitic worms as well as to measure fat content of stool in case of malabsorption.	Stool sample is collected in a sterile container and sent to lab for test.
22.	**Urine routine and microscopy**	In this test urine is examined under microscope for abnormal cells like pus cell or red cells or WBC's. Also enzymatic reactions are done to detect infection and bacterial activity.	In this test mid-stream urine sample is collected in a sterile container and sent to the lab.
23.	**Blood/Urine/ Sputum/CSF culture**	In this test the particular sample is cultured in a suitable medium to increase the activity of the particular infective organism present in the blood or urine or other tissue fluid.	Appropriate sample is collected in a sterile container and sent to the lab for the test.
24.	**D-Dimer**	In this test we measure the substance that is released when a blood clot breaks up. This test is done in case of pulmonary embolism, DVT.	Usually by inserting a needle into the vein of the arm and withdrawing blood, collecting it in a blood vial and sending to lab for the test.
25.	**Diagnostic peritoneal lavage (DPL)**	In this test we can detect the present of blood within the abdominal cavity especially in patients with suspected abdominal injury and are unstable or free fluid can be taken, sent to the lab for testing for infection or malignant cells	In this test a needle is inserted in the abdominal cavity and fluid aspirated it could be clear or blood colored; sample is sent for examination.

26.	**ABG**	In this test the blood levels of oxygen, CO_2, pH and bicarbonate are measured to determine the level of blood gases from the artery. It also helps to show how well the lung and kidney are functioning in maintaining the acid base levels of the body as well as the gas exchange in the lungs.	Usually by inserting a needle into the artery of the arm/wrist radial artery commonly and withdrawing blood, collecting it in a blood vial and sending to lab for the test.
27.	**Serum Lactate**	Lactic acid is normally produced by muscle cells and RBC. When the oxygen supply is low to the tissues they undergo anaerobic metabolism to produce lactate. An imbalance in the production and clearance of lactic acid can increase these levels e.g. in liver dysfunction.	Usually by inserting a needle into the vein/artery of the arm and withdrawing blood, collecting it in a blood vial and sending to lab for the test.
28.	**Endoscopy/ Colonoscopy/ Sigmoidoscopy/Anoscopy**	In this test a flexible long tube with a camera (endoscope) at its end is used to take pictures and see any abnormalities of the internal hollow organs e.g. stomach (Gastroscopy) or food pipe (esophagoscopy) or part of small intestine (upper GI endoscopy), rectum (anoscopy), lower part of large intestine, rectum and anus (sigmoidoscopy), entire large intestine, rectum and anus (colonoscopy). In this test various instruments can also be passed through the endoscope e.g. to biopsy the tissue of the organs an instrument with small clipper is passed to take sample of tissue through the endoscope. It can also be used for therapeutic purposes.	The patient made to lie in a position and anaesthetic sprayed at the patient's throat which is made numb before insertion of the endoscope. The patient is also prepared before a procedure by keeping the patient in fasting state.

29.	**Cystoscopy**	In this test we visualize the urethra and urinary bladder by looking through a flexible viewing tube with a light and camera at its end (cystoscope)	In this test small amount of anaesthetic jelly is applied over the endoscope before insertion and then camera attached to endoscope takes videos and pictures.
30.	**Biopsy**	In this test a sample of tissue is taken and examined under a microscope to see the microscopic structural details of the organ and detect any abnormalities e.g cancer.	It is usually done by cutting a sample of tissue from the affected part by using a specialized needle or tissue clipper e.g skin or liver tissue and stained with dye, then examined under a microscope to look at microscopic structural tissue changes usually used as confirmatory test as it allows definitive diagnosis.
31.	**Mammography**	In this test low dose X-rays are used to check for abnormal areas of the breast.	In this test the woman's breast is placed over an X ray plate and top and side views of the breast are captured over the X ray film to look for tissue abnormalities and helps in early detection of breast cancer.
32.	**Nuclear isotopic scan (e.g. HIDA scan)**	In these test harmless radioactive materials are given which on entering the body emit radiation, and these radiations are captured to produce images of internal structures and look for their functional activity.	In this test small amount of radioactive material are either given by mouth, as part of meal or drink or injected in vein.

33.	**Laparoscopy**	In this procedure examination of the abdominal cavity is done using an endoscope to look at any organ in the abdominal cavity, take tissue samples and even do surgery.	In this procedure the patient is under general anaesthesia, the appropriate area of skin is washed with an antiseptic, small incision is made around the navel and endoscope passed.
34.	**B-hcg (Beta-hcg)**	In this test we measure for the level of hormone produced by the placenta (sac supporting the fetus in uterus) during pregnancy.	Usually by inserting a needle into the vein of the arm and withdrawing blood, collecting it in a blood vial and sending to lab for the test. Levels of this hormone can also be tested in urine.
35.	**Barium Study**	In this test we can examine the contours and lining of the digestive tract and also look for erosions, ulcers, blockages and tumors due to abnormal accumulation of barium in the digestive tract.	In this test the person swallows the barium in a flavoured liquid mixture or as barium coated food. It looks white on the X-ray and outlines the digestive tract. It is eventually passed in the stool, and appears as chalky white.
36.	**C- Reactive Protein**	In this test we measure this protein which is normally produced by the liver but is present in trace amounts in the blood however in case of acute inflammation (infection, coronary artery disease) its level rises in the blood.	Usually by inserting a needle into the vein of the arm and withdrawing blood, collecting it in a blood vial and sending to lab for the test.
37.	**HLA B-27**	In this test we look for this protein coated on the WBCs. If this protein is higher than permissible limit, the patient may have higher propensity to autoimmune joint disease	Usually by inserting a needle into the vein of the arm and withdrawing blood, collecting it in a blood vial and sending to lab for the test.

38.	**PCR**	In this test we amplify the single copy or few copies of DNA of an organism to millions of copies which help in detection of infectious agents and the discrimination of non-pathogenic (non disease causing) from pathogenic strains (disease causing) by virtue of specific genes, It helps in their rapid and specific diagnosis.	It is a molecular biology test in which a blood sample is obtained by inserting a needle into the vein of the arm and send to lab for special testing.
39.	**Echocardiography**	In this test one uses ultrasound waves to see the structure and activity of heart by measuring its wall motion and amount of blood being pumped out of the heart with each beat into great vessels.	In this test the transducer probe is place over the skin of the chest which sends sound waves into the body tissue and these waves bounce off the structures in the body tissues which are then reflected back to the transducer which coverts these signals into images
40.	**Coronary Angiography**	In this test one can obtain the patency and images of coronary artery which supplies the oxygen rich blood to heart muscle. In this test we can detect blockages in the artery as well as narrowing which can be treated with different modalities.	In this test a thin catheter is inserted through the artery of the arm or leg till it reaches the coronary artery, following the path via fluoroscopy (continuous X-ray). After the catheter tip is in place dye is injected into the coronary arteries which helps to outline them.
41.	**Manometry**	In this test we measure the pressure within various parts of GI tract, it helps to diagnose movement disorders of the gastro intestinal tract in patients with structurally normal picture.	In this test a catheter containing pressure transducers is passed through the mouth or esophagus and the readings help to determine whether the contractions are normal or not.

42.	**Cardiac Troponins**	In this test we measure the level of cardiac proteins which are released in the blood stream only when the heart muscle is damaged or dead. Most commonly measured are Troponin I/T or CK-MB	Usually by inserting a needle into the vein of the arm and withdrawing blood, collecting it in a blood vial and sending to lab for the test.
43.	**BNP/pro-BNP**	In this test we measure the substance which is released by the heart in response to changes in the heart lower chambers which occur when it is in failure or it worsens.	Usually by inserting a needle into the vein of the arm and withdrawing blood, collecting it in a blood vial and sending to lab for the test.
44.	**Pulmonary Function Test**	In this test one can measure the capacity of lung to hold air, its ability to exchange oxygen and carbon dioxide, and its ability to move air in and out with each breath. This helps in determining the type and severity of lung disease.	This test can be carried out using a device called spirometer or body plethysmography with gas dilution.
45.	**Electronystagmography**	In this test one can determine the function of the inner ear and brain responsible for maintaining balance, position by assessing the movement of eyes in response in response to input from ear and brain.	In this test electrodes (sensors) are placed over the eye muscles and then various manoeuvres are done (moving objects in front of eye) and then eye movements are noted for abnormal movements.
46.	**Audiometry**	In this test we measure the hearing for sound intensity and pitch and also tonal purity. It helps to diagnose the type and severity of hearing loss.	This test is done using automatic or manual audiometers, the subjects ears are then tested through a range of frequencies and hearing level recorded for each frequency.

47.	**Holter monitoring**	In this test the patients heart rhythm is monitored over 24 hours for any abnormality which was absent on resting ECG. It also helps us to know the frequency of abnormal rhythms over 24 hours.	In this test the electrodes are placed over the chest and connected to a small recording device which records data over 24hrs and then analyzed using computer.
48.	**Otoscopy**	In this test we use a device called otoscope to visualize the external auditory canal and the tympanic membrane (ear drum) to look for any abnormalities such as infection.	Otoscope is inserted into the external ear to visualize the ear canal and ear drum.
49.	**Tonometry**	In this test we can measure the pressure within each eye and it helps to diagnose glaucoma and monitor its treatment.	In this test we can use a non-contact air puff tonometer to measure the pressure in each eye. The amount of time it takes to flatten the cornea is measured as intraocular pressure.
50.	**Sleep Studies**	In this test we determine information about sleep stages as well as quality of sleep. It helps to diagnose various sleep disorders such as obstructive sleep apnea and others.	In this test patient is asleep and we monitor the brain's electrical activity as well as eye movements, heart rate, muscle activity and breathing. The combined data is then analyzed for patterns of specific disorders e.g. narcolepsy
51.	**Periodic Acid Schiff Staining**	PAS staining is used to diagnose conditions with increased concentration of carbohydrate. The test is usually done on tissues obtained from the body and analysed under a microscope. Some conditions diagnosed with PAS staining are: Glycogen storage disorders, Adenocarcinomas, Ewing's sarcoma, Paget's Disease of the Breast and α-1 an-titrypsin deficiency.	The Periodic Acid in PAS stain acts by breaking up the bonds between two carbon atoms in the carbohydrate and converting it into an aldehyde. This aldehyde then reacts with the Schiff stain to give a purple-magenta colour. Diastase, an enzyme that breaks up glycogen is also frequently used.

52.	**Gram Staining**	While a gram stain does not give a definite answer to which organism it may be, it helps us in the initial classification which helps narrow down the diagnosis. It is also faster than culture which may take longer. The principle of Gram staining is based on the property of individual cell walls namely the presence of a peptidoglycan layer in the cell wall. When the dye is infused, cells that retain the colour are called Gram positive (also presence of peptidoglycan call wall) and those that do not are called Gram negative. It must be remembered that not all bacteria can be grouped in this manner. These are called Gram variable or Indeterminate groups.	1) Heat fixation of specimen 2) Application of Crystal Violet 3) Addition of Iodide 4) Rapid addition of ethanol or acetone 5) Control-staining with Carbol-Fuschin
53.	**Ziehl Neelson Staining**	While a Ziehl-Neelson does not give a definite answer to which organism it may be, it helps us in the initial classification which helps narrow down the diagnosis. Appropriate treatment may then be initiated. There are very few Acid Fast organisms. This coupled with the clinical symptoms generally renders further testing unnecessary. Acid fast organisms contain lipids in their cell walls called mycolic acids that makes it difficult to perform Gram stain on.	1) Heat fixation of specimen 2) Application of Carbol Fuschin 3) Addition of mild solution of hydrochloric acid and isopropyl alcohol 4) Stain with methylene blue

54.	**Cold Agglutinin**	All humans have antibodies with the tendency to hemolyse RBCs. The relative concentration of these, however, is small. Patients with cold agglutinin disease have a higher concentration of these antibodies which precipitate at lower temperatures (in winter months) and lead to clinically significant lysis of RBCs. This is activated through the complement pathway which forms the membrane attack complex. If sufficient membrane attack complex is formed, it leads to more pores on the RBC surface and subsequently intravascular lysis. If not enough membrane attack complex is formed, they get deposited on the surface of the RBC which marks it for phagocytosis. Either way, the RBC gets functionally removed from circulation.	Usually by inserting a needle into the vein of the arm and withdrawing blood, collecting it in a blood vial and sending to lab for the test.

55.	**MRCP**	The bile ducts (which carry bile) and the pancreatic duct (which carry pancreatic enzymes), join together before entering the duodenum. If there is blockage in this system, it will lead to increase back pressure and clogging. Magnetic Resonance Cholangiopancreatico-graphy or MRCP is a process that helps us to visualize these ducts and evaluate for any pathologies. While similar in function to ERCP, it is less non-invasive and is coming up in a huge way for diagnostic purposes. MRCP is used to diagnose pathologies that block the common bile duct or pancreatic duct. These may include but are not restricted to: Gallstones Pancreatitis Cholangitis Tumors Strictures Sclerosis Sphincter of Oddi dysfunction While ERCP is mostly used for therapeutic purposes, MRCP is used for diagnostic purposes.	When a person is put in a high powered magnetic field, the hydrogen atoms that are naturally present in his body redirect the alignment which is read by the machine and can be analysed. This same principle is used in MRCP where the hydrogen atoms in the fluid normally present in the ductal systems realign themselves and the common bile duct and pancreatic duct may be visualized. This is non-invasive.
56.	**Urine pregnancy test**	In pregnancy, after the sperm and ovum combine, the resultant mass (known as zygote) travels to the uterus and implants itself in the wall, a process known as implantation. Initially corpus luteum and later on the placenta secretes β-HCG for the propagation and preservation of the pregnancy.	β-HCG is excreted in the urine and is measured as a part of Urine Pregnancy Test. As the hormone is not secreted under any other conditions, its mere presence is almost confirmatory for pregnancy. The test may also be used to monitor the progress of pregnancy as the β-HCG levels should serially rise over time.

57.	**Creatine kinase**	The types of creatine kinase are: CK-B- Brain type, CK-M- Muscle type. It is the muscle type that is routinely tested. An increased creatine kinase points to muscle damage. Some common inferences that may be drawn are: Myocardial infarction (mostly replaced by troponin), Rhabdomyolysis, Muscular dystrophy. Creatine kinase, after an insult to the muscle, increases in 4-8 hours. It reaches a maximum in 12-24 hours and then falls back to the normal range in 3-4 days.	Usually by inserting a needle into the vein of the arm and withdrawing blood, collecting it in a blood vial and sending to lab for the test.
58.	**Creatinine**	Creatine is produced in the liver and taken to the various organs where it undergoes reactions to form creatine phosphate. This cycle goes on and new creatine is frequently replenished. It is then converted to creatinine and transported to the kidney via blood where it is excreted in the urine. Testing of creatinine is done in in blood and urine. If it rises in blood, it signifies that the kidney is not filtering properly and that renal failure has started. If it rises in urine, it signifies over filtration and this is the sign of kidney disease.	Usually by inserting a needle into the vein of the arm and withdrawing blood, collecting it in a blood vial and sending to lab for the test.
59.	**Fibrinogen**	Fibrinogen, once converted to fibrin helps in the formation of clots. It may also be associated with cardiovascular disease. A congenital deficiency of fibrinogen may lead to bleeding manifestations. Correction by infusion of fresh frozen plasma or cryoprecipitate may be necessary	Usually by inserting a needle into the vein of the arm and withdrawing blood, collecting it in a blood vial and sending to lab for the test.

60.	**Follicle stimulating hormone**	FSH acts as a precursor hormone acting on the reproductive system, thus catalysing further reactions. It helps in maturation of germ cells, the cells that lead to the formation of sex hormones and products required for reproduction. It induces the formation of inhibitory hormones. It helps in ovulation. It helps in the maturation of sperm. Variations in FSH level may be noted as a feature of certain pathology. Some conditions are: HIGH FSH: 1) Premature menopause 2) Turners syndrome 3) Klienfelter's syndrome 4) Systemic Lupus Erythematosus LOW FSH: 1) Polycystic ovarian syndrome 2) Kallmann Syndrome 3) Hyperprolactinemia 4) Gonadotropin deficiency The list is not exhaustive	Usually by inserting a needle into the vein of the arm and withdrawing blood, collecting it in a blood vial and sending to lab for the test.

61.	**Lutenizing Hormone**	Luteinizing hormone generally functions as a precursor hormone acting on the sex organs to produce its various effects.
		In males, it acts on the Leydig cells of the testes and produces testosterone.
		In females, it acts on the theca cells and stimulates estradiol production. The LH surge during menstruation (a peak mid-way in the menstrual cycle) is the point where ovulation takes place and the corpus luteum that remains behind starts secreting progesterone. The progesterone is needed to prepare the endometrium for implantation of the ovum.
		Thus, LH levels may be used as a marker of ovulation.
		HIGH LH:
		   1) Premature menopause
		   2) Turners syndrome
		   3) Klienfelter's syndrome
		   4) Systemic Lupus Erythematosus
		LOW LH:
		   1) Polycystic ovarian syndrome
		   2) Kallmann Syndrome
		   3) Hyperprolactinemia
		   4) Gonadotropin deficiency
		The list is not exhaustive.
			Usually by inserting a needle into the vein of the arm and withdrawing blood, collecting it in a blood vial and sending to lab for the test.

62.	**Rheumatoid Factor**	Rheumatoid factor is an auto-antibody, i.e. an antibody produced by the body against its own cells that generally target the articular tissue. It is elevated in many of the rheumatoid diseases. Rheumatoid factor is usually used to confirm the presence of an autoimmune disease. It is found to be elevated in the following diseases: Rheumatoid arthritis, SLE, Sjörgren's disease, Primary Biliary Cirrhosis, Systemic Sclerosis, Sarcoidosis, Dermatom-yositis. This list is not all inclusive or exhaustive in any manner and includes a lot more diseases. It must however be kept in mind that rheumatoid factor may not be used to confirm the presence of any of these diseases.	Usually by inserting a needle into the vein of the arm and withdrawing blood, collecting it in a blood vial and sending to lab for the test.
63.	**Prothrombin Time**	The coagulation pathways in a human have three distinct pathways, the intrinsic or contact activation pathway, the extrinsic pathway and the common pathway. The extrinsic pathway is controlled by the extrinsic factors. Prothrombin time or PT is used to detect abnormalities and monitor the effects anticoagulants have on the extrinsic pathway.	Usually by inserting a needle into the vein of the arm and withdrawing blood, collecting it in a blood vial and sending to lab for the test.

64.	**Activated Partial Thromboplastin Time**	Coagulation pathways in a human have three distinct pathways: intrinsic or contact activation pathway, extrinsic pathway and common pathway. The intrinsic pathway is controlled by the intrinsic factors. Activated Partial Thromboplastin time or APTT is used to detect abnormalities and monitor the effects anticoagulants have on the intrinsic pathway. It is called 'partial' as tissue factor is not used for this test.	Usually by inserting a needle into the vein of the arm and withdrawing blood, collecting it in a blood vial and sending to lab for the test.
65.	**Basal Metabolic Profile**	Basal metabolic panel, BMP or a complete metabolic panel is a set of seven to eight investigations, obtained as a blood report that is universally ordered as one of the most common routine tests. It is used to evaluate the metabolic status of the body. It gives us a general idea about the electrolyte levels, acid-base balance, kidney function (sometimes) and glucose. A basal metabolic panel, as the name suggests, helps establish a baseline on the metabolic values. This assists us in both diagnosing a disease if present and monitoring the effects of therapy. Some commonly checked values in BMP and their normal values are: Na^+-sodium-135-145mEq/L K^+-potassium- 3.5-5mEq/L Cl^-chloride- 97-107mEq/L $HCo3^-$Bicarbonate- 22-28mEq/L Blood Urea Nitrogen-7-20mg/dl Creatinine- 0.8-1.4mg/dl Glucose- 90-120mg/dl The values given here are	Usually by inserting a needle into the vein of the arm and withdrawing blood, collecting it in a blood vial and sending to lab for the test.

		rounded off for ease in USMLE exams and patient reference and may vary slightly from the actual normal values. The comprehensive metabolic panel also includes liver function tests.	
66.	**Anti-Thyroid Antibodies**	Anti-thyroid auto antibodies are autoantibodies produced by the body that have their target of action on a part of the thyroid gland. The resultant thyroid becomes hypo-functional. Two common diseases associates with TPO are: 1) Graves disease 2) Hashimoto's thyroiditis	Usually by inserting a needle into the vein of the arm and withdrawing blood, collecting it in a blood vial and sending to lab for the test.
67.	**Cryoglobulins**	Cryoglobulins are proteins that are precipitated at low temperatures. They mainly consist of immunoglobulins and when precipitated, tend to clump together blocking the microvasculature and leading to gangrene. They may be associated with various diseases.	Usually by inserting a needle into the vein of the arm and withdrawing blood, collecting it in a blood vial and sending to lab for the test.
68.	**ESR**	Erythrocyte sedimentation rate, ESR or Westergen's test is a common test routinely done in clinical practice. It is the rate at which red blood cells sediment in a period of one hour. ESR is a non-specific marker of inflammation and is raised in a number of conditions. It must also be mentioned that while depicting inflammation, ESR is not confirmatory for any one disease. Any inflammatory process may cause the elevation of ESR by forming fibrinogens that chunk the RBC's together.	Usually by inserting a needle into the vein of the arm and withdrawing blood, collecting it in a blood vial and sending to lab for the test.

This chunked RBC cluster is termed Roleaux. It may also rise as a result of abnormal globulins.

Some common causes where an increased ESR may be noted are:
1) Pregnancy
2) Autoimmune conditions
3) Anemia
4) Cancers such as lymphoma and multiple myeloma
5) Kawasaki's Disease [1]
6) Inflammatory Bowel Disease
7) A reduced ESR may be noted in
8) Polycythemia
9) Hyperviscosity
10) Leukemia
11) Sickle Cell Anemia [1]

69.	**Glycaemic Load**	On intake of food, the blood glucose rises. This is mainly due to the breakdown of carbohydrates to sugars. This phenomenon may be measured by the glycaemic load. Simply put, it measures the rise in glucose after food intake. The more the glycaemic load, the greater chances of increased blood sugar levels.	Usually by inserting a needle into the vein of the arm and withdrawing blood, collecting it in a blood vial and sending to lab for the test.
70.	**Glycaemic Index**	On intake of food, the blood glucose rises. This is mainly due to the breakdown of carbohydrates to sugars. This phenomenon is measured by the glycemic index discovered by Dr.Wolever and Dr.Jenkins. Simply put, it measures the rise in glucose after food intake and represents it on a scale of 0-100. The more the glycemic index, the greater chances of increased blood sugar levels.	Usually by inserting a needle into the vein of the arm and withdrawing blood, collecting it in a blood vial and sending to lab for the test.

72.	**RDW**	An RDW or red cell distribution width measures the range of variation of red blood cell volume. Some diseases cause an increase in the RDW and subsequent increase in size of the cell. This is known as anisocytosis. It must be remembered that the term width is not used in its usual 2D meaning but as distribution width. The term signifies change in volume not diameter. It is calculated as a part of the complete blood count or CBC. Some conditions diagnosed by RDW are: 1) Anemia with normal RDW- Thalassemia, High RDW may be seen in: Iron deficiency anemia 2) Folate deficiency anema 3) Vitamin B12 deficiency anemia 4) Hemorrhage	Usually by inserting a needle into the vein of the arm and withdrawing blood, collecting it in a blood vial and sending to lab for the test.
73.	**Renal Function Tests**	A renal function panel, as the name suggests, helps establish a baseline on the kidney function. This assists us in both diagnosing a disease if present and monitoring the effects of therapy. Some commonly checked values in RFT and their normal values are: Blood Urea Nitrogen-7-20mg/dl Creatinine- 0.8-1.4mg/dl Glucose- 90-120mg/dl Blood Urea Nitrogen: Creatinine ratio-10:1-20:1 Na^+-sodium-135-145mEq/L K^+-potassium- 3.5-5mEq/L Cl^--chloride- 97-107mEq/L $HCo3^-$Bicarbonate- 22-28mEq/L The values given here are	Usually by inserting a needle into the vein of the arm and withdrawing blood, collecting it in a blood vial and sending to lab for the test.

		rounded off for ease in USMLE exams and patient reference and may vary slightly from the actual normal values.	
74.	**Thrombin time**	The coagulation pathways in a human have three distinct pathways, the intrinsic or contact activation pathway, the extrinsic pathway and the common pathway. The common pathway ends with the conversion of fibrinogen to fibrin clots in the presence of Thrombin. Defects in this conversion are targeted by the Thrombin test. It is used to diagnose disorders of coagulation and to find defects in the fibrinolytic pathway.	Usually by inserting a needle into the vein of the arm and withdrawing blood, collecting it in a blood vial and sending to lab for the test.
76.	**TSH**	TSH or thyroid stimulating hormone is a hormone secreted by the pituitary gland in response to the thyroid releasing hormone from the hypothalamus. It helps to regulate the release of hormones from the thyroid gland. Measurement of TSH helps us to determine if a thyroid pathology is primary or secondary. By convention, an increase or decrease in the thyroid hormones from the thyroid itself (T4 and T3) should be accompanied by an opposite response in the TSH due to feedback loop inhibition. If the same trend is seen in both (eg. An increase in both) will suggest a secondary pathology in the pituitary or hypothalamus.	Usually by inserting a needle into the vein of the arm and withdrawing blood, collecting it in a blood vial and sending to lab for the test.

77.	**ERCP**	The bile ducts (which carry bile) and the pancreatic duct (which carry pancreatic enzymes), join together before entering the duodenum. It therefore stands to reason that any blockage in this transit system will lead to increased back pressure and clogging of the ducts. Endoscopic Retrograde Cholangiopancreaticography or ERCP is a process that helps us to visualize these ducts and evaluate for any pathologies. ERCP is used to diagnose pathologies that block the common bile duct or pancreatic duct. These may include but are not restricted to: 1) Gallstones 2) Pancreatitis 3) Cholangitis 4) Tumors 5) Strictures 6) Sclerosis 7) Sphincter of Oddi dysfunction 8) Pseudocysts [1] However, with the advent of less invasive procedures such as MRCP and Endoscopic Ultrasound, ERCP is preferred for therapeutic procedures such as: 1) Sphincterotomy and dilatation of strictures 2) Gall bladder stone removal 3) Stent placement	An endoscope is inserted into the intestine until the point where the bile and pancreatic ducts open into the duodenum. A catheter is passed into the duct and a dye is injected which travels along the ducts and helps in the visualization of biliary pathway, gall bladder and pancreas [2]. The therapeutic intervention may then be performed.
78.	**Eticholanolone**	Eticholanolone or 3α-hydroxy-5β-androstan-17-one is a metabolite of testosterone that is found in the urine. It is a 17-ketosteroid. It is usually found in the sulphate salt form. It is	Usually by inserting a needle into the vein of the arm and withdrawing blood, collecting it in a blood vial and sending to lab for the test.

		also known as 5-isoandrosterone. Eticholanolone once formed has a wide range of functions like: 1) It stimulates release of Interleukin-1 from leukocytes and incites fever. 2) It is also involved in leucocytosis. Eticholanolone through its effect on the immune system may be used in the evaluation of: 1) Cancer 2) Androgenic alopecia 3) Adrenal Cortex Function 4) Bone marrow performance It is also known to be an anti-epileptic though application in current pharmacology has yet to be evaluated.	
79.	**Hematocrit**	Hematocrit is the volume percentage of Red Blood Cells (RBC'S) in blood. It signifies the amount of oxygen available to the tissues as it is the function of haemoglobin (and by extension RBC) to carry oxygen. It is calculated as a part of the complete blood count or CBC. A hematocrit defines the amount of oxygen available to the tissues. These may be decreased (anemia) or elevated (polycythemia). Some conditions where variations in haemoglobin may be seen are: 1) Lowered: Anemia, Leukamia, Pregnancy 2) Increased: Elevated landscapes, Sleep apnea, Polycythemia Rubra Vera, Dehydration	Usually by inserting a needle into the vein of the arm and withdrawing blood, collecting it in a blood vial and sending to lab for the test.
80.	**MCH**	MCH or mean corpuscular	Usually by inserting a needle

		haemoglobin is the average mass of haemoglobin per red blood cell in a given sample of blood. It is reduced in hypochromic anemias. It is a part of the complete blood count or CBC	into the vein of the arm and withdrawing blood, collecting it in a blood vial and sending to lab for the test.
		MCH is used to determine the average mass of haemoglobin in a red blood cell in a given sample. This in turns helps us to determine if a sample is hypochromic or has less hemoglobin, a condition very commonly seen in Iron deficiency anemias.	
81.	**MCHC**	Subtle differences exist between MCH and MCHC. While MCH is the hemoglobin per red blood cell in a given sample, MCHC is the concentration of hemoglobin in a given volume of packed RBC. It is calculated by dividing haemoglobin by hematocrit and is a part of the complete blood count or CBC. MCHC is used to determine the concentration of hemoglobin in a red blood cell in a given sample of packed RBC. This in turns helps us to determine if a sample is hypochromic or has less hemoglobin, a condition very commonly seen in iron deficiency anemias. Normochromic anemias may be seen in macrocytic anemias while hyperchromic anemias may be seen in sickle cell disease. People with cold agglutinins may report a high MCHC as the RBC's tend to clump together and suggest a wrong value.	Usually by inserting a needle into the vein of the arm and withdrawing blood, collecting it in a blood vial and sending to lab for the test.
82.	**MCV**	MCV or mean corpuscular volume is the volume of an RBC	Usually by inserting a needle into the vein of the arm and

		obtained by multiplying the volume of the blood with the hematocrit and dividing for both reduced MCV and increased MCV. MCV is used to determine the volume of the RBC, whether it is macrocytic or microcytic. This helps narrow down diagnosis. Some common causes where an increased MCV may be noted are: ✓ Vitamin B12 deficiency anemia ✓ Folate deficiency anemia A reduced MCV may be noted in ✓ Iron deficiency anemia ✓ Thalassemia ✓ Sideroblastic anemia	withdrawing blood, collecting it in a blood vial and sending to lab for the test.
83.	T_3	Triiodothyronine has a lot of functions in the body predominantly responsible for maintaining the basal metabolic rate. It is the active form of the hormone. Measurement of T_3 helps determine if a patient is hyper- or hypothyroid.	Usually by inserting a needle into the vein of the arm and withdrawing blood, collecting it in a blood vial and sending to lab for the test.
84.	T_4	Thyroxine has a lot of functions in the body predominantly responsible for maintaining the basal metabolic rate. Measurement of T_4 helps determine if a patient is hyper- or hypothyroid.	Usually by inserting a needle into the vein of the arm and withdrawing blood, collecting it in a blood vial and sending to lab for the test.

Section I

Recap or Recall

Repeat to Remember,
Remember to Repeat
~John Medina

Section I – Recap or Recall

How to memorize associated symptoms?

Nervous system

Headache

Blurring of vision	Glaucoma, Giant Cell Arteritis, Migraine
Double vision	SAH, Sinus venous thrombosis
Hearing Loss	TMJ dysfunction, Acoustic neuroma, Meningitis
Tearing of eyes and rhinorrhea	Cluster headache
Worst headache of my life	Subarachnoid hemorrhage
Worse on intake of cheese, wine, chocolate or OCPs	Migraine
Abnormal vision/smell preceding headache (Aura)	Migraine
Early morning headache	Space occupying lesion (Brain tumor), Raised ICP (Pseudotumor cerebri), COPD (CO_2 retention)
After the weekend/holiday(more in the afternoon)	Tension type headache
Numbness and tingling in upper limbs	Cervical arthritis/spondylosis

Symptoms/Signs	Diagnosis	Test
Headache+Blurring vision		
Headache+ Double vision		
Headache+ Hearing loss		
Headache+Tearing of eyes and rhinorrhea		
Headache+Worst headache		
Headache+Worse on intake of cheese, wine, chocolate or OCPs`		
Headache+Abnormal vision/smell preceding headache (Aura)		
Headache+Early morning headache		
Headache+After the weekend/ holiday (more in the afternoon)		
Headache+Numbness and tingling in upper limbs		

Loss of consciousness

Symptoms/Signs	Diagnosis	Test
Loss of consciousness+ Warmth, sweating and lightheadedness		
Loss of consciousness+During cough, urination, defecation or laughter		
Loss of consciousness+ jerky movements		
Loss of consciousness+Loss of bowel or bladder control		
Loss of consciousness+ Post-ictal weakness/ confusion		
Loss of consciousness+Focal neurological deficit		

Dizziness

Symptoms/Signs	Diagnosis	Test
Dizziness+Vertigo (spinning sensation)		
Dizziness+Tinnitus and hearing loss		
Dizziness+Worsens on lying down or rolling over in bed		
Dizziness+Ear fullness		
Dizziness+Sweating and LOC		
Dizziness+Lightheadedness		
Dizziness+Drugs		
Dizziness+Blurring of vision/ painful vision		

Numbness and Tingling

Glove and stocking pattern	Peripheral neuropathy/ metabolic (diabetes mellitus)
Associated dizziness, bloating/ abdominal fullness, erectile dysfunction, orthostatic hypotension	Autonomic neuropathy, Diabetes mellitus
Single limb numbness and tingling	Radiculopathy, multiple sclerosis
Hypopigmented rash with tingling and dumbness	Leprosy
Back pain	Lumbar stenosis, Lumbar disc herniation, multiple myeloma
Perioral tingling	Hypocalcemia, panic attack

Symptoms/Signs	Diagnosis	Test
Numbness and tingling+Glove and stocking pattern		
Numbness and tingling+Associated dizziness, bloating/ abdominal fullness, erectile dysfunction, orthostatic hypotension		
Numbness and tingling+Single limb numbness and tingling		
Numbness and tingling+Hypopigmented rash with tingling and dumbness		
Numbness and tingling+Back pain		
Numbness and tingling+Perioral tingling		

Muscle weakness

Worsening in the evening	Myasthenia gravis
Improves by evening	Lambert Eaton Syndrome
Ascending muscle paralysis	Guillain-Barré Syndrome (GBS), Tick Paralysis
Descending muscle paralysis	Botulism
Remitting and relapsing type	Multiple sclerosis, Transverse myelitis
Hemiparesis	Stroke/ TIA
Restlessness at night	Restless leg syndrome
Muscle weakness with loss of temperature and pain in upper limbs	Syringomyelia
Loss of bowel and bladder control with muscle weakness	Cauda equine syndrome, GBS
Loss of sensation, muscle function	Traumatic nerve injury

Symptoms/Signs	Diagnosis	Test
Muscle Weakness+Worsening in the evening		
Muscle Weakness+Improves by evening		
Muscle Weakness+Ascending muscle paralysis		
Muscle Weakness+Descending muscle paralysis		
Muscle Weakness+Remitting and relapsing type		
Muscle Weakness+Hemiparesis		
Muscle Weakness+Restlessness at night		
Muscle Weakness+Muscle weakness with loss of temperature and pain in upper limbs		
Muscle Weakness+Loss of bowel and bladder control with muscle weakness		
Muscle Weakness+Loss of sensation, muscle function		

Tremors

Intentional tremors	Essential tremors
Resting tremors	Parkinsonism
Jaundice	Alcoholic liver disease, Liver failure (Hepatic encephalopathy)
Caffeine intake	Caffeine induced tremors
Shortness of breath/ cough	COPD, CO_2 narcosis
Abnormal gait	Cerebellar disorders, Parkinson disease

Symptoms/Signs	Diagnosis	Test
Tremors+Intentional tremors		
Tremors+Resting tremors		
Tremors+Jaundice		
Tremors+Caffeine intake		
Tremors+Shortness of breath/ cough		
Tremors+Abnormal gait		

Seizures

Loss of Consciousness	Complex partial seizure, GTCS
No LOC	Partial seizure
High fever in children (Age < 5years)	Febrile seizure
Neck rigidity with fever	Meningitis, Encephalitis
h/o Alcoholism/benzodiazepine abuse	Withdrawal seizure
Illicit drug abuse	Cocaine induced
Blank stare	Absence seizure
Pre-seizure aura (visual/auditory/foul smell/ focal neurological symptoms	Encephalitis
No postictal weakness or loss of bowel and bladder control	Convulsive syncope

Symptoms/Signs	Diagnosis	Test
Seizures+Loss of Consciousness		
Seizures+No LOC		
Seizures+High fever in children (Age < 5years)		
Seizures+Neck rigidity with fever		
Seizures+h/o Alcoholism/benzodiazepine abuse		
Seizures+Illicit drug abuse		
Seizures+Blank stare		
Seizures+Pre-seizure aura (visual/ auditory/foul smell/ focal neurological symptoms		
Seizures+No Postictal weakness or loss of bowel and bladder control		

Confusion

Vomiting and diarrhea	Metabolic cause of delirium, chronic renal disease
Elderly patient	Drug induced, Diabetic complication, electrolyte imbalance
Muscle weakness/ focal neurological signs	Stroke, TIA
Postictal weakness	Seizures
Memory loss	Dementia

Symptoms/Signs	Diagnosis	Test
Confusion+Vomiting and diarrhea		
Confusion+Elderly patient		
Confusion+Muscle weakness/ focal neurological signs		
Confusion+Postictal weakness		
Confusion+Memory loss		

Memory Loss

Acute onset memory loss with confusion and violent behaviour	Drug induced, metabolic, infections
Rapid onset (weeks to months) with myoclonus	Creutzfeldt-Jakob disease
Stepwise worsening	Vascular dementia, multiple strokes, heart disease
Parkinson-like features	Lewy-body dementia
Associated change in behaviour, psychosis	Pick's disease (fronto-temporal dementia)
Loss of orientation to time, place, person and situation and anosognosia	Alzheimer disease
Pseudodementia (patient complains of forgetfulness) plus depressive symptoms (DIGEST P CAPSULE)	Major Depression
h/o Head injury	Retrograde (old memories)/anterograde (new memories) amnesia

Symptoms/Signs	Diagnosis	Test
Acute onset memory loss with confusion and violent behaviour		
Memory loss+Rapid onset (weeks to months) with myoclonus		
Memory loss+ Stepwise worsening		
Memory loss+ Parkinson-like features		
Memory loss+ Associated change in behaviour, psychosis		
Memory loss+ loss of orientation to time, place, person and situation and anosognosia		
Patient complains of forgetfulness+ depressive symptoms		
Memory loss+ h/o Head injury		

Loss of Vision

Painful Loss of vision	Glaucoma, Uveitis, keratitis, optic neuritis (Multiple sclerosis)
Painless Loss of vision	Complete retinal vein occlusion (CRVO), Complete retinal artery occlusion (CRAO), Vitreous hemorrhage, retinal detachment
Tunnel vision, blurring of vision	Glaucoma, MS
Photophobia (unilateral/bilateral)	Uveitis, Keratitis
Eye swelling	Orbital cellulitis

Symptoms/Signs	Diagnosis	Test
Painful Loss of vision		
Painless Loss of vision		
Tunnel vision, blurring of vision		
Loss of vision+Photophobia (unilateral/bilateral)		

Hearing Loss

Ear pain and discharge	Chronic Suppurative Otitis media (CSOM)/ Acute Suppurative Otitis media (ASOM), Malignant otitis externa
Vertigo and tinnitus	Meniere's disease, vestibular neuronitis, Sensorineural hearing loss (SNHL)
Ear fullness	Meniere's disease
Headache/Jaw pain	TMJ dysfunction
Alcohol/NSAIDS/Loop diuretics/ Aminoglycosides/Chemotherapy	SNHL
Hearing loss to particular frequencies	Presbycusis (Age related)
h/o Noise pollution, ear trauma, war/factories	Traumatic hearing loss

Symptoms/Signs	Diagnosis	Test
Hearing loss+ Ear pain and discharge		
Hearing loss+ Vertigo and tinnitus		
Hearing loss+ Ear fullness		
Hearing loss+ Headache/Jaw pain		
Hearing loss+ Alcohol/NSAIDS/Loop diuretics/Aminoglycosides/ Chemotherapy		
Hearing loss+ Hearing loss to particular frequencies		
Hearing loss+ h/o Noise pollution, ear trauma, war/factories		

Cardiovascular System

Chest pain

Shortness of breath	Myocardial Infarction (MI), Pulmonary Embolism (PE), Acute CHF, Acute exacerbation of COPD
Dizziness/Syncope	Aortic stenosis, Arrhythmia, Aortic dissection
Excessive sweating	MI, arrhythmia
Palpitation	MI, arrhythmia, mitral or aortic regurgitation
Hemoptysis	Acute PE, Mitral stenosis
Tearing pain radiating to the back	Aortic dissection
Chest pain worsens on inspiration	Pleuritis, pericarditis, musculoskeletal pain (costochondritis)
Chest pain improves on bending forward	Pericarditis
Fever	Infective endocarditis (Other stigmata like Osler's node, Roth's spot, Janeway lesions, Hematuria may also be present.
h/o Sudden deaths in family	Hypertrophic Obstructive Cardiomyopathy (HOCM)

Symptoms/Signs	Diagnosis	Test
Chest pain+ Shortness of breath		
Chest pain+ Dizziness/ Syncope		
Chest pain+ Excessive sweating		
Chest pain+ Palpitation		
Chest pain+ Hemoptysis		
Chest pain+ Tearing pain radiating to the back		
Chest pain+ Chest pain worsens on inspiration		
Chest pain+ Chest pain improves on bending forward		
Chest pain+ Fever		
Chest pain+ h/o Sudden deaths in family		

Palpitation

Sweating, tremors, anxiety	Panic attacks, excessive caffeine intake and hyperdynamic states like severe anemia, hyperthyroidism, wet beri beri, mitral/aortic regurgitation
Irregular palpitation	Cardiac arrhythmia, HOCM, Atrial fibrillation, Atrial flutter
Dizziness/ Syncope	Arrhythmia
Chest pain	MI, COPD
Shortness of breath	Arrhythmia, MI
Tremors/ weight loss/sweating	Hyperthyroidism, panic attack
h/o blood loss, malnutrition	Anemia
h/o drug intake	Cocaine use, excessive caffeine intake
Post-palpitations diuresis	Arrhythmia leading to left ventricular dysfunction and raised atrial pressures causing it to release natriuretic peptide. This leads to excretion of water and sodium.

Symptoms/Signs	Diagnosis	Test
Palpitation+ Sweating, tremors, anxiety		
Palpitation irregular		
Palpitation+ Dizziness/ Syncope		
Palpitation+ Chest pain		
Palpitation+ Shortness of breath		
Palpitation+ Tremors/weight loss/sweating		
Palpitation+ h/o blood loss, malnutrition		
Palpitation+ h/o drug intake		
Palpitation+ Post-palpitations diuresis		

Respiratory System

Shortness of breath

Orthopnea/Paroxysmal Nocturnal dyspnea (PND)	Cardiac cause of shortness of breath (Left ventricular failure, cardiogenic pulmonary edema)
Chest pain	Venous-Thromboembolism (VTE), COPD, MI, Acute MR, pleuritis
Leg pain	VTE
Wheezing	Asthma, COPD, Exercise induced asthma, Heart failure
Sneezing, Postnasal drip, rhinorrhea, nasal stuffiness	URI, Allergic rhinitis, Flu, Sinusitis
Cough	Bronchitis, asthma, COPD, heart failure, Sinusitis
Fever	Pneumonia, Bronchitis
Weight loss	Tuberculosis, Lung cancer, COPD
Phlegm	Chronic bronchitis (teaspoon), Bronchiectasis (cupful), heart failure (Pink frothy), Aspergillosis (black colored)
Hemoptysis	Tuberculosis, cancer, aspergillosis, pulmonary embolism, mitral stenosis, AV fistula

Symptoms/Signs	Diagnosis	Test
Orthopnea (SOB while lying down) / Paroxysmal Nocturnal dyspnea (PND)(SOB during sleep)		
Shortness of breath+ Chest pain		
Shortness of breath+ Leg pain		
Shortness of breath+ Wheezing		
Shortness of breath+ Sneezing, Postnasal drip, rhinorrhea, nasal stuffiness		
Shortness of breath+ Cough		
Shortness of breath+ Fever		
Shortness of breath+ Weight loss		
Shortness of breath+ Phlegm		
Shortness of breath+ Hemoptysis		

Sore Throat

Fever, myalgia, cough, nasal stuffiness	Flu
Skin rash, joint ache, hematuria	Streptococcal pharyngitis
Ulcers in the throat	Coxsackie virus infection/ herpangina
Loss of appetite	Infectious mononucleosis, Acute HIV
Dysphagia, change in voice, fever	Retropharyngeal abscess
Acid reflux, cough, halitosis	GERD, Zenker's diverticulum

Symptoms/Signs	Diagnosis	Test
Sore throat+ Fever, myalgia, cough, nasal stuffiness		
Sore throat+ Skin rash, joint ache, hematuria		
Sore throat+ Ulcers in the throat		
Sore throat+ Loss of appetite		
Sore throat+ Dysphagia, change in voice, fever		
Sore throat+ Acid reflux, cough, halitosis		

Snoring

Weight gain, cold intolerance, dry skin or constipation	Hypothyroidism
Excessive daytime symptoms	Obstructive Sleep apnea (OSA)
Excessive daytime symptoms, change in voice and dysphagia	Central sleep apnea/ bulbar palsy
h/o Recurrent tonsillitis	Adenoid/tonsillar hypertrophy
Shortness of breath	Secondary pulmonary hypertension due to Chronic OSA

Symptoms/Signs	Diagnosis	Test
Snoring+ Weight gain, cold intolerance, dry skin or constipation		
Snoring+ Excessive daytime symptoms		
Snoring+ Excessive daytime symptoms, change in voice and dysphagia		
Snoring+ h/o Recurrent tonsillitis		
Snoring+ Shortness of breath		

Gastrointestinal System

Abdominal Pain

Nausea/vomiting	Pancreatitis, Gastroenteritis, Acute appendicitis, Acute bowel obstruction.
Hematemesis	Peptic Ulcer, Esophageal Varices
Diarrhea	Gastroenteritis, Carcinoid Syndrome, Lactose Intolerance
Bloody Diarrhea	Intussusception, Acute mesenteric ischemia, Shigella/Yersinia/Campylobacter/Salmonella/ Hemorrhagic E.Coli infection
Weight loss	Malabsorption, GI Malignancy, Mesenteric Ischemia, Gastric Ulcer, Pancreatitis.
Increases with food intake, increases with fatty food	Gallstones, Pancreatitis, Gastric Ulcer, Mesenteric ischemia.
Decreases with food intake	Duodenal Ulcer
Radiates to the back	Pancreatitis, Duodenal Ulcer, Abdominal Aortic Aneurysm, Hodgkin's Lymphoma, Pyelonephritis, Renal Cell carcinoma
Loud Bowel Sounds	Small Bowel Disease, Partial obstruction, Enteric Fever, Malabsorption
Bleeding PV, Menstrual Problems	Ectopic Pregnancy, PID, Endometriosis
Painful Defection	Rectal disease

Symptoms/Signs	Diagnosis	Test
Abdominal pain+ Nausea/vomiting		
Abdominal pain+ Hematemesis		
Abdominal pain+ Diarrhea		
Abdominal pain+ Bloody Diarrhea		
Abdominal pain+ Weight loss		
Abdominal pain+ Increases with food intake, increases with fatty food		
Abdominal pain+ Decreases with food intake		
Abdominal pain+ Radiates to the back		
Abdominal pain+ Loud Bowel Sounds		
Abdominal pain+ Bleeding PV, Menstrual Problems		
Abdominal pain+ Painful Defection		

Dysphagia

Eating solids and liquids	Achalasia
Eating solids>liquids	Mechanical obstruction : Esophageal Cancer, Schatzki ring , Plummer-Vinson Syndrome
GERD	Zenker's Diverticulum, Schatzki ring, Scleroderma, CREST syndrome, Barrett's Esophagus
Weight loss	ALS, Esophageal Cancer
Change of voice	Zenker's Diverticulum, Schatzki Ring
Brainstem lesions	CSA, ALS

Symptoms/Signs	Diagnosis	Test
Dysphagia+ Eating solids and liquids		
Dysphagia+ Eating solids>liquids		
Dysphagia+ acid reflux		
Dysphagia+ Weight loss		
Dysphagia+ Change of voice		
Dysphagia+ Brainstem lesions		

Weight Loss

h/o laxative abuse, diets pills, excessive exercising, restricted eating habits	Anorexia Nervosa
Night sweats	TB, Cancer
Palpitations, sweating, cold/heat intolerance	Hyperthyroidism
Flushing, Hypertension, palpitations	Pheochromocytoma
Polyuria, polydypsia	DM
Abdominal Pain	Malabsorption, GI Malignancy, Mesenteric Ischemia, Gastric Ulcer, Pancreatitis

Symptoms/Signs	Diagnosis	Test
Weight loss+ h/o laxative abuse, diets pills, excessive exercising, restricted eating habits		
Weight loss+ Night sweats		
Weight loss+ Palpitations, sweating, cold/heat intolerance		
Weight loss+ Flushing, Hypertension, palpitations		
Weight loss+ Polyuria, polydypsia		
Weight loss+ Abdominal Pain		

Vomiting

h/o nausea	Gastroenteritis, Pregnancy, Chemotherapy, Intestinal Obstruction
no h/o nausea	Increased Intracranial pressure
Abdominal pain	Gastroenteritis, Intestinal Obstruction, Malabsorption, GI malignancy, Pancreatitis, Appendicitis, Cholecystitis.
Weight loss	Gastric Ulcer, Mesenteric Ischemia, Obstruction, GI Malignancy
Dysphagia	Zenker's Diverticulum, Esophageal obstruction (Achalasia, Malignancy, Schatzki Ring, PVS)
Diarrhea	Gastroenteritis, Malabsorption

Symptoms/Signs	Diagnosis	Test
Vomiting+ h/o nausea		
Vomiting+ no h/o nausea		
Vomiting+ Abdominal pain		
Vomiting+ Weight loss		
Vomiting+ Dysphagia		
Vomiting+ Diarrhea		

Diarrhea

Fever, Bloody diarrhea	Bacterial Enteritis (Campylobacter species, EHEC, Salmonella, Shigella, Entamoeba histolytica)
h/o recent antibiotic use	Clostridium difficile infection
h/o Diarrhea alternating with constipation	IBS
Malabsorption, rash, arthritis	Celiac disease, IBD
h/o travel to an endemic area	ETEC, Giardiasis
h/o mucus with blood, vomiting	C.difficile infection,
Crampy abdominal pain	Campylobacter infection
h/o step-ladder fever, chills, weakness	Salmonella infection
Flushing, wheezing	VIPoma, Carcinoid syndrome
Laxative abuse, weight loss	Anorexia nervosa

Symptoms/Signs	Diagnosis	Test
Bloody Diarrhea+ Fever		
Diarrhea+ h/o recent antibiotic use		
h/o Diarrhea alternating with constipation		
Diarrhea+ Malabsorption, rash, arthritis		
Diarrhea+ h/o travel to an endemic area		
Diarrhea+ h/o mucus with blood, vomiting		
Diarrhea+ Crampy abdominal pain		
Diarrhea+ h/o step-ladder fever, chills, weakness		
Diarrhea+ Flushing, wheezing		
Diarrhea+ Laxative abuse, weight loss		

Jaundice

Itching	Gallstones, Pancreatic Cancer
H/o travel to an endemic area	Hepatitis A, Hepatitis E
Pregnancy	Intrahepatic Cholestasis of Pregnancy
h/o drugs	OCPs, Amiodarone, Methyldopa, Halothane, Isoniazid, Chlorpromazine, Anabolic steroids
H/o hair loss, alcohol, sleep disturbances, testicular atrophy, spider nevi	Liver cirrhosis, Liver Failure, Hepatic Carcinoma
Non specific symptoms	Autoimmune Hepatitis

Symptoms/Signs	Diagnosis	Test
Jaundice+ Itching		
Jaundice+ H/o travel to an endemic area		
Jaundice+ Pregnancy		
Jaundice+ h/o drugs		
Jaundice+ H/o hair loss, alcohol, sleep disturbances, testicular atrophy, spider nevi		
Jaundice+ Non specific symptoms		

Bloody Vomiting

Symptoms	Diagnosis
Nausea, black stools, feeling of fullness after meals	Gastritis
Abdominal pain, light headedness, melena	Esophageal varices
Loss of appetite, epistaxis, jaundice, weight loss, ascites, edema	Cirrhosis
Abdominal pain, retching, fatigue, weight loss	GI Cancer (stomach/esophageal)
Abdominal pain, bloating, decrease in pain after meals	Duodenal Ulcer
Abdominal pain, weight loss, appetite changes, chest pain	Peptic Ulcer
Abdominal pain, easy bruising, jaundice, weight loss	Liver cancer
Dysphagia, sore throat, hoarseness of voice, abdominal pain, heart burn	Esophagitis

Symptoms/Signs	Diagnosis	Test
Bloody vomiting+ Nausea, black stools, feeling of fullness after meals		
Bloody vomiting+ Abdominal pain, light headedness, melena		
Bloody vomiting+ Loss of appetite, epistaxis, jaundice, weight loss, ascites, edema		
Bloody vomiting+ Abdominal pain, retching, fatigue, weight loss		
Bloody vomiting+ Abdominal pain, bloating, decrease in pain after meals		
Bloody vomiting+ Abdominal pain, weight loss, appetite changes, chest pain		
Bloody vomiting+ Abdominal pain, easy bruising, jaundice, weight loss		
Bloody vomiting+ Dysphagia, sore throat, hoarseness of voice, abdominal pain, heart burn		

Bloody Stools

Black colored stools (Melena)	GE varices, Mallory-Weiss syndrome, gastritis, bleeding gastric ulcer, trauma
Mucus and abdominal pain	C.difficile infection
Malabsorption, bloody diarrhea, arthritis, uveitis, skin rash, weight loss	IBD
Severe abdominal pain	Mesenteric ischemia
Painful defecation with streaks of blood on stool	Anal fissure
Painless fresh blood	Diverticulosis, hemorrhoids, IBD, intestinal infection

Symptoms/Signs	Diagnosis	Test
Bloody stools(black colored)		
Bloody stools+ Mucus and abdominal pain		
Bloody stools+ Malabsorption, bloody diarrhea, arthritis, uveitis, skin rash, weight loss		
Bloody stools+ Severe abdominal pain		
Bloody stools+ Painful defecation with streaks of blood on stool		
Bloody stools+ Painless fresh blood		

Fatigue with Pallor

Blood Loss	Anemia, GI bleed (Upper/Lower)
Weight gain	Hypothyroidism, muscle weakness, chronic fatigue syndrome, Depression
Weakness	Anemia, fibromyalgia, Hep C/Hep B

Symptoms/Signs	Diagnosis	Test
Fatigue with pallor+ blood loss		
Fatigue with pallor+ weight gain		
Fatigue with pallor+ weakness		

Endocrine System

Polyuria (Increased passage of urine>2.5 L/day)

Increased hunger, increased thirst, weight loss, visual changes	Diabetes Mellitus
Headaches	Pituitary tumor
Head injury	Diabetes Insipidus
h/o drugs intake	Diuretics, Demeclocycline, caffeine, water pills, ethanol, lithium
Excessive water ingestion	Primary polydypsia
Increased frequency, painful urination	UTI
h/o hesitancy	BPH

Symptoms/Signs	Diagnosis	Test
Polyuria+ Increased hunger, increased thirst, weight loss, visual changes		
Polyuria+ Headaches		
Polyuria+ Head injury		
Polyuria+ h/o drugs intake		
Polyuria+ Excessive water ingestion		
Polyuria+ Increased frequency, painful urination		
Polyuria+ H/o hesitancy		

Weight gain

Excessive eating, inactivity	Overeating, immobility
Heat/cold intolerance, weakness, rough/dry skin, constipation, decreased libido	Hypothyroidism
h/o sadness, stress, sleep disturbances, loss of interest, suicidal thoughts	Depression
Moonface, fat around neck (buffalo's hump), purple/pink striae around abdomen	Cushing's syndrome
Headache, lethargy, diplopia, blurred vision	Insulinoma
Menstrual changes, hirsutism, infertility, acne	PCOS
Missed periods, morning sickness	Pregnancy

Symptoms/Signs	Diagnosis	Test
Weight gain+ Excessive eating, inactivity		
Weight gain+ Heat/cold intolerance, weakness, rough/dry skin, constipation, decreased libido		
Weight gain+ H/o sadness, stress, sleep disturbances, loss of interest, suicidal thoughts		
Weight gain+ Moonface, fat around neck (buffalo's hump), purple/pink striae around abdomen		
Weight gain+ Headache, lethargy, diplopia, blurred vision		
Weight gain+ Menstrual changes, hirsutism, infertility, acne		
Weight gain+ Missed periods, morning sickness		

Neck Mass

Symptoms/Signs	Diagnosis
Heat/cold intolerance, weight gain, dry skin	Hypothyroidism
Weight loss, palpitations, exophthalmos, tremors	Hyperthyroidism, Grave's Disease
Weight loss	Cancer, Lymphoma, HIV, TB
Chronic cough, lymphadenopathy, weight loss	TB
Draining sinuses, mass moves with swallowing	Thyroglossal cyst, branchial cyst
Difficulty breathing/eating	Retrosternal thyroid
h/o hoarseness of voice, weight loss	Cancer
Difficulty in neck movement, abnormal neck movement	Torticollis (TIP: Always do an X-Ray to rule out TB)
Halitosis, h/o undigested food on pillow in the morning	Zenker's diverticulum

Symptoms/Signs	Diagnosis	Test
Neck mass+ Heat/cold intolerance, weight gain, dry skin		
Neck mass+ Weight loss, palpitations, exophthalmos, tremors		
Neck mass+ Weight loss		
Neck mass+ Chronic cough, lymphadenopathy, weight loss		
Neck mass+ Draining sinuses, mass moves with swallowing		
Neck mass+ Difficulty breathing/eating		
Neck mass+ H/o hoarseness of voice, weight loss		
Neck mass+ Difficulty in neck movement, abnormal neck movement		
Neck mass+ Halitosis, h/o undigested food on pillow in the morning		

Musculoskeletal System

Knee Pain

h/o early morning pain, crepitus, bony enlargement	Osteoarthritis
h/o early morning stiffness lasting >1 hr, stiffness in PIP and MCP joints	Rheumatoid arthritis
Worsened on going down the stairs	Meniscal injury
Redness of joint, chills and fever, recent h/o flu, GI infection	Septic arthritis
h/o accident/fall, swelling, immobility/difficulty in movement	Ligament injury, Fracture, dislocation
Playing sports like football and basketball	Jumper's knee - Tendonitis
h/o kneeling for long time, sweeping floors while sitting	Bursitis

Symptoms/Signs	Diagnosis	Test
Knee pain+ H/o early morning pain, crepitus, bony enlargement		
Knee pain+ H/o early morning stiffness lasting >1 hr, stiffness in PIP and MCP joints		
Knee pain+ Worsened on going down the stairs		
Knee pain+ Redness of joint, chills and fever, recent h/o flu, GI infection		
Knee pain+ H/o accident/fall, swelling, immobility/difficulty in movement		
Knee pain+ Playing sports like football and basketball		
Knee pain+ H/o kneeling for long time, sweeping floors while sitting		

Ankle Pain

Early morning pain on standing up, after resting	Plantar fasciitis
h/o accident, trauma, fall, twisting, swelling, bruising	Sprain, Calcaneal fracture
Old age, morning stiffness, crepitus, bony enlargement	Osteoarthritis
Medial side pain	Bony spur
Increases on squeezing calves	Achilles tendon rupture
h/o fever, swelling, injury, long standing, excessive movement	Tenosinovitis

Symptoms/Signs	Diagnosis	Test
Ankle pain+ Early morning pain on standing up, after resting		
Ankle pain+ H/o accident, trauma, fall, twisting, swelling, bruising		
Ankle pain+ old age, morning stiffness, crepitus, bony enlargement		
Ankle pain+ medial side pain		
Ankle pain+ Increases on squeezing calves		
Ankle pain+ H/o fever, swelling, injury, long standing, excessive movement		

Elbow Pain

h/o fall, swelling, bruising, difficulty moving	Injury, trauma, dislocation, fracture, olecranon bursitis (pain at tip of elbow)
Fever, swelling, inflammation post abrasion	Cellulitis
Worsened with shaking hands, opening jars, door knobs, playing golf/tennis	Tennis elbow (lateral), Golfer's elbow (medial) - synovitis

Symptoms/Signs	Diagnosis	Test
Elbow pain+ H/o fall, swelling, bruising, difficulty moving		
Elbow pain+ Fever, swelling, inflammation post abrasion		
Elbow pain+ Worsened with shaking hands, opening jars, door knobs, playing golf/tennis		

Shoulder Pain

Stiffness, swelling, difficulty moving	Frozen shoulder, Arthritis (osteo and rheumatoid)
h/o fall, swelling, immobility	Trauma, fracture, dislocation
Pain on lifting arm above head, on combing hair, reaching behind the back	Rotator cuff injury
Headache, jaw pain, scalp tenderness, GCA	Polymyalgia Rheumatica
RTA, neck pain, stiffness, dizziness	Whiplash injury
Fever, redness, swelling	Septic arthritis
Numbness and tingling on medial side of arm and forearm	Thoracic outlet syndrome

Symptoms/Signs	Diagnosis	Test
Shoulder pain+ Stiffness, swelling, difficulty moving		
Shoulder pain+ h/o fall, swelling, immobility		
Shoulder pain+ Pain on lifting arm above head, on combing hair, reaching behind the back		
Shoulder pain+ Headache, jaw pain, scalp tenderness, GCA		
Shoulder pain+ RTA, neck pain, stiffness, dizziness		
Shoulder pain+ Fever, redness, swelling		
Shoulder pain+ Numbness and tingling on medial side of arm and forearm		

Back Pain

Excessive exercising, accident, fall	Trauma, muscle sprain
Fever, tenderness	TB
Decreases with cycling, bending forward	Spinal stenosis
Bowel and bladder incontinence	Cauda Equina Syndrome
Increases with extending the back	Disc herniation
BPH, old age, urgency, frequency	Prostate cancer mets to spine
Swelling, fever	Abscess

Symptoms/Signs	Diagnosis	Test
Back pain+ Excessive exercising, accident, fall		
Back pain+ Fever, tenderness		
Back pain+ Decreases with cycling, bending forward		
Back pain+ Bowel and bladder incontinence		
Back pain+ Increases with extending the back		
Back pain+ BPH, old age, urgency, frequency		
Back pain+ Swelling, fever		

Urology and Reproductive System

Bloody Urine

Urgency, frequency, burning	UTI, stones, BPH
Fever	Pyelonephritis, cystitis
Flank pain	Pyelonephritis, stones
Difficulty urination	BPH, Cystitis
Fever, sore throat, microscopic hematuria	Glomerulonephritis, IgA nephropathy, Strep infection, Diabetic, Viral
Weight loss, smoking	Transitional cell carcinoma, Kidney cancer, prostate cancer
Hemoglobinuria	Sickle cell anemia, Alport syndrome
h/o blow/injury	Accident, injury to kidney, contact sports
h/o drug intake	Cyclophosphamide, Penicillin, Rifampin, Heparin, Aspirin
Myoglobinuria	Excessive exercise, Trauma, Burns
Consumption of beetroot	Diet related
Rashes, bruises	HUS, ITP, HSP

Symptoms/Signs	Diagnosis	Test
Bloody urine+ Urgency, frequency, burning		
Bloody urine+ Fever		
Bloody urine+ Flank pain		
Bloody urine+ Difficulty urination		
Bloody urine+ Fever, sore throat, microscopic hematuria		
Bloody urine+ Weight loss, smoking		
Bloody urine+ Hemoglobinuria		
Bloody urine+ H/o blow/injury		
Bloody urine+ H/o drug intake		
Bloody urine+ Myoglobinuria		
Bloody urine+ consumption of beetroot		
Bloody urine+ Rashes, bruises		

Burning Urination

Urgency, vaginal discharge	STD (Chlamydia, gonorrhea), Bacterial infection of Urinary tract, Cystitis
Hematuria	Bladder Cancer, UTI, Stones
Dysuria, frequency, urgency,	UTI, Stones, Cystitis
Dysuria, old age, incomplete voiding	BPH

Symptoms/Signs	Diagnosis	Test
Burning urination+ Urgency, vaginal discharge		
Burning urination+ Hematuria		
Burning urination+ Dysuria, frequency, urgency,		
Burning urination+ Dysuria, old age, incomplete voiding		

Incontinence

Flank pain	Stone, UTI
Lower abdominal pain, urgency, frequency	Cystitis, UTI
Amenorrhea	Pregnancy
Old age	Normal phenomenon due to muscle weakness, menopause, BPH
Hemiplegia	Stroke
Bradykinesia, tremors, rigidity	Parkinson's disease
Headache	Brain tumor
h/o accident, back pain	Spinal injury
Weight loss, urgency, frequency, dysuria	Prostate Carcinoma
Polyuria, polydypsia	Diabetes
Low back pain, feeling of fullness in lower abdomen, dysuria	Uterine Prolapse
Diet	Alcohol, caffeine, spicy food, corn syrup, carbonated drinks

Symptoms/Signs	Diagnosis	Test
Incontinence+ Flank pain		
Incontinence+ Lower abdominal pain, urgency, frequency		
Incontinence+ Amenorrhea		
Incontinence+ Old age		
Incontinence+ Hemiplegia		
Incontinence+ Bradykinesia, tremors, rigidity		
Incontinence+ Headache		
Incontinence+ Weight loss, urgency, frequency, dysuria		
Incontinence+ Polyuria, polydypsia		
Incontinence+ H/o accident, back pain		
Incontinence+ Low back pain, feeling of fullness in lower abdomen, dysuria		
Incontinence+ Diet		

Lower Abdominal Pain

Infrequent bowel movements, hard stools, bloating	Constipation
Nausea, vomiting, fever	Gastroenteritis, appendicitis, diverticulitis
2 weeks after LMP	Ovulation pain
Irregular periods/spotty, nausea, vomiting	Ovarian cyst
Dysuria, frequency, urgency, hematuria	Kidney infection, Kidney stones
Missed periods, spotting	Ectopic pregnancy
Coinciding with menses	Dysmenorrhea, endometriosis

Symptoms/Signs	Diagnosis	Test
Lower abdominal pain+ Infrequent bowel movements, hard stools, bloating		
Lower abdominal pain+ nausea, vomiting, fever		
Lower abdominal pain+2 weeks after LMP		
Lower abdominal pain+ irregular periods/spotty, nausea, vomiting		
Lower abdominal pain+ dysuria, frequency, urgency, hematuria		
Lower abdominal pain+ Missed periods, spotting		
Lower abdominal pain+ Coinciding with menses		

Pregnancy

Increased nausea, vomiting	Hyperemesis Gravidarum, morning sickness
Spotting	Miscarriage (threatened abortion/complete abortion)
Passage of vesicular mass per vagina	GTN, Molar pregnancy
Spotting, severe abdominal pain	Ectopic pregnancy
h/o multiple miscarriages	APLA syndrome, other autoimmune diseases
High blood sugar	GDM
High BP	Hypertension, Gestational Hypertension

Symptoms/Signs	Diagnosis	Test
Pregnancy+ increased nausea, vomiting		
Pregnancy+ Spotting		
Pregnancy+ Passage of vesicular mass per vagina		
Pregnancy+ spotting, severe abdominal pain		
Pregnancy+ H/o multiple miscarriages		
Pregnancy+ high blood sugar		
Pregnancy+ high BP		

Unable to Conceive

Headache, milky discharge from nipples, vision changes	Pituitary tumor (prolactinoma)
Weight gain, fatigue, cold/heat intolerance, amenorrhea	Hypothyroidism
h/o long duration of drugs intake	OCPs, Norplant
No h/o menses	Genetic diseases (Turner's syndrome), imperforate hymen, Androgen insensitivity syndrome, 5-alpha reductase deficiency
Irregular menses, hirsutism, weight gain, acne	PCOS
Abdominal pain, h/o chlamydia/gonorrhea infection	PID

Symptoms/Signs	Diagnosis	Test
Unable to conceive+ Headache, milky discharge from nipples, vision changes		
Unable to conceive+ Weight gain, fatigue, cold/heat intolerance, amenorrhea		
Unable to conceive+ H/o long duration of drugs intake		
Unable to conceive+ No h/o menses		
Unable to conceive+ Irregular menses, hirsutism, weight gain, acne		
Unable to conceive+ abdominal pain, h/o chlamydia/gonorrhea infection		

Erectile Dysfunction

Smoking	PVD, Leriche's syndrome
Polydypsia, polyuria, polyphagia	DM
increased BP	CVS, HTN, stroke
Tremors, bradykinesia, rigidity	Parkinson's disease
Headaches, nipple discharge	Pituitary tumor(prolactinoma)
Difficulty in getting an erection, painful erection	Peyronie's disease, Penile fracture, cavernous fibrosis
h/o Drug intake	Anabolic steroids (hypogonadism), antihypertensives, antipsychotics, antidepressants.
Neurological disease	Spinal cord lesions, brain stem lesions, MS

Symptoms/Signs	Diagnosis	Test
Erectile dysfunction+ Smoking		
Erectile dysfunction+ polydypsia, polyuria, polyphagia		
Erectile dysfunction+ increased BP		
Erectile dysfunction+ Tremors, bradykinesia, rigidity		
Erectile dysfunction+ Headaches, nipple discharge		
Erectile dysfunction+ Difficulty in getting an erection, painful erection		
Erectile dysfunction+ h/o Drug intake		
Erectile dysfunction+ neurological disease		

Vaginal Bleeding

h/o previous amenorrhea, abdominal pain	Miscarriage, ectopic pregnancy
h/o LMP 2 weeks ago	Mid-cycle ovulation bleeding
h/o irregular menses, hirsutism, acne, weight gain	PCOS
h/o bleeding after intercourse, douching	PID
Excessive bleeding during menses	Uterine fibroids
h/o uterine prolapse or polyp	Carcinoma cervix, uterine, vagina
post-menopausal	Vaginal atrophy, cancer, polyps, endometrial hyperplasia, post-menopausal hormonal therapy

Symptoms/Signs	Diagnosis	Test
Vaginal bleeding+ h/o previous amenorrhea, abdominal pain		
Vaginal bleeding+ h/o LMP 2 weeks ago		
Vaginal bleeding+ h/o irregular menses, hirsutism, acne, weight gain		
Vaginal bleeding+ h/o bleeding after intercourse, douching		
Vaginal bleeding+ excessive bleeding during menses		
Vaginal bleeding+ h/o uterine prolapse or polyp		
Vaginal bleeding+ post-menopausal		

Pain During Sex (Dyspareunia)

Old age	Vaginal atrophy
h/o surgery, trauma	Childbirth, pelvic surgery, sexual abuse
h/o spasm	Vaginismus
Amenorrhea	Imperforate hymen, vaginal agenesis
Dysmenorrhea	Endometriosis, uterine fibroids
Stress, depression, anxiety	Psychological factors
h/o skin diseases	Eczema
h/o drugs	Antidepressants, antihypertensive drugs, antihistamines, OCPs

Symptoms/Signs	Diagnosis	Test
Pain during sex+ Old age		
Pain during sex+ H/o surgery, trauma		
Pain during sex+ H/o spasm		
Pain during sex+ Amenorrhea		
Pain during sex+ Dysmenorrhea		
Pain during sex+ Stress, depression, anxiety		
Pain during sex+ H/o skin diseases		
Pain during sex+ H/o drugs		

Psychiatry

Depressed Mood

Dry skin, constipation	Hypothyroidism
Changes in sleep, appetite, weight, death/suicidal ideation	Major Depressive disorder
Depressed mood <2 months after the death of a loved one	Normal Bereavement
Depressed mood with irritability, anxiety, appetite changes, breast tenderness, joint swelling/bloating weight gain	PMS
Depressed mood with alternating mood to mania characterized by grandiosity, flight of ideas and increased activity	Bipolar disorder
Mood swings from mild depression to emotional highs for more than 2 years	Cyclothymia
Depressed mood for at least 2 years in adults and 1 year in adolescents and children, poor appetite and concentration, feeling of helplessness and transient euthymic episodes of up to 2 months during the course if dysthymia	Dysthymia

Symptoms/Signs	Diagnosis	Test
Depressed mood+ Dry skin, constipation		
Depressed mood+ Changes in sleep, appetite, weight, death/suicidal ideation		
Depressed mood+ Depressed mood <2 months after the death of a loved one		
Depressed mood+ Depressed mood with irritability, anxiety, appetite changes, breast tenderness, joint swelling/bloating weight gain		
Depressed mood+ Depressed mood with alternating mood to mania characterized by grandiosity, flight of ideas and increased activity		
Depressed mood+ Mood swings from mild depression to emotional highs for more than 2 years		
Depressed mood+Depressed mood for at least 2 years in adults and 1 year in adolescents and children, poor appetite and concentration, feeling of helplessness and transient euthymic episodes of up to 2 months during the course if dysthymia		

Hallucinations

Anxiety, suspiciousness, social withdrawal, ongoing unusual thoughts and beliefs	Psychosis
Behavioral symptoms like flattened affect, catatonia, violent behaviour, positive, negative symptoms	Schizophrenia
Excessive alcohol intake, anxiety, agitation, irritability, delirium, delusions, nightmares, restlessness	Delirium tremens
Throbbing, pulsating headaches with nausea, vomiting, extreme sensitivity to light	Migraines
Fluctuations in cognition, attention, alertness, behavioral and mood symptoms, impaired thinking	Lewy Body Dementia
Increased appetite, difficulty solving problems, decreased coordination and concentration, insomnia, irritability, anxiety	Marijuana abuse
Excessive daytime drowsiness, sudden loss of muscle tone, sleep paralysis	Narcolepsy
Jerky movements, tingling, dizziness, loss of consciousness, biting the tongue, loss of bladder and bowel control	Seizure disorder

Symptoms/Signs	Diagnosis	Test
Hallucinations+ Anxiety, suspiciousness, social withdrawal, ongoing unusual thoughts and beliefs		
Hallucinations+ Behavioral symptoms like flattened affect, catatonia, violent behaviour, positive, negative symptoms		
Hallucinations+ Excessive alcohol intake, anxiety, agitation, irritability, delirium, delusions, nightmares, restlessness		
Hallucinations+ Throbbing, pulsating headaches with nausea, vomiting, extreme sensitivity to light		
Hallucinations+ Fluctuations in cognition, attention, alertness, behavioral and mood symptoms, impaired thinking		
Hallucinations+ Increased appetite, difficulty solving problems, decreased coordination and concentration, insomnia, irritability, anxiety		
Hallucinations+ Excessive daytime drowsiness, sudden loss of muscle tone, sleep paralysis		
Hallucinations+ Jerky movements, tingling, dizziness, loss of consciousness, biting the tongue, loss of bladder and bowel control		

Insomnia

Snoring with excessive day time sleepiness	Sleep apnea
Sleep paralysis, hypnagogic and hypnopompic hallucinations	Narcolepsy
h/o Alcohol/Drug abuse, depressed mood, withdrawal symptoms	Substance abuse
Fatigue, dehydration/malaise, headache, indigestion, lack of concentration, irritability, muscle pain, recent travel from different time zone	Jet Lag
Exophthalmos, palpitations, weight loss, excessive sweating, heat intolerance	Hyperthyroidism
Irresistible urge to move the legs, leg cramps, restlessness, uncomfortable tingling and burning	Restless leg syndrome
Excessive day time sleepiness, unintended dozing, impaired mental acuity, irritability, reduced performance and accident proneness	Shift work sleep disorder

Symptoms/Signs	Diagnosis	Test
Insomnia+ Snoring with excessive day time sleepiness		
Insomnia+ Sleep paralysis, hypnagogic and hypnopompic hallucinations		
Insomnia+ H/o Alcohol/Drug abuse, depressed mood, withdrawal symptoms		
Insomnia+ Fatigue, dehydration/malaise, headache, indigestion, lack of concentration, irritability, muscle pain, recent travel from different time zone		
Insomnia+ Exophthalmos, palpitations, weight loss, excessive sweating, heat intolerance		
Insomnia+ Irresistible urge to move the legs, leg cramps, restlessness, uncomfortable tingling and burning		
Insomnia+ Excessive day time sleepiness, unintended dozing, impaired mental acuity, irritability, reduced performance and accident proneness		

Anxiety

Restlessness, fatigue, concentration problems, irritability, muscle tension, sleep disturbances	Generalized Anxiety Disorder (GAD)
Fear triggered by specific stimulus or situation (e.g. heights, fire or insects etc.)	Specific phobias
Intense fear and avoidance of negative public scrutiny, public embarrassment, humiliation/social interaction	Social phobias/ Anxiety
Trembling, shaking, confusion, dizziness, nausea/difficulty breathing, chest tightness, feeling of impending doom.	Panic disorder
Following certain behaviors to relieve anxiety (Obsessions and Compulsions) Patient knows it is not right and has trouble dealing with it. (Ego dystonic)	Obsessive Compulsive Disorder (OCD)
Flashbacks, nightmares, sleep disturbances, aggression, agitation, anger, general discontent, guilt, hopelessness. h/o of trauma, sexual assault or obnoxious insult in the past.	Post-Traumatic Stress Disorder (PTSD)

Symptoms/Signs	Diagnosis	Test
Anxiety+ Restlessness, fatigue, concentration problems, irritability, muscle tension, sleep disturbances		
Anxiety+ Fear triggered by specific stimulus or situation (e.g. heights, fire or insects etc.)		
Anxiety+ Intense fear and avoidance of negative public scrutiny, public embarrassment, humiliation/social interaction		
Anxiety+ Trembling, shaking, confusion, dizziness, nausea/difficulty breathing, chest tightness, feeling of impending doom.		
Anxiety+ Following certain behaviors to relieve anxiety (Obsessions and Compulsions) Patient knows it is not right and has trouble dealing with it. (Ego dystonic)		
Anxiety+ Flashbacks, nightmares, sleep disturbances, aggression, agitation, anger, general discontent, guilt, hopelessness. H/o of trauma, sexual assault or obnoxious insult in the past.		

Dehydration

Nausea, Vomiting	Gastroenteritis, Intussusception, Meckel's Diverticulum
Diarrhea	Gastroenteritis(Viral/bacterial) Celiac disease(Malabsorption) Inflammatory Bowel disease, IBS
Polyuria, Polydipsia, Weight Loss	DM/DI,DKA
Excessive sweating in hot weather	Hyperthermia/electrolyte disturbances

Symptoms/Signs	Diagnosis	Test
Dehydration+ Nausea, vomiting		
Dehydration+ Diarrhea		
Dehydration+ Polyuria, polydipsia, weight loss		
Dehydration+ Excessive sweating in hot weather		

Seizures

High fever	Febrile seizures
Jerky movements of the body with incontinence of urine and stools	GCTS
Blank staring	Absence seizures
Headache, neck stiffness, fever	Meningitis
Diarrhea	Electrolyte disturbances

Symptoms/Signs	Diagnosis	Test
Seizures+ High fever		
Jerky movements of the body with incontinence of urine and stools		
Seizures+ Blank staring		
Seizures+ Headache, neck stiffness, fever		
Seizures+ Diarrhea		

Enuresis

Excessive thirst, urination, dehydration, high blood sugar	DM, DI
Burning micturition	UTI
Incontinence with recurrent UTIs	Vesicoureteral reflux
Nerve damage	Spina-bifida
Unfamiliar social situations, angry parents, overwhelming family events such as the birth of a brother/sister	Anxiety

Symptoms/Signs	Diagnosis	Test
Enuresis+ Excessive thirst, urination, dehydration, high blood sugar		
Enuresis+ Burning micturition		
Enuresis+ Incontinence with recurrent UTIs		
Enuresis+ Nerve damage		
Enuresis+ Unfamiliar social situations, angry parents, overwhelming family events such as the birth of a brother/sister		

Wheezing

Symptoms	Diagnosis
SOB, chest tightness, cough, getting worsened by particular season/allergies	Asthma
Hives, itching, feeling of warmth, weak rapid pulse, nausea, vomiting, diarrhea, dizziness/fainting	Anaphylaxis
Runny and stuffy nose, cough, slight fever, difficulty breathing	Bronchiolitis, cold(allergies)
Fever, chills, cough, chest pain, SOB, fatigue, nausea, vomiting, diarrhea	Pneumonia
Congested/runny nose, dry cough, low grade fever, sore throat, mild headache. In severe cases, it can lead to a lower respiratory tract illness, cyanosis, severe cough, difficult breathing	RSV or Bronchiolitis or Pneumonia
Atypical crying/irritability, apnea, failure to thrive(poor appetite), sore throat, recurrent pneumonitis	Pediatric GERD

Symptoms/Signs	Diagnosis	Test
Wheezing+ SOB, chest tightness, cough, getting worsened by particular season/allergies		
Wheezing+ Hives, itching, feeling of warmth, weak rapid pulse, nausea, vomiting, diarrhea, dizziness/fainting		
Wheezing+ Runny and stuffy nose, cough, slight fever, difficulty breathing		
Wheezing+ Fever, chills, cough, chest pain, SOB, fatigue, nausea, vomiting, diarrhea		
Wheezing+ Congested/runny nose, dry cough, low grade fever, sore throat, mild headache In severe cases, it can lead to a lower respiratory tract illness, cyanosis, severe cough, difficult breathing		
Wheezing+ Atypical crying/irritability, apnea, failure to thrive (poor appetite), sore throat, recurrent pneumonitis		

Fever

Cough, SOB, Chest pain	Pneumonia
Headache, neck stiffness, nausea, vomiting, chills	Meningitis, brain abscess
Runny nose, sore throat, malaise, rash	Viral infections
Diarrhea, poor appetite, dehydration	Viral/bacterial gastroenteritis
Stridor, sore throat, difficult and painful swallowing, drooling, anxious	Epiglottitis
Bone pain, nausea, vomiting	Osteomyelitis
Burning micturition, polyuria, bloody urine	UTI, Renal stones
Joint pain	Septic arthritis, JRA

Symptoms/Signs	Diagnosis	Test
Fever+ Cough, SOB, Chest pain		
Fever+ Headache, neck stiffness, nausea, vomiting, chills		
Fever+ Runny nose, sore throat, malaise, rash		
Fever+ Diarrhea, poor appetite, dehydration		
Fever+ Stridor, sore throat, difficult and painful swallowing, drooling, anxiety		
Fever+ Bone pain, nausea, vomiting		
Fever+ Burning micturition, polyuria, bloody urine		
Fever+ Joint pain		

Section J

Medications

Section J - Common Medications

Ophthalmic Alpha Agonists

- ✓ Alphagen P
- ✓ Brimonidine

ACE inhibitors
- ✓ Fosinopril
- ✓ Monopril
- ✓ Quinapril
- ✓ Accupril
- ✓ Ramipril
- ✓ Altace
- ✓ Trandolapril
- ✓ Mavik
- ✓ Moexipril
- ✓ Univasc
- ✓ Perindopril
- ✓ Aceon

Anti- Diabetic

- ✓ Metformin
- ✓ Glucophage

Insulin
- ✓ Humalog
- ✓ Humulin
- ✓ Lantus

NSAIDs

- ✓ Celebrex
- ✓ Celecoxib
- ✓ Advil
- ✓ Ibuprofen

Nasal Corticosteroids

- ✓ Nasonex
- ✓ Mometasone furoate
- ✓ Rhinocort Aqua
- ✓ Budesonide
- ✓ Nasacort AQ
- ✓ Triamcinolone acetonide
- ✓ Veramyst
- ✓ Fluticasone furoate
- ✓ Omnaris, Zetonna
- ✓ Ciclesonide
- ✓ Patanase
- ✓ Olopatadine

Colony Stimulating Factors

- ✓ Neupogen
- ✓ Granix

Drugs for Urinary Incontinence

- ✓ Sanctura
- ✓ Trospium
- ✓ Vesicare
- ✓ Solifenacin
- ✓ Detrol
- ✓ Tolterodine
- ✓ Toviaz
- ✓ Fesoterodine
- ✓ Oxybutynin

Antianxiety

- ✓ Xanax
- ✓ Alprazolam

Antidepressants

- ✓ Pristiq
- ✓ Desvenlafaxine

Alzheimer's Disease

- ✓ Namenda

Drugs for heart failure

- ✓ Coreg
- ✓ Carvedilol

Calcium regulator

- Fortical
- Calcitonin
- Cardizem
- Diltiazem
- Xifaxan Rifamixin
- Megace ES
- Megestrol
- Hectorol
- Doxercalciferol
- Prolense
- Bromfenac

Proton Pump Inhibitors

- Prevacid
- Lansoprazole
- Aciphex
- Rabeprazole
- Nexium
- Esoprazole
- Prilosec
- Omeprazole
- Dexilant
- Dexlansoprazole

Lipid lowering drugs

- Crestor
- Rosuvastatin
- Livalo
- Pitvastatin
- Altoprev
- Lovastatin ER
- Simvastatin
- Vytorin
- Ezetimibe/Simvastatin
- Lescol
- Fluvastatin

Incretin like mimetic interchange

- Byetta, Bydureon
- Exenatide
- Victoza
- Liraglutide

Prostaglandin Analogue Interchange

- Lumigan
- Bimatoprost
- Zioptan
- Tafluprost
- Rescula
- Unoprostone

Interferon Beta products

- Betaseron
- Interferon beta-1b

Drugs for Osteoporosis

- Boniva
- Ibadronate
- Binosto
- Alendronate

Angiotensin Receptor Blockers

- Atacand
- Candesartan
- Avapro
- Irbesartan
- Micardis
- Telmisartan
- Teveten
- Eprosartan
- Benicar
- Olmesartan
- Edarbi
- Azilsartan
- Diovan
- Valsartan
- Atacand HCT
- Candesartan/HCTZ
- Avalide Irbesartan/HCTZ
- Micardis HCT
- Telmisartan/HCTZ
- Teveten HCT
- Eprosartan/HCTZ
- Benicar HCT
- Olmesartan/HCTZ
- Edarbyclor
- Azilsartan/chlorthalidone
- Diovan HCT
- Valsartan/HCTZ

Drugs for Asthma

- Flovent HFA
- Fluticasone
- Symbicort
- Budesonide/Formoterol
- Dulera
- Formoterol/Mometasone

Antibiotics

- Vancocin
- Vancomycin Capsules
- Amoxicillin
- Amoxil, Polymox, Trimox
- Cephalexin
- Keflex, Keftabs

BPH drugs

- Rapaflo
- Silodosin
- Avodart
- Dutasteride
- Uroxatral
- Alfuzosin

Dopamine Agonist

- Mirapex
- Pramipexole
- Ropinirole

B-agonist nebulizers

- Xopenex
- Levalbuterol
- Proair, Proventil HFA, Ventolin
- Albuterol HFA

Drugs in CKD

- Renagel, Renvela
- Sevelamer

Cholinesterase Inhibitors

- Exelon
- Rivastigmine
- Razadyne
- Galantamine
- Donepezil

Fibrate Interchange

- Antara, Tricor
- Fenofibrate
- Trilipix
- Fenofibric acid

Topical Antiseptic

- Bactroban
- Mupirocin
- Altabax
- Retapamulin
- Bactroban Nasal
- Mupirocin Nasal

Section K

Practice Cases

Section K – Practice Cases

Case 1

Miss Joey Casablanca, 19-year-old female patient comes with chest pain.

Vitals:
HR - 112 beats per minute
BP - 110/70 mm of HG
Pulse Ox - 92%
RR - 16 respirations per minute

Notes: Do a focused clinical examination.

Case Summary: This clinical scenario is of a panic attack. SP should present with sharp chest pain. Panic attacks can be due to work or abuse at home.

Challenging Question: Do you think I am going to die?

Associated Symptoms:

- Palpitations (heart making funny sensations)
- Tremors & Shaking
- Sweating
- Fear of impending doom
- Fear of losing control
- Shortness of breath

Examinee: Must ask these questions and examine patient;

- Evaluate for heart problems
- Evaluate for lungs problems
- Evaluate for thyroid problems

The examinee must diagnose this case as: Panic Attack

Case 2

Miss Georgy Abraham, 29-year-old female comes with swelling in the legs.

Vitals:
HR - 92 beats per minute
BP - 110/70 mm of hg
Pulse Ox - 92%
RR - 21 respirations per minute

Notes: Do a focused physical, history and clinical scenario.

Case Summary: This patient may have problems with skin (cellulitis); deep veins (clots in the legs), thrombosis, and superficial veins thrombosis.

Challenging Question: "Doc. Can you give me a water pill? I have gained water weight and I have a hot date tonight."

Associated Symptoms:

- Pain in legs
- Legs go numb
- Have a hard time walking

Examinee: Must ask these questions and examine patient;

These questions must be asked:

- H/O Travel
- H/O Diabetes
- H/O Trauma
- H/O Heart Disease
- H/O Liver Failure
- H/O Kidney Failure
- Family history of clots must be asked

Examinee must examine patients:

- Legs
- Back
- Heart
- Lungs
- JVD should be checked

The examinee must diagnose this case as: Hepatojugular Reflux

Case 3

Miss Courtney Walsh, 35-year-old female comes with acid reflux.

Vitals:
HR - 92 beats per minute
BP - 110/70 mm of hg
Pulse Ox - 92%
RR - 16 respirations per minute

Notes: Do a focused clinical exam.

Case Summary: SP should present this case by the associated symptoms.

Challenging Question: "Doc. My husband does not want to kiss me because I have bad breath. Do you have anything stronger than Prilosec?"

Associated Symptoms:

- Bad taste in mouth early in the morning
- Wheezing
- Family history of esophageal cancer
- Cough in the middle of the night
- Heartburn
- Hoarseness in mouth.

Examinee: Must ask these questions and examine patient;

These questions must be asked:

- Stress and worries

Examinee must examine patients:

- Tongue for cobble-stoning

The examinee must diagnose this case as: Acid reflux

Case 4

Mrs. Angelina Cole, 42-year-old female, comes with burning pain while passing urine.

Vitals:
HR - 92 beats per minute
BP - 110/70 mm of hg
Pulse Ox - 92%
RR - 16 respirations per minute

Notes: Do a focused clinical exam.

Case Summary: SP should present this case by the associated symptoms.

Challenging Question: "Doc. I get repeating infections. Do you think my husband is cheating on me?"

Associated Symptoms:

- Burning while urinating

Examinee: Must ask these questions and examine patient;

These questions must be asked:

- Burning pain
- Blood
- How frequent?
- Urgency
- Incontinence
- Retention
- Nausea
- Abdominal pain
- Pregnancy

Examinee must examine patients:

- Suprapubic tenderness and CVA tenderness

The examinee must diagnose this case as: UTI

Case 5

Miss Laura Gabitzee, 26-year-old female comes with acne on face.

Vitals:
HR - 92 beats per minute
BP - 110/70 mm of hg
Pulse Ox - 92%
RR - 16 respirations per minute

Notes: Dandruff, OCP and family h/o acne, depression

Case Summary: SP should present this case by the associated symptoms.

Challenging Question: "Can you prescribe me Accutane?"

Associated Symptoms:

- Discharge from acne

Examinee: Must ask these questions and examine patient;

These questions must be asked:

- H/O tanning beds
- Family history of acne
- Make sure to ask about depression
- Pregnancy
- Liver disease
- Alcohol intake

Examinee must examine patients:

- Skin and examine head for dandruff

The examinee must diagnose this case as: acne

Case 6

Mrs. Tiffany Roads, 29-year-old female comes to the office with vaginal discharge.

Vitals:
HR - 92 beats per minute
BP - 110/70 mm of hg
Pulse Ox - 92%
RR - 16 respirations per minute

Notes: Turn this clinical scenario to an abusive relationship.

Case Summary: SP should present troubled emotion, fear and trust issues towards men.

Challenging Question: "Doc. My husband is forcing me to have sex with him. What should I do?"

Associated Symptoms:

- Itching
- Burning

Examinee: Must ask these questions and examine patient;

These questions must be asked:

- Amount   Normal Vagina: 1-4   Abnormal: N/A
- Blood-   +
- Color/consistent   White or transparent   Thick
- Duration   Mid-menstrual
- Exit
- Frequency
- Redness-+
- Swelling-+
- Pain-+
- Color of the area-red
- Functional -can't pee

Examinee must examine patients:

- No Pelvic exam but mention in the note

The examinee must diagnose this case as: Vaginal Discharge

Case 7

Mrs. Tricia Vanstensal, 47-year old female comes with shortness of breath.

Vitals:
HR - 92 beats per minute
BP - 110/70 mm of hg
Pulse Ox - 92%
RR - 22 respirations per minute

Notes: Do a focused clinical exam.

Case Summary: SP should present this case by the associated symptoms. Occupation, work in factory and are exposed to harmful fumes

Challenging Question: "Doc. My employer is not buying masks! I want to sue him."
(Don't encourage lawsuits to other health care providers, as you don't know the story from both sides)

Associated Symptoms:

- Shortness of breath - while taking deep breaths
- Coughing
- Chest pain

Examinee: Must ask these questions and examine patient;

These questions must be asked:

- Occupation Hazards

Examinee must examine patients:

-

The examinee must diagnose this case as: Restrictive or Obstructive Lung Disease

Case 8

Mrs. Charlie Ray, 26-year old female comes with eating disorder and her face is badly bruised.

Vitals:
HR - 92 beats per minute
BP - 110/70 mm of hg
Pulse Ox - 92%
RR - 16 respirations per minute

Notes: This is a clinical scenario of intimate partner violence.

Case Summary: SP should present this case with heightened emotions and self-hate.

Challenging Question: "I don't want to talk about this. I am happily married. I am a faithful Christian wife and God wants us to be together forever."

Associated Symptoms:

- Scars and Sinuses

Examinee: Must ask these questions and examine patient;

These questions must be asked:

First Aid for MOTHERS

- F - Firearms or weapons in home
- O - Alcohol or drugs in home
- M - Money Issues
- Other issues - kids, work, not spending enough time with spouse
- T - Threats
- H - Hit, slapped or kicked
- E - Exit plan
- R - Relationship inside the home/outside the home
- S - Suicidal

Examinee must examine patients:

- Bruises should be documented and measured. Site and side of the bruises is key.

The examinee must diagnose this case as: Abuse patient

Case 9

Mrs. Liana Keffer, 27-year old female comes with tooth ache and could not sleep at night.

Vitals:
HR - 92 beats per minute
BP - 110/70 mm of hg
Pulse Ox - 92%
RR - 16 respirations per minute

Notes: Do a focused clinical scenario - DOCTOR AID @ PM

Case Summary: SP should present this case with pain - Life isn't good. SP does not have dental insurance.

Challenging Question: "Doc. Can I get a slip so I don't have to go into work?"

Associated Symptoms:

> Fever, Chills, headaches

Examinee: Must ask these questions and examine patient;

These questions must be asked:

> Questions about the acid reflux must be asked

Examinee must examine patients:

> HEENT

The examinee must diagnose this case as: Dental Abscess

Case 10

Mrs. Elliot Stevens, 51-year old female comes for a normal routine physical examination and she found a lump on the right breast.

Vitals:
HR - 92 beats per minute
BP - 110/70 mm of hg
Pulse Ox - 92%
RR - 16 respirations per minute

Notes:

Case Summary: SP should present this case with fear of having cancer.

Challenging Question: "Doc. Do you think this could be cancer?"

Associated Symptoms:

- Pain
- Discharge
- Nodes (Lymph Node swelling)

Examinee: Must ask these questions and examine patient;

These questions must be asked:

- Family H/O breast cancer or other cancers

Examinee must examine patients:

-

The examinee must diagnose this case as: Breast cancer

NOTES -

Section L
Patient Notes

Section L – Patient Notes

How to create a good patient note?

History is broken down into the following 6 categories:

1- Chief complaint;
2- History of Present Illness;
3- Review of Systems;
4- Past Medical History, Family History and Social History
5- Examination
6- Assessment and Plan

It is important to document the chief complaint. It should be a concise statement describing the symptoms, problem, and diagnosis, follow up and/or refill of the medications.

History of presenting illness (HPI) should be presented in detailed fashion using the Vital Checklist for the pain or the non-pain symptoms. A brief HPI should have one to three elements and extended HPI will consist of at least 4 elements. The brief or extended HPI is not only useful for billing and coding purposes but also to form an assessment and plan the further coarse of action.

In the USMLE course, you must always take an extended history and try to extract as much history you can as this will help you to nail the problem and narrow the differential diagnosis. We propose that by using Vital Checklist[1]—Life isn't Good, **D.O.C.T.O.R aid @ PM** you will be able to narrow differential diagnosis and this will further help you to order precise tests for that clinical problem. Most importantly it will prevent you from ordering unnecessary tests. This will not only save health care dollars but patients will not be exposed to harmful radiations and unnecessary blood work.

Narrowing differential diagnosis will help you to educate, activate and engage with the patient in a more meaningful way. As a health care provider you will be connected to the patient.

Review of systems using Vital Checklist's **G.H.A.L.E.N and G.H.U.L.A.M** approach will help you to link more associated symptoms to the chief complaint and history of presenting illness.

For example, if you get a clinical scenario of patient with snoring in a patient who is obese. Your first thought is to write diagnosis of obstructive sleep apnea and obviously you are correct about the diagnosis. However, patients who are morbidly obese have separate code in International Classification of Diseases-10 (ICD-10).

> Why it is important to document separately all the morbidities?
> How will it help the patient and patient safety?

It is not only important from a billing and coding standpoint but it is important from statistic collection and comparison with other demographic regions. This will allow the correct allocation of funds and will help epidemiologist to target specific population group.

In clinical case scenario of snoring, these are the questions you are going to ask

	Do Snoring	CI	PI
D	☐ **D**aytime Sleepiness		
O	☐ **O**besity		
S	☐ **S**noring		
N	☐ **N**egative pressure in the pharynx		
O	☐ L**o**w Oxygen and increase in Carbon dioxide		
R	☐ **R**estlessness		
I	☐ **I**mpotence		
N	☐ **N**octuria		
G	☐ Blood **G**as and **G**ERD		
Ci=Caregiver initials Pi- Patient Initials			

Copyright 2016: Harpreet Singh MD, FACP

In this clinical scenario, these diagnoses can be added:

1- Obstructive Sleep Apnea
2- Morbid Obesity (If you have BMI)
3- Metabolic Syndrome (If you have lab values)
4- Nocturia
5- Atrial Fibrillation (If you have EKG or you do a good clinical examination)
6- Hypoxia (If you have low oxygen)
7- Hypercapnia (If you have blood gas results)

The morbidity of this patient increases with other associated syptoms and if this patient is hospitalized, he will need more resources—bariatric bed, telemetry and frequent pulse oxygen evaluation. This increases the Case Mix Index.

He may have bradycardia or tachycardia and therefore asking questions of palpitations become very important. Not only that when you have daytime somnolence, it is important to evaluate for narcolepsy. Patients might be fatigued and may have restless leg syndrome. Patient who have sleep apnea stand more chance of having cardiovascular event and non-alcoholic steato-hepatitis or fatty liver. They might have mild elevation of liver enzymes and therefore ordering the blood work becomes important or doing an EKG and ordering ultrasound of right upper quadrant becomes important.

Furthermore, asking questions about Past Medical History, Family History and Social History with help of this Vital Checklist tool—**What if PAMS Family SHOUTS vaccinate 'em** will help you to extract more answers for the general history. If this sleep apnea patient drinks alcohol, he can get exacerbation of the symptoms, which can be deleterious to the health of the patient. You must counsel this patient on strict cessation of alcohol. In real life clinical scenario, electronic health records have made our life easy and you may not need a checklist for past, family and social history. When you are a medical student you must not to skip this exercise. As explained earlier in the book, it is important to make mental models and prevent cognitive tunneling.

In Step 2 Clinical Skills exam, diagnosis of clinical problems is not complex as they are usual straightforward clinical scenarios and therefore documenting the correct clinical diagnosis is important. This can be done only when you have a complete picture of the patient and therefore paying close attention to the vital signs and examination is of great help. This will help with the medical decision-making. Try to document as many abnormalities as you can in the exam. Even if you see minor scars and sinuses, you must document those as this will help to reach the accurate diagnosis.

In this clinical scenario of sleep apnea, it is important to look into the nose and mouth for crowding of the upper airways. If you can find a tape measure, it is good idea to measure the neck size as if this is above 17 inches or larger in males or 16 inches or larger in female, you will a higher chance of having sleep apnea.

In USMLE Step 2 CS exam, it is mentioned to do focus examination. In ICD-10 and real life it is important to understand the difference between different types of examinations. *A problem focused examination* means that you must document one body area and system. To get to the level of **EXPANDED** *problem focused examination* detailed examination of 2-4 body areas or systems must be included and that must have the affected area. After this level is the *detailed examination* and *comprehensive level* where you must include 5-7 body systems and 8 or more body areas respectively. In the USMLE exam, it is next to impossible to reach to detailed examination and comprehensive level because of the time constraints. On numerous occasions, we have told medical students coming to our workshop to focus on counseling and do only one system examination. However, if you are trained properly, you can manage 2-4 body systems in three and half minutes.

The most important aspect of the Step 2 CS exam is to communicate. Medical students have a habit of coming out of the room when they have completed their clinical scenarios before the stipulated time of 15 minutes. We despise this practice, as more time you spend with the patient, more you will develop trust. If you have nothing else to discuss, draw pictures and try to explain in layman terms.

Once you have collected all the history point and done good examination you will have 10 minutes to write a patient note. Most students fear that they will not be able to finish the patient note in timely fashion as failing in the patient note, means failing in the exam.

How can you make sure that you pass this segment?

With good typing speed, you will be able to complete the patient note. Writing a patient note is tact. However, never cut down on face-to-face time to complete patient note. If you are slow in typing, then practice patient notes but never exit the patient examination room in 12 or 13 minutes.

On October 1st, 2015, International Classification of Diseases-10 was implemented in American healthcare. This is different from ICD-9 in following aspects:

ICD-9	ICD-10
➢ 3-5 characters	➢ 3-7 characters
➢ 14,000 codes	➢ 69,000 codes
➢ No details	➢ Laterality and severity information
➢ Need multiple codes for a case	➢ Use combination codes to describe manifestation in a single code
➢ Based on outdated (more than 35 years) medical terminology	➢ Updated medical terminology

It is important to point out the fact that in the patient note it is important to document right and left and not mention the abbreviation "R" or "L" as they result in errors. In ICD-10, progression, previous episodes and laterality and associated symptoms are important. ICD-10 helps to transmit information in a single code, which helps in planning the treatment. In the USMLE exam, it is important to mention if you have right shoulder pain or left shoulder pain. Never just mention shoulder pain in the diagnosis section. This brings us to assessment and planning the treatment.

In a patient with sleep apnea, you will often encounter hypertension and this may affect the heart. Unless you know the anatomy and physiology, you will not be able to order the correct investigations. Patients, who have sleep apnea, have daytime somnolence, have obesity and snore. When they sleep, pharyngeal dilator muscles collapse under the force of gravity thus retaining CO^2 and preventing O^2 from diffusing. When the patient is hypoxic, blood vessels vasodilate to provide blood to the important organs. This leads to stimulation of the carotid body and release of sympathetic hormones causing vasoconstriction for adequate perfusion. This release of sympathetic hormones raises the blood pressure in the systemic circulation and also blood pressure is increased in pulmonary circulation. Once pulmonary hypertension ensues, it causes right heart failure and swelling in the legs. This is the reason that you must order BNP and echocardiography. An increase in the pressure in the atrial chamber will release atrial natriuretic peptide causing nocturia.

[1] A. B. Haynes, T. G. Weiser, W. R. Berry, S. R. Lipsitz, A. H. Breizat, E. P. Dellinger, *et al.*, "A surgical safety checklist to reduce morbidity and mortality in a global population," *N Engl J Med,* vol. 360, pp. 491-9, Jan 2009.

Examples of Patient Notes

Patient Note 1- Corrected Patient Note

HPI: Mr Davis, 21 yo M, truck driver by profession c/o Sore throat since 2 weeks.

Positive History should be written first and all symptoms should be described separately.
Sudden in onset, gradually worsening, with no aggravating or relieving factors. The pt. did not take any medication for it. It is associated with fever, but did not record it (or subjective feeling of fever), more in the morning, relieved with Tylenol. Pt. also complains of difficulty swallowing and speaking and a 5Lbs weight loss in 2 weeks. Also c/o LUQ abdomen pain, 4/10 severity, non-radiating, no aggravating or relieving factors. .

This is followed by negative history to rule out other system involvement
No headaches, facial pain, runny nose, cough, chest pain, shortness of breath, nausea, vomiting, bowel or urinary complains. His girlfriend has similar complaints 2 weeks back.
ROS: None except above
PMH: **(always inquire about the type of antibiotic and duration of course)**
h/o Gonorrhea 4 months back, treated with intramuscular ceftriaxone and azithromycin (or one injectable antibiotic and one oral antibiotic, unable to recall)

PSH: None
Current Medications: Tylenol for fever
FH: No h/o DM, HTN or any cancer
SH: student, **Alcohol use**→be more precise- consumes alcohol twice weekly, mostly beer, CAGE- 0/4, Smokes 1 PPD since 6 yrs, multiple sexual partners, prefers both men and women, no contraceptives (unprotected)
GPE: patient in mild distress
Vitals: Temp: 99.4, Pulse- 100/min, BP- 110/70mm of Hg or rest WNL
AO* 3
HEENT: **(Positive findings described first for easy understanding of the patient note)**
Mild pharyngeal erythema, with pustular exudates. Lymphadenopathy +(LNP- localized or generalized?)
NCAT, PEERLA, EOMI, no edema, icterus,
CVS: RRR, S1, S2 heard, no murmurs, gallops
Respi: B/l Air entry present, normal to percussion
Abd: soft, non distended, mild tendernessLUQ, (Be very careful of right and left)
BS+, Splenomegaly+
Neuro- within normal limits

D/D

History	P/E
Infectious Mononucleosis	Fever
Sore throat	Lymphadenopathy +

LUQ Abd pain	LUQ Tenderness
h/o similar symptoms in girlfriend	Splenomegaly +

History	P/E
Viral/Bacterial Pharyngitis	Fever
Fever	Swollen Nodes
Sore throat	Pharyngeal erythema
Swelling in Neck	

History	P/E
HIV	Lymphadenopathy
H/o wt loss	Fever
multiple sexual partners	
unprotected sexual intercourse	

Investigations

CBC, ESR, Monospot test, HIV, Abd USG, Throat Swab, Genital swab

Patient Note 2 - Corrected Patient Note

HPI: A 55yo G2P2 F c/o sudden onset, gradually worsening, burning, intermittent, right upper quadrant pain, 7/10 severity, relieved by food, antacids, milk, worsens with fatty meals. Non radiating, currently taking maalox, ibuprofen.
Assoc. with nausea +, vomiting + one time at am, sour, yellow, non-bloody vomitus.
No h/o -fever -, chest discomfort-, SOB -, skin changes -, - bowel and bladder changes, weight change -, appetite NL, insomnia -
OB/GYN: LMP; 3 weeks back, regular monthly cycles, menarche 13yo, Normal flow and duration
PMH: UTI one year back Rx with Nitrofurantoin **(Specify if known).**
h/o arthritis of joints, taking ibuprofen
PSH: 2 C-Section Allergies: NKDA
FH: father died of pancreatic CA at 55 yo, no h/o DM or HTN
SH: smoking-, EtOH -, illicit drugs-, sexually active with husband, uses contraception

PHYSICAL EXAMINATION:
GA: appears in pain
VS: WNL
HEENT: NCAT, PEERLA, EOMI, no pallor edema, icterus, lymphadenopathy
Abdomen: BS + all 4Q, tympanic notes + all 4Q, Soft, ND, tenderness + RUQ, guarding -, rebound tenderness -, Murphy's sign +, no organomegaly, CVA NT
CVS: S1, S2 +, RRR, no murmur, rubs, gallops
RS: clear to auscultation B/L, normal percussion findings
CNS: moves all 4 limbs equally, CN grossly intact

D/D

History	P/E
Peptic Ulcer Disease	Epigastric tenderness
Abdomen pain	
Relieved by Maalox	
Burning type of pain	

History	P/E
Cholecystitis	RUQ tenderness
RUQ Abdomen pain, intermittent	Murphy's sign +
Worsens after fatty food	
Vomiting	

History	P/E
NSAID induced Gastritis	Epigastric tenderness
Abdomen pain	
h/o ibuprofen use	

Investigations
CBC, ESR, Rectal exam, stool occult blood, H.pylori stool antigen, Urine b-hCG, S.Bilirubin (Direct and Indirect) AST/ALT/ALP, USG Abdomen, UGI endoscopy, CT Abdomen

Patient Note 3-Corrected Patient Note

HPI: A 46 yo M % sudden onset of retrosternal chest pain while sleeping at 5am, 7/10 severity, pressure like, constant pain that radiates to Left arm and jaw. Lasted for 30 minutes.
-% previous episodes of similar chest pain in milder form 2-3 times/week, each episode lasting for 5-10 mins, aggravated by taking stairs, exercise and heavy meal.
-Associated with SOB + during the pain episode, sweating +,
No h/o nausea-, cough-, aggravating and relieving factors -, exercise-
ROS: negative except as above
Meds: Maalox, diuretics   All: NKDA
PMH: HTN 5 yrs uncontrolled, Rx with diuretics (non-compliant); GERD 10 yrs back treated with Maalox; high cholesterol, poor compliance with diet control
FH: dad lung Ca died at 72 yo, mom alive and has GERD, No h/o HTN or DM in the family
SH: smokes 1ppd for 25 yrs, stopped 3 months back because of doctor's advice; social drinker→2-3 beers over weekend or parties, CAGE-0/4; uses cocaine once a week, last used it yesterday afternoon, sexually active with girlfriend, uses contraception

PHYSICAL EXAMINATION
GA: pt appears in distress
VS: BP 165/85, RR 22, HR 90
Neck: No JVD, no bruits, no lymphadenpathy
CVS: PMI not displaced; no palpable thrill/murmur/tenderness; S1, S2 +; RRR; no murmurs, rubs, gallops;
RS: CTA B/L
GI: BS+
CNS: grossly intact, obeys commands
Ext: Edema -, peripheral pulses + and symmetric

D/D

History	P/E
Myocardial infarction	High BP
Pressure like retrosternal chest pain	
Radiating to left jaw + arm	
High cholesterol and uncontrolled HTN	

History	P/E
Cocaine induced MI	RUQ tenderness
h/o recent Cocaine abuse	High BP
Pressure like retrosternal chest pain	
Radiating to left jaw	

History	P/E
GERD	
Epigastric pain	
Previous h/o GERD	

Diagnostic Study/Studies
CBC, ECG, CPK, CPK-MB, Tropnin T, MBP, Transthoracic Echo, Coronary Angiogram, UGI Endoscopy

Patient Note 4-Corrected Patient Note

HPI: Hx obtained from mother, who is also the legal guardian of the child. Pt is a 7mo baby boy with fever (rectal temp 101F, measured at home) with sudden onset and continuous since last night, partially relieved by Tylenol syrup. Fever was associated with tiredness, runny nose, SOB, rapid breathing, irritability, excessive sleepiness, decreased activity, excessive crying, difficulty in swallowing, decreased feeding (refused BF since last night)
Negative history- -No h/o cough, noisy breathing, rash, ear pulling, eye rubbing, bowel/bladder disturbances, chills, nausea/vomiting
Sick contact: 3 yo older brother had URTI 2 weeks ago.
ROS: negative except as above
Birth history: FT NVD, uncomplicated pregnancy
UTD on vaccines, last checkup one month back
Development appropriate for age, weight/height normal
Diet: BF + vitamins prescribed by doctors + Baby Food TID (In transition from exclusive breast feed to solid food)
PMH-Non contributory,
PSH- Non contributory,
Allergies- Non contributory,
Medications- Syrup Tylenol
Family History- Elder brother had UTI 2 weeks back,
Social History- attended daycare, no h/o sick contacts at daycare

PHYSICAL EXAMINATION:
Unable to perform as the child is at home.

D/D

History	P/E
Pneumonia	
Fever	
Rapid breathing	
Excessive sleepiness	

History	P/E
UTI	
Fever	
H/o older brother with UTI	
Difficulty in swallowing	

History	P/E
Meningitis	
Fever	
Excessive Sleepiness	
Irritable	

Investigations
Physical examination, **CBC, ESR, Blood culture, CXR PA view, Otoscopy, Throat swab, LP- CSF Analysis, cell count and culture.**

To get your patient note corrected,

please contact hi@vitalchecklist.com

Practice Material[1]: How to create and share a template for the patient note using Google docs

- Most students have a Gmail account but if you don't one have then make an account in Gmail.
- Start a new document
- Change the name from Untitled document to Case-1—Name of the problem with which presented—your name
- Click on the tab named 'TABLE' and this is the seventh tab on the table.
- Holding or hovering the mouse over the TABLE will give you a choice to select one vertical and 20 horizontal rows.
- On the first line write your case name.
- The second line should be left blank for this line which we have taken from the USMLE website [1]
- The third horizontal row is a box for history writing. Make sure you always write a chief complaint of the patient followed by HPI. This should follow past medical and surgical history. Never forget to mention the review of systems, family history, social history, sexual history, vaccination, travel and sick contact history.
- Following this leave a blank row or a box for a physical examination.
- After you have written a physical exam, you will find this:
  - Lines 1 /15 Characters: 950
- Then there are three horizontal rows, which are highlighted in turquoise blue, yellow and turquoise blue. In these horizontal rows, you can write the diagnosis according to the clinical presentation. During Step 2 CS test, you must be able to support your diagnosis with history findings and physical exam findings. In the patient note, you have separate rows for these findings but in Google docs, we inserted another table with two columns and three rows.
- Last but not the least; we have rows for the diagnostic studies.

After you have completed your patient note, you can get your patient note checked by sharing with our experts at hi@vitalchecklist.com

As we get many patient notes for correction, we try to help everybody but have time constraints. We will prioritize the students who have enrolled in our workshop. I hope you will understand.

Good luck.

Case

HISTORY: Describe the history you just obtained from this patient. Include only information (pertinent positives and negatives) relevant to this patient's problem(s)

Chief complaint

History of presenting illness

PMH and Surgical history

ROS

FH

SH

Sexual History

Vaccination, Travel and Sick contacts

Lines: Total Line-15 **Characters:** 950

PHYSICAL EXAMINATION: Describe any positive and negative findings relevant to this patient's problem(s). Be careful to include *only* those parts of examination you performed in *this* encounter.

Physical Examination

Lines: Total Line-15 **Characters:** 950

Diagnosis 1→	
History Findings	Physical Exam Findings

Diagnosis 2→	
History Findings	Physical Exam Findings

Diagnosis 3→	
History Findings	Physical Exam Findings

DIAGNOSTIC STUDIES:

[1] (2016, June 29th). *Patient Note Entry Form.* Available: http://www.usmle.org/practice-materials/step-2-cs/patient-note-practice2.html

Investigations based on Symptoms

Nervous System

Headache

- CT head without contrast
- MRI is more sensitive and demonstrates white matter lesions (MS) posterior fossa lesions, seller lesions, cranio-cervical junction lesions and congenital anomalies.
- CT Angiography or Magnetic resonance angiography (if blood is present in the subarachnoid space or parenchyma)
- Lumbar Puncture
- XRAY of the Cervical Spine
- CT Scan of the Sinus
- CBC, CMP, Magnesium, Phosphorous, PT, INR, UA
- ESR, CRP
- BETA-Hcg (if child bearing woman)

Loss of Consciousness

- CT Scan of the brain without contrast
- MRI of the brain
- EKG, (May need holter monitor or event monitor)
- Carotid ULTRASOUND
- ECHO
- CBC, CMP, Magnesium, Phosphorous, UA, Pro BNP
- EEG
- BETA-Hcg (if child bearing woman)

Dizziness

- CT Scan of the brain without contrast
- MRI of the brain
- EKG, (May need Holter monitor or event monitor)
- Carotid ULTRASOUND
- ECHO
- CBC, CMP, Magnesium, Phosphorous, UA, Pro BNP
- URINE Sodium, Serum Osmolality and Urine Osmolality (Hyponatremia)
- BETA-Hcg (if child bearing woman)

Numbness and Tingling

- XRAY of the lumbosacral area (if lower extremity)
- XRAY of the Cervical Spine (if upper extremity)
- Vitamin b12 level
- CT scan without contrast (Stroke)
- MRI (Multiple Sclerosis)
- CBC, CMP, Magnesium, Phosphorous
- Ionized Calcium, PTH
- HBA1c and Microalbuminuria
- Nerve conduction study and EMG
- Beta HCG (if child bearing woman)

Muscle Weakness

- CT Scan of the Brain
- MRI of the Brain with contrast
- MRI of the lumbosacral area
- Vitamin B12 level
- Iron Panel, Zinc level (Restless legs)
- Lyme titers (Tick bites)
- LP, Nerve conduction and EMG (GBS)
- Acetylcholine Receptor Antibody, Anti Musk Antibody, EMG (Myasthenia Gravis)
- Voltage gated calcium channel antibodies, CT Scan of thorax, Bronchoscopy, PET scan and Edrophonium (Tensilon) Test
- Beta HCG (if child bearing woman)

Tremors

- CT Scan of the brain
- MRI of the brain
- ABG
- Urine Copper 24 hour
- Alcohol level
- Sleep Apnea testing
- Genetic Testing
- CBC, CMP, Magnesium, Phosphorous
- Ionized Calcium, PTH
- Urine Drug Screen
- Beta HCG (if child bearing woman)

Seizures

- CT scan of the brain
- MRI of the brain
- CBC, CMP, Magnesium, Phosphorous, UA
- Blood culture
- PT, INR
- Lumbar Puncture
- EEG
- Urine Drug screen
- Beta HCG (if child bearing woman)

Confusion

- CT scan of the brain
- MRI of the brain
- CBC, CMP, Magnesium, Phosphorous, UA, ABG
- Blood culture
- PT, INR
- Lumbar Puncture
- EEG
- Urine Drug screen
- Beta HCG (if child bearing woman)
- Urine sodium, urine osmolality and serum osmolality

Memory Loss

- CT Scan of the brain
- MRI of the brain with and without contrast
- CBC, CMP, Magnesium, Phosphorous, UA, ABG
- Blood culture
- PT, INR
- Lumbar Puncture
- EEG
- Urine Drug screen
- Beta HCG (if child bearing woman)
- Urine sodium, urine osmolality and serum osmolality
- Vitamin B12 level, TSH, Free T4, T3, TPO and TG
- HIV
- Lyme titers
- Urine Copper 24 hour

Loss of Vision

- CBC, CMP
- UA
- Visual Field
- Intraocular Pressure
- Retinal Examination

Hearing Loss

- CBC
- CMP
- Pneumoscopy
- Audiology testing

Cardiovascular System

Chest Pain

- **Vital Signs**

(Does the patient have tachycardia or tachypnea, low BP, high BP or low pulse ox?)
- **EKG**→STEMI or Non-STEMI→ Cardiology; Go to the next step do Chest XRAY
- **Chest Xray**- Evaluate for Pneumothorax, Aortic Dissection, Pneumonia and Heart Failure→ May need confirmation with **CT Scan** and **ECHO**→**Pro-BNP and serial Pro-BNP**
- IF chest X-RAY is non-diagnostic → **cardiac markers** are positive→ Acute coronary syndrome
- IF chest X-RAY is non-diagnostic → cardiac markers are negative→ This is not acute coronary syndrome; Seek other diagnosis
- IF chest X-RAY is non-diagnostic → **D-Dimer** is positive→**V/Q scan, CT-Angio and Ultrasound** of the legs→Pulmonary Clots→Treat
- IF chest X-RAY is non-diagnostic → D-Dimer is negative and low pretest probability of pulmonary embolism→ seek another diagnosis
- If chest Xray and EKG are non-diagnostic; cardiac markers and d-dimer are negative→ **bedside ultrasound** to evaluate for tamponade or pericarditis.

Once the life threatening cause of chest pain is ruled out; next step
- **Stress EKG**
- **Stress echocardiography**

- **Stress myocardial perfusion imaging**
- **Pharmacologic myocardial perfusion imaging**

Pharmacological agents are preferred if patient is not able to exercise, have left bundle branch block, ventricular paced rhythm.
Vasodilator pharmacologic agents are contraindicated in the following conditions:

A	**A**sthma	Pronounced active broncho-spastic airway disease
B	**B**lood Pressure	Significant hypotension
C	**C**oronary Syndrome	Unstable or complicated acute coronary syndrome
D	**D**ead Pacemaker	Sick sinus syndrome and high-degree atrio-ventricular block

Palpitations

- CBC, CMP, magnesium and phosphorous
- TSH, free T4, T3, TPO and TG
- Urine Drug Screen
- Iron panel
- Beta HCG pregnancy test
- Twelve-lead EKG
- Echocardiography→ May need stress testing also.
- Holter monitor
- Loop event recorders
- Electrophysiologic testing

Respiratory Disease

Shortness of Breath

- **CBC, CMP, ABG** → Anemia, metabolic and respiratory acidosis and/or alkalosis→respiratory depression
- **Magnesium level** →Hypo-magnesium→Muscle weakness→respiratory depression
- **Magnesium level**→Hyper-magnesium→Neuromuscular toxicity, hypotension and bradycardia→respiratory depression
- **Phosphorous level**→ Remember ATP→Adenosine tri-phosphate→Cardiac myocyte contractility is dependent on the phosphate→heart failure when the phosphate concentration falls below 1mg/dl. Diaphragm also weakens when phosphate levels are low leading to respiratory failure.
- **Chest X-ray**

- **TSH, free T4, T3**
- **ECG**
- **Pro-BNP**
- **Ambulatory Pulse OX**
- **Spirometer**→airflow limitation with reduced FEV1/FVC→ think of COPD (irreversible) or asthma (reversible) with reduced FVC→ if reduced DLCO think of emphysema or bronchiolitis
- **Lung volume**→no airflow limitation with normal FEV1/FVC→think of restrictive lung disease→ if reduced DLCO think of interstitial lung disease; If normal DLCO think of neuromuscular disorders
- **High resolution CT** if interstitial Lung disease is diagnosed. HRCT may also be used for tumors and airway obstruction
- **Echocardiography** helps to differentiate between heart failure with reduced ejection fraction and heart failure with preserved ejection fraction
- **Doppler Echocardiography** for pulmonary artery hypertension

Cough

- Medications-ACE inhibitor should be stopped
- Chest XRAY
- PPD testing
- Blood culture and sputum culture
- Spirometry
- CT SCAN of the Sinus
- EGD and biopsy
- Lung volume
- HRCT
- Bronchoscopy
- Echocardiography

Sore throat

- Rapid Strep testing
- Throat culture
- DNA Probe
- CBC, CMP, with manual differential
- Helicobacter Pylori stool antigen testing
- HIV Elisa testing
- Blood culture

(No cough- Group A Streptococcus; Cough- Can be anything)

Snoring

- Home Sleep Apnea Testing
- Polysomnogram
- TSH, Free T4, T3
- CT Scan of the sinus

Gastrointestinal System

Abdominal Pain

- CBC, CMP, Magnesium and Phosphorous
- Lactic Acid
- Lipase and Amylase
- Beta HCG in childbearing woman
- Stool test-Ova and Parasite, Stool leukocyte, FOBT, Helicobacter Stool antigen testing
- Celiac Panel
- Iron Panel
- UA
- Ultrasound
- CT scan of the abdomen and pelvis with PO and IV contrast

IF cancer is suspected
- CEA
- CA19-9
- CA-125
- ELISA testing

More invasive testing
- EGD
- Colonoscopy
- Capsule Endoscopy
- ERCP
- MRCP

Dysphagia

- EGD

- Barium Swallow
- Motility studies
- CBC, CMP, Mag and Phosphorous
- Iron panel
- Stool studies
- ANA, Rheumatoid Factor; SSA and SSB

Weight Loss

- Same as the abdominal pain
- PPD

Vomiting

- Same as the abdominal pain

Diarrhea

- CBC, CMP, Mag, Phosphorous
- Lactic acid
- Lipase and Amylase
- Stool test Ova and Parasite, Stool WBC, FOBT
- Pancreatic elastase
- Clostridium difficile Toxin Assay
- Breath test

Jaundice

- Due to problems in the blood→CBC and Urine Test, Bilirubin→ Prehepatic
- Due to problems in the Liver→ LFT→Intrahepatic or Posthepatic
- Due to the problems in the bile duct→Alkaline Phosphatase and GGT are high→Post-hepatic
- Due to the problems compressing the bile duct from outside→Alkaline Phosphatase and GGT are high→Post hepatic
- Due to problems in the bone→Alkaline Phosphatase high with normal GGT
- No elevation of GGT or Alkaline phosphatase but mild elevation of liver enzymes→ An easy way to remember is by remembering children books: The Cat in the Hat or is it "The Fat Cat MEOW in the Hat!"

In daily practice, you will get many patients with mild elevation of liver enzymes, don't start ordering expensive tests right from the get go.

The Cat in the Hat or "The Fat Cat MEOW in the Hat!"		
	The Fat Cat Meow	
Initial Evaluation		
T	**T**herapy and treatment	Urine Drug Screen
H	**H**epatitis and **H**emochromatosis	HBsAg, anti-HBs, anti-HBc, anti-HCV; Fe/TIBC >45 percent
E	**E**thanol	AST/ALT ratio > 2/1
Fat	**Fat**ty Liver	Liver Ultrasound
Second Line Evaluation		
C	**C**eliac Disease	Celiac Panel
A	**A**utoimmune Hepatitis	ANA; anti-smooth muscle antibodies [ASMA]
T	**T**hyroid	TSH, Free t4, t3, TPO and TG
Third Line evaluation		
M	**M**uscle problems	Creatinine kinase
E	**E**ndocrine-Adrenal insufficiency	8am cortisol and plasma ACTH
O	**O**thers	Alpha 1 Antitrypsin deficiency
W	**W**ilson Disease	Serum ceruloplasmin
Lastly		
	Liver biopsy	

Reference:

www.uptodate.com

Castillo, N. E., Vanga, R. R., Theethira, T. G., Rubio-Tapia, A., Murray, J. A., Villafuerte, J., . . . Leffler, D. A. (2015, 07). Prevalence of Abnormal Liver Function Tests in Celiac Disease and the Effect of a Gluten-Free Diet in the US Population. *Am J Gastroenterol The American Journal of Gastroenterology, 110*(8), 1216-1222. doi:10.1038/ajg.2015.192

Daniel, S. (1999, 10). Prospective evaluation of unexplained chronic liver transaminase abnormalities in asymptomatic and symptomatic patients. *The American Journal of Gastroenterology, 94*(10), 3010-3014. doi:10.1016/s0002-9270(99)00507-9

Skelly, M. M., James, P. D., & Ryder, S. D. (2001, 08). Findings on liver biopsy to investigate abnormal liver function tests in the absence of diagnostic serology. *Journal of Hepatology, 35*(2), 195-199. doi:10.1016/s0168-8278(01)00094-0

Bloody Vomiting

- CBC, CMP, Magnesium, and Phosphorous
- Helicobacter Pylori Antigen stool testing
- EGD
- PT and PTT

- INR
- EKG
- Troponin and BNP
- Lactic acid
- Lipase and Amylase
- EGD

Bloody Stools

- CBC, CMP, Magnesium, and Phosphorous
- Helicobacter Pylori Antigen stool testing
- EGD
- PT and PTT
- INR
- EKG
- Troponin and BNP
- Lactic acid
- Lipase and Amylase
- EGD
- Clostridum Diffcile toxin assay
- Stool Ova and Parasite
- Stool WBC
- Stool Pancreatic elastase

Fatigue with Pallor

- CBC, CMP, Magnesium, and Phosphorous
- Helicobacter Pylori Antigen stool testing
- EGD
- PT and PTT
- INR
- EKG
- Troponin and BNP
- Lactic acid
- Lipase and Amylase
- EGD
- Clostridum Diffcile toxin assay
- Stool Ova and Parasite
- Stool WBC
- Stool Pancreatic elastase
- TSH, FREE T4, T3
- Hepatitis Panel
- Sedimentation Rate, CRP

Endocrine System

Polyuria

Key Concepts before you order tests:
1. Glucose out→Water out (Diabetes Mellitus has osmotic induced polyuria)
2. Water in = Water out (Diabetes Insipidus) Primary Psychogenic Polydipsia
3. Less Water in < More Water out→Due to Brain issues (Central Diabetes Insipidus)
4. Less Water in < More Water out → Due to Kidney issues (Genetic Nephrogenic Diabetes Insipidus) → Mutations in the AVPR2 gene encoding the ADH receptor V2; mutations in the aquaporin-2 (water channel) gene.
5. Less Water in < More Water out → Due to Kidney issues (Acquired Nephrogenic Diabetes Insipidus) → Lithium and Hypercalcemia

Tests to be ordered

- CBC, CMP
- Plasma Osmolality
- Urine Osmolality
- Water restriction test (make sure patient is not high risk)
- Plasma ADH and Urine ADH

Weight gain

- CBC, CMP, UA
- Hba1c, Microalbuminuria
- TSH, Free T4, T3
- 8am cortisol and ACTH
- FSH, LH, Estrone
- Testosterone
- CRP
- Beta HCG

Neck Mass
- CBC with manual difference
- TSH, free T4, T3
- HIV
- Sedimentation rate, CRP,
- Blood culture
- CMV and EBV
- HIV

- PPD
- Antibodies to Ro/SSA and Ro/SSB
- Ultrasound
- CT scans of the Neck
- MRI for the soft tissues

Musculoskeletal System

Knee pain

- CBC, CMP,
- Sedimentation rate, CRP
- Joint Fluid Aspirate (this should be written in the patient note)
- X-rays
- MRI of the Knee

Ankle Pain

- CBC, CMP,
- Sedimentation rate, CRP
- Joint Fluid Aspirate (this should be written in the patient note)
- X-rays
- MRI of the Ankle

Elbow pain

- CBC, CMP,
- Sedimentation rate, CRP
- Joint Fluid Aspirate (this should be written in the patient note)
- X-rays
- MRI

Shoulder pain

- CBC, CMP,
- Sedimentation rate, CRP
- X-rays
- MRI

Back Pain

- CBC, CMP,
- Sedimentation rate, CRP
- X-rays
- MRI

Urology and Reproductive System

Bloody urine

- CBC, CMP
- UA, C3, C4,
- Hepatitis Panel
- C-ANCA and P-ANCA
- Urine cytology
- Urine Culture
- Kidney Ultrasound
- Cystoscopy

Burning Urination

- CBC, CMP
- UA
- Urine cytology
- Urine Culture
- Kidney Ultrasound
- Cystoscopy
- Beta HCG

Incontinence

- CBC, CMP
- UA
- Urine cytology
- Urine Culture

- Kidney Ultrasound
- Cystoscopy
- Xrays of the lumbosacral spine
- CT scan of the brain
- MRI of the brain and neck
- Beta HCG

Lower abdominal pain

- CBC, CMP
- UA
- Urine cytology
- Urine Culture
- Beta HCG
- Ultrasound
- CT scan of abdomen and pelvis

Pregnancy

- CBC, CMP
- UA
- Urine cytology
- Urine Culture
- Beta HCG
- Ultrasound
- Iron level
- PT and INR

Unable to conceive

- CBC, CMP
- UA
- TSH, Free T4, T3
- FSH, LH
- Ultrasound- Pelvic and Transvaginal Ultrasound
- Genetic testing
- Male sperm analysis
- MRI of the brain with contrast

Erectile Dysfunction

- CBC
- CMP
- HBA1c
- Vitamin B12 level
- Lumbosacral xrays
- MRI of the Brain
- Arterial Plethysomography
- TSH, free T4, T3
- Urine drug screen

Vaginal Bleeding

- CBC, CMP
- UA
- Urine cytology
- Urine Culture
- Beta HCG
- Iron level
- PT and INR
- TSH, Free T4, T3
- FSH, LH
- Ultrasound- Pelvic and Transvaginal Ultrasound
- Pap smear

Pain During Sex

- CBC, CMP
- UA
- Urine cytology
- Urine Culture
- Beta HCG
- Iron level
- PT and INR
- TSH, Free T4, T3
- FSH, LH
- Ultrasound- Pelvic and Transvaginal Ultrasound
- Pap smear

Psychiatry

Depressed Mood

- CBC, CMP
- UA
- Urine cytology
- Urine Culture
- Beta HCG (in woman)
- Iron level
- PT and INR
- TSH, Free T4, T3
- FSH, LH
- Urine drug screen

Hallucinations

- CBC, CMP
- UA
- Urine cytology
- Urine Culture
- Beta HCG (in women)
- Iron level
- TSH, Freet4, t3
- Urine drug screen
- CT scan of the brain
- MRI of the Brian

Insomnia

- CBC, CMP
- UA
- Urine cytology
- Urine Culture
- Beta HCG (in woman)
- Iron level
- TSH, Free T4, T3
- Urine drug screen
- Obstructive Sleep apnea testing
- FSH and LH

Anxiety

- CBC, CMP
- UA
- Urine cytology
- Urine Culture
- Beta HCG (in woman)
- Iron level
- TSH, Free T4, T3
- Urine drug screen
- Obstructive Sleep apnea testing
- FSH and LH

Dehydration

- CBC, CMP, UA
- Urine Osmolality
- Stool test Ova and Parasite
- Stool Leukocytes
- Stool culture
- Pancreatic elastase

Seizures

- CBC, CMP, UA
- Blood culture
- CT scan of the brain
- PT/INR
- Lumbar puncture
- CSF analysis
- Urine culture

Enuresis

- CBC, CMP, UA
- HBA1c
- Urine Micro albuminuria
- Urine osmolality
- Urine sodium
- Xrays of the lumbosacral region
- Ultrasound of the bladder
- Cystoscopy

Wheezing

- CBC, CMP
- Allergy testing
- Chest Xray
- Sputum culture
- Spirometry
- Lung volumes

Fever

- CBC, CMP, UA
- Blood culture
- Urine Culture
- CSF Culture
- Chest Xray
- Sed rate
- CRP
- CT Scan of the abdomen and pelvis (depends on the symptoms)
- CT scan of the brain (depends on the symptoms)
- White Blood Scan (if cannot find the source of infection)

NOTES:

Section M

Vital Checklist Workshop & Health Care Strategy

Section M – Vital Checklist Workshop and Health Care Strategy

Enroll in Vital Checklist Workshop

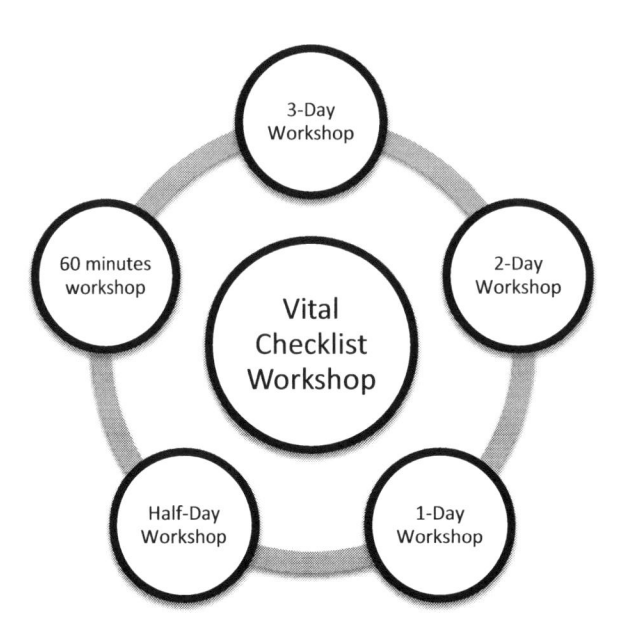

- 3-Day Workshop
- 2-Day Workshop
- 1-Day Workshop
- Half-Day Workshop
- 60 minutes workshop

Vital Checklist Workshop

Who benefits and how do they benefit?

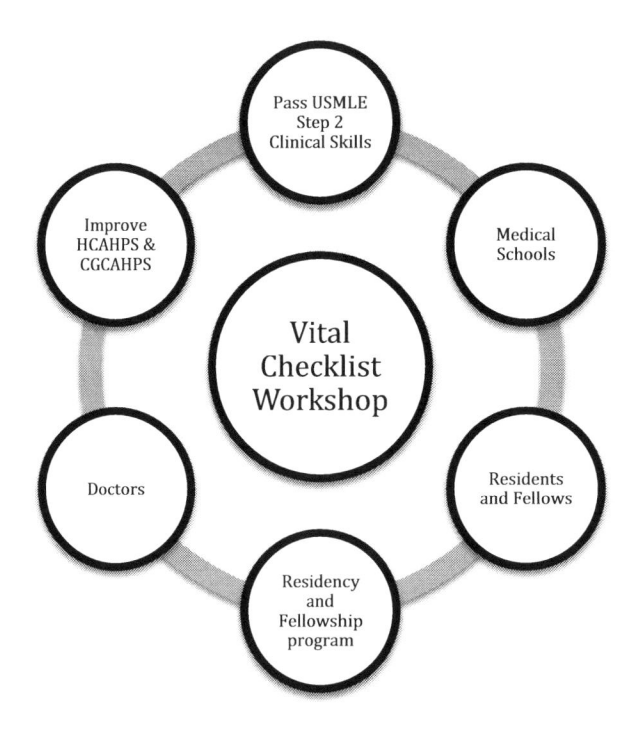

- Pass USMLE Step 2 Clinical Skills
- Medical Schools
- Residents and Fellows
- Residency and Fellowship program
- Doctors
- Improve HCAHPS & CGCAHPS

Vital Checklist Workshop

Shortage of doctors! Medical practices are being disrupted. We need more physician assistants and nurse practitioners.

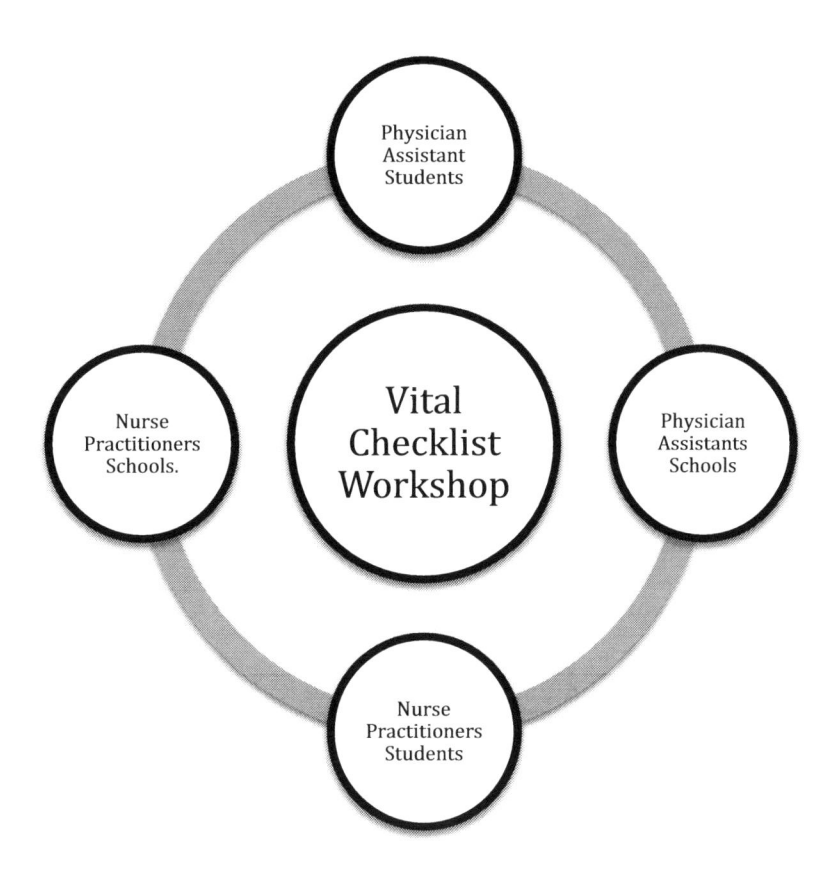

- Physician Assistant Students
- Nurse Practitioners Schools.
- **Vital Checklist Workshop**
- Physician Assistants Schools
- Nurse Practitioners Students

Invite Dr.Harpreet Singh and his team to conduct Vital Checklist Workshop at your hospital, clinic, residency, fellowship, medical school, physician assistant or medical assistant school.

Dr.Harpreet Singh also conducts wellness seminars under www.icrush.org and has developed innovative tools and techniques to help his patients. His vision is "healthcare knowledge at fingertips." His mission "early to diagnose, early to treat makes patients healthy, wealthy and wise." Let's "Flip the Healthcare." Invite Dr.Singh to give a health talk in your community, church or a business.

You can listen to Dr.Harpreet Singh every Saturday at 7pm on WBRN radio show—Talk Medicine.

If you would like to have a second opinion or become his patient you can call or email him at drsingh@vitalchecklist.com

Vital Checklist Workshop for Medical Students and Medical Schools

Vital Checklist Workshop for Medical Students and Medical Schools

- ➢ Our Immediate Goal: Pass USMLE Step 2 Clinical Skills on the first attempt
- ➢ Long Term Goal: Build a solid foundation and improve Consumer Assessment of Health Care Providers and Systems (CAHPS) Survey.[1]

Patients have 15 minutes in the clinic and about 30 minutes in the hospital for discussing the discharge instructions and while health caregivers have years/decades in training about the diseases. However, when it comes to educating the patient, health caregivers check the box in the electronic health system after giving a pamphlet to the patient. Is a pamphlet going to educate the patient? Some patient will read the pamphlet diligently, but the most patient will trash it, store it, shred it or leave it in the car trunk. If we need to educate, activate and engage the patient we need to develop trust and this will only happen when you sit with the patient and explain the disease process. We have two ears and one tongue and they should be used proportionately to listen to the patients. At Vital Checklist Workshop, we teach medical students how to pay attention to all the non-verbal and verbal cues of the patients.

After listening to the patients, we firmly believe that two-dimensional diagrams and Vital Checklist can speed up the process of teaching patients and make the life easier for the patients. Many students have commended this approach and have passed the exam with flying colors. Our coaching process emulates Tony Robbins Immersion Coaching methodology where we expose the medical student to the standardized patient so that they can make the mistakes in the Vital Checklist Workshop and improve. We employ The Training Effect[2] curve, which explains how the advantage of consistent and spaced repetition leads to overcoming one bottleneck at a time—clinical skills, communications skills or patient note writing.

We have extended principles of the neuroplasticity and synaptic pruning. Synaptic pruning deletes the weaker synaptic connections, while it keeps the stronger connections. If you learn wrong clinical skills techniques, it becomes a habit, which is hard to remove from your clinical practice. At Vital Checklist Workshop, we will help to prune the bad techniques by immersing and coaching correct clinical practice. We see many students doing knee reflex never expose quadriceps muscle and are just looking for the knee jerk. Not paying attention to the quadriceps contraction is a wrong way to do the test.

Research has shown the growth of the posterior part of the Hippocampus in London taxi drivers[3] and structural change[4] in the jugglers who acquired new juggling skills. This explains that the brain is plastic and it can change and grow when you train. This tenet of neuroplasticity is what we use at Vital Checklist Workshop.

Once you have passed the clinical skills exam, you can use the same techniques in your electives, externships, internships and residency to score well in your CAHPS score leading to more patient satisfaction and this improving patient experience. This in turn leads to more goodwill for the health caregivers leading to job satisfaction for the providers.

References:

[1] C. A. H. P. S. program.". (2016, July 1st). *About CAHPS | Agency for Healthcare Research & Quality.* Available: http://www.ahrq.gov/cahps/about-cahps/index.html

[2] T. Robbins. (2016, April 25th). *The Training Effect | Personal Development | Tony Robbins.* Available: https://www.tonyrobbins.com/coaching/training-effect/

[3] E. A. Maguire, D. G. Gadian, I. S. Johnsrude, C. D. Good, J. Ashburner, R. S. Frackowiak, *et al.*, "Navigation-related structural change in the hippocampi of taxi drivers," *Proc Natl Acad Sci U S A,* vol. 97, pp. 4398-403, Apr 11 2000.

[4] B. Draganski, C. Gaser, V. Busch, G. Schuierer, U. Bogdahn, and A. May, "Neuroplasticity: Changes in grey matter induced by training," *Nature,* vol. 427, pp. 311-312, 2004-01-22 2004.

Vital Checklist Workshop for Physician Assistant, Nurse Practitioners, Physician Assistant Schools and Nurse Practitioner Schools

Gross Domestic Product (GDP) spent on healthcare has increased from 7 percent in 1970 to 16 percent in 2007. As per CMS, healthcare share of the GDP is going to increase to 19.6 by 2024.

Clayton M. Christensen, a Professor of Business Administration at the Harvard Business School, writes in his book-The Innovators Prescription, that healthcare is moving from intuitive medicine to precision medicine. With technology, we can pinpoint the disease with superior accuracy. Because of this superior accuracy even physician assistants and nurse practitioners can take good care of the patients at low cost. This disruption of providing low-cost care by employing nurse practitioner (NPs) or physician assistant (PAs) is the need of the hour. Even the NPs and PAs can start antibiotics as per the sensitivity of blood cultures, fix things by the radiological findings or give anesthesia to the patients as per the pre-calculated doses. With the shortage of doctors, the need for PAs and NPs will grow. Not only this, as we move to value-based care— health, wellness and disease prevention model, their demand will increase. Even though the increase in precision medicine is growing, we still need to develop strong communication and clinical skills to connect with the patient and develop trust with them. The trust development is what patient experience is, and this translates into Consumer Assessment of Health Care Providers and Systems (CAHPS) survey.

The problem we may face in the clinical experience is when the PAs/NPs (Physician extenders) are not matched up with the physicians because the number of years in training are far less. The question that looms on us is, "Are two years of physician assistant school enough to get trained while physicians spend more than a decade to get trained?"

Time is the major constraint for the physician extenders, as they have to learn voluminous amount of medical knowledge in limited time.

	Schooling and Training Medical Fields	Schooling and Training Surgical Fields	Schooling, Training & Specialization in medical field (Cardiology, GI)	Schooling, Training & Specialization in surgical field	PAs
Number of years in training for physicians					
Undergraduate	4 years	4 years	4 years	4 years	4 years
Medical School	4 years	4 years	4 years	4 years	2 years of PA school
Residency	3 years or 4 years	5 years	3 years	5 years	
Fellowship			3 years	2 years	
Super specialization			1 or 2 years		
Total years	**11 or 12 years**	**13 years**	**15 or 16 years**	**15 years**	**6 years**

Before they immerse themselves into evaluating patients in the second year of their PAs school, should physician extenders get proper clinical training like medical students are getting?

Should there be a Clinical Skills Exam for Physician Assistants and Nurse Practitioners?

If PAs and NPs are running disease prevention clinics or practicing healthcare on an independent basis, should they be trained in communication and clinical skills? We are not sure about the clinical skills exam as this will already increase the burden on physician extenders and expense of training for another exam; however, they are the front line providers impacting CAHPS scores. If providing health care services is teamwork, then it is not the PA'\s or NPs fault for the misdiagnosis, the fault lies on the system. Rather than spending millions on technology, we should have devoted people that are physician extenders. Why have technology companies failed to bring the down the costs and provide higher-quality care?

The answer lies in the fact that most healthcare companies focus on processes or technology without paying close attention to the people. As Marcus Lemonis of The Profit on CNBC says, People First, Process Second and Profit will follow automatically. Until you train people and change the culture from the roots, nothing can change.

Our hope with the Vital Checklist Workshop is that we not only teach medical students but also coach physician extenders who will be an important to extend the technological advances at the lower costs. The trust development starts with good communication and clinical skills as they become important fit where CAHPS survey are measured.

Praise for Dr. Harpreet Singh's Vital Checklist Workshop

Dr. Harpreet Singh's clinical course is a godsend for students who want to improve their clinical skills. My impression is that it was initially designed to train medical students who needed help passing their Step 2 CS test- but what I really think is that it should be offered to anyone seeking to enhance their clinical skills- even those who have already graduated!

Each day he focuses on 3 main areas:

1) He has created Vital Checklist (mnemonics) and really has a full system for facilitating learning and inspiring clinical confidence through order and mental speed- he does all of this while still keeping it fun.

2) He has students practice with model patients- the model patients progressively plant pitfalls and allow students to build confidence in the mnemonic system and through their own ability to circumvent the challenges and/or improve their speed,

3) He coaches- if you have ever had a really good coach, you know what I mean by this, he watches the students, studies their patterns, and personally addresses areas that require improvement and relax in areas where they already exhibit leadership.

Through this system he creates an environment of enthusiasm, open communication, and collaboration (A much healthier learning environment than the perpetual performance anxiety, masked insecurity, and ruthless competition that many medical programs and seminars perpetuate). Dr. Singh reconnects students to the deep mission of putting the patient at the center of healthcare; and I think that is his secret. Even the lecture session, and his brilliant mnemonic system are about non-judgment -(giving the same quality care to every patient every time), and about education (explaining and educating as a kind of treatment, more important than any sort of drug or referral).

I was a student of Dr. Singh's, over 2 year ago, and you can probably see, that I am still inspired. It is not just the facts and mnemonics that are important, it is also the coaching, that he allows his students to connect to medicine with the best parts of themselves, that is the component that makes his courses last beyond the course, beyond the testing, and even last well into one's own professional life.

~John Smieska PA-C

"In all of my discussions and interactions with Dr Singh, it is evident that he has tremendous passion to medicine and patient care. His commitment, compassion and empathy is the greatest gift that he shares with his patients and students...He is a great role model for rising and well-experienced providers. It is a privilege to witness and experience his passion... "

~Christine Khamis

Certificate of Appreciation from GVSU-2009

IN APPRECIATION

Grand Valley State University
College of Health Professions

Recognizes

Harpreet Singh, MD

by appointment to the
CLINICAL FACULTY
Physician Assistant Studies
for dedication and professionalism
in precepting our students

2008

Carl Piersma, R.Ph., PA-C
Clinical Coordinator
Physician Assistant Studies

Jeffery Libra, MD
Medical Director
Physician Assistant Studies

Wallace D. Boeve, Ed.D, PA-C
Program Director
Physician Assistant Studies

Certificate of Appreciation from GVSU-2009

IN APPRECIATION

Grand Valley State University
College of Health Professions

Recognizes

Harpreet Singh, MD

by appointment to the
CLINICAL FACULTY
Physician Assistant Studies
for dedication and professionalism
in precepting our students

2009

Carl Piersma, R.Ph., PA-C
Clinical Coordinator
Physician Assistant Studies

Jeffery Libra, MD
Medical Director
Physician Assistant Studies

Wallace D. Boeve, Ed.D, PA-C
Program Director
Physician Assistant Studies

Vital Checklist Workshop for Tele-health and Health Caregivers

Good empathetic communications are the cornerstone of any health discussions. Exchange of medical information between the patient and the health caregiver via technology is a key to the success of telemedicine. As we cannot examine the patient during a tele-health conversation, it is of paramount importance to collect complete history from patients and health caregivers.

Patient consultations via video conferencing, transmission of radiological images, vital signs monitoring, and patient education, and appointment with the health caregivers all depend on communication skills.

We at Vital Checklist Workshop have developed tools (checklists and touch-points) for healthcare givers so as to get a good history. In this day and age of global health and where technology is bridging the gap, we should develop a system of communicating with patients.

Dr. Harpreet Singh consults with the patients globally via Skype with his innovative Vital Checklist methodology. Following that he explains to the patient the next course of action. His explanations in layman language are easy to understand and difficult to forget.

In USMLE Step 2 Clinical Skills, medical students get a phone case and mostly that involves a pediatrics clinical scenario. It is very important for the student to pay close attention on the presenting complaint, history of presenting complaint, review of the systems and form an assessment and plan for patients. It is always a good idea to ask the family history of sick contacts or similar problems. There is a limitation of what you can do over the phone from an examination standpoint. At least, as health caregivers, we can talk politely and listen to the patient. Listening to the patient and giving your ear is what patients want and is half the battle.

Recently radiological clinical scenario has been added as one of the cases where students have to interpret the images.

Whether it is Step 2 Clinical Skills test or telemedicine, in both scenarios trust will only develop when you have excellent communication skills and you can form a rapport with the patient. Let's start talking to the patient empathetically and start teaching patients patiently.

	Love Communicating with patients Telephone or Tele health Encounter **Remember with HISWEPT ™**
H	☐ Hello ☐ Hello from _____.
I	☐ Introduce ☐ Did you introduce yourself?
S	☐ Survey the chief concern and listen; Then summarize ☐ Summarize the previous data, symptoms and problems
W	☐ Worries ☐ Any worries-depression/anxiety/Insurance coverage/side effects of medications/ refill of the medications
E	☐ Evaluate and Explain ☐ Try to evaluate the situation and see if patient needs to be seen
P	☐ Plan it! ☐ Plan the assessment
T	☐ Treatment, Disposition and Thank You ☐ Treat the patient; tell the disposition and Thank you the patient.

2016 © Harpreet Singh MD, FACP | Vital Checklist | (iCrush)

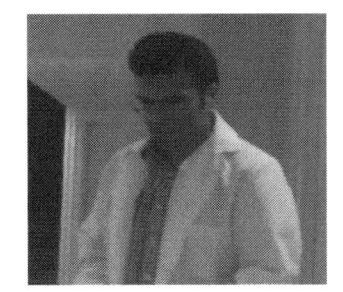

Putting yourself in your patients' shoes

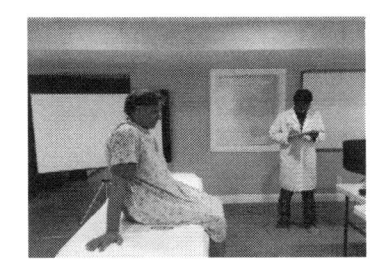

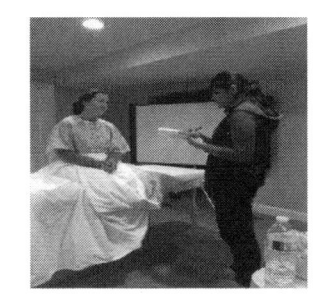

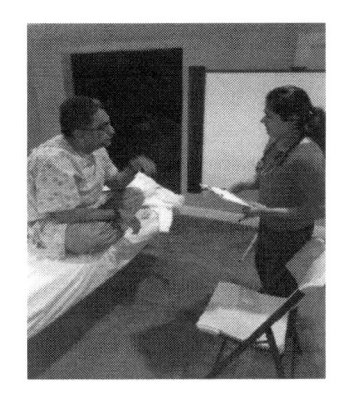

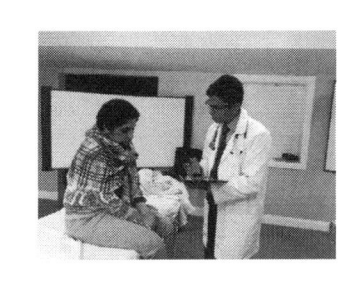

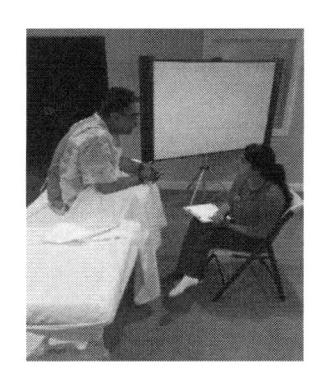

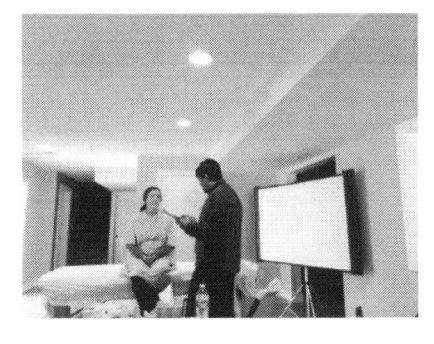

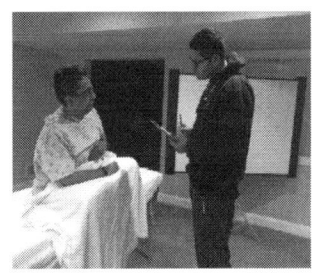

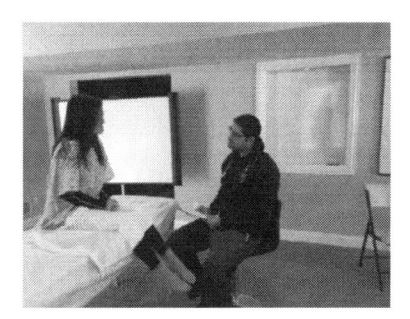

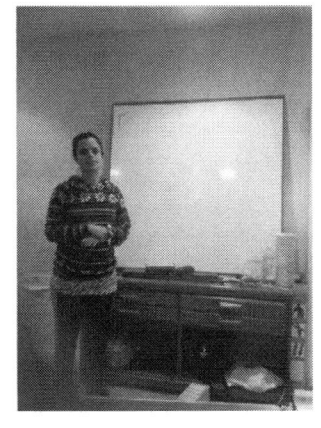

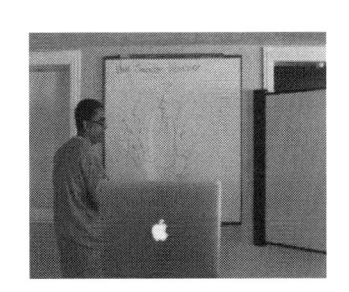

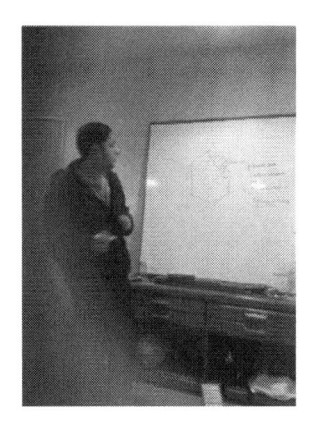

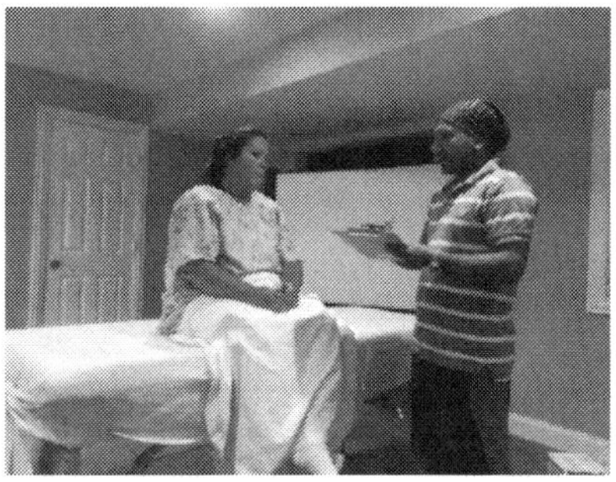
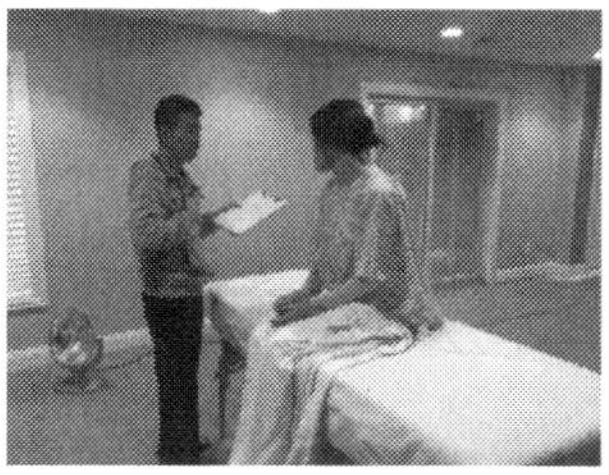
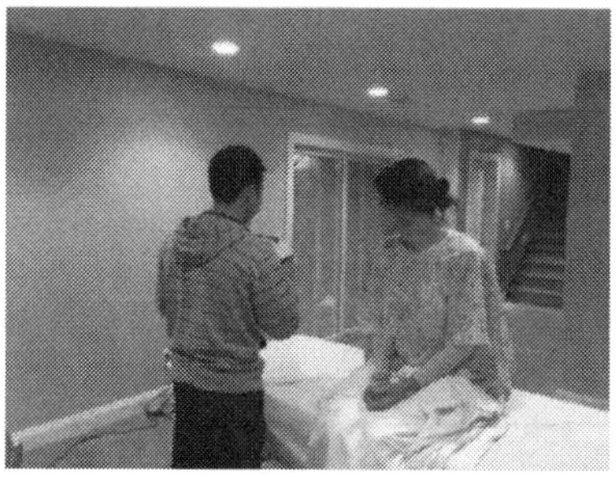
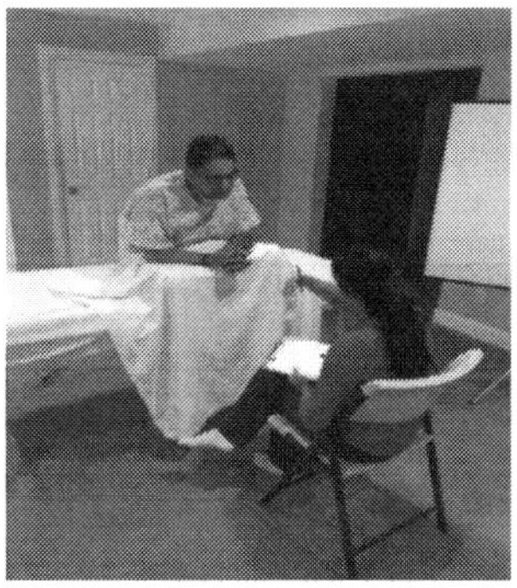
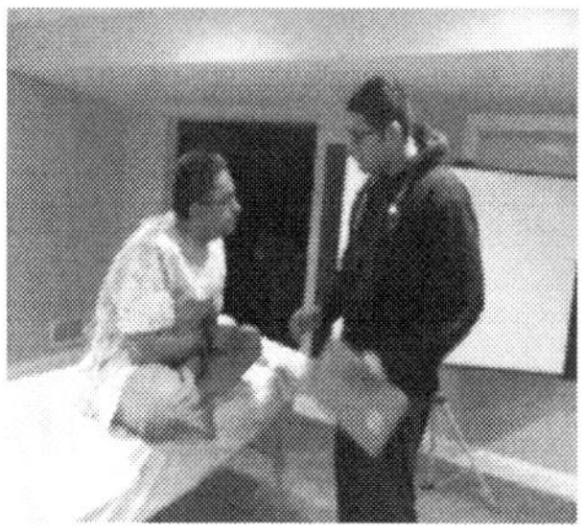
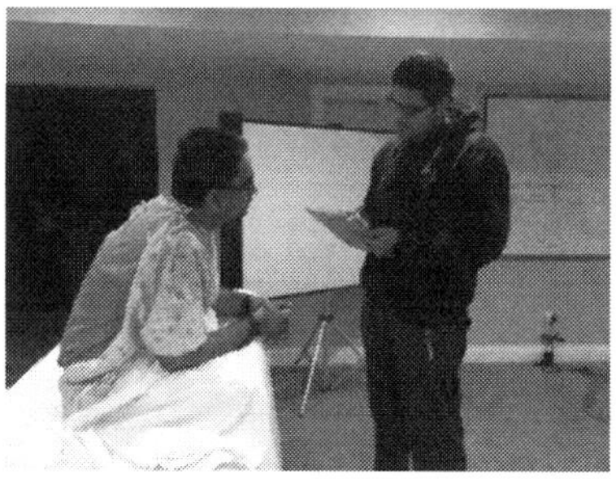
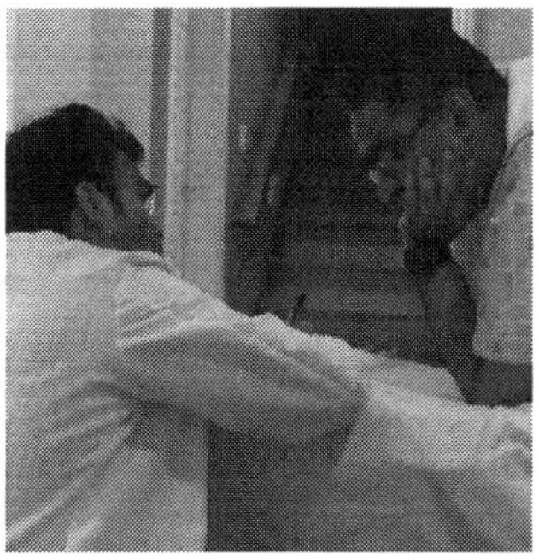
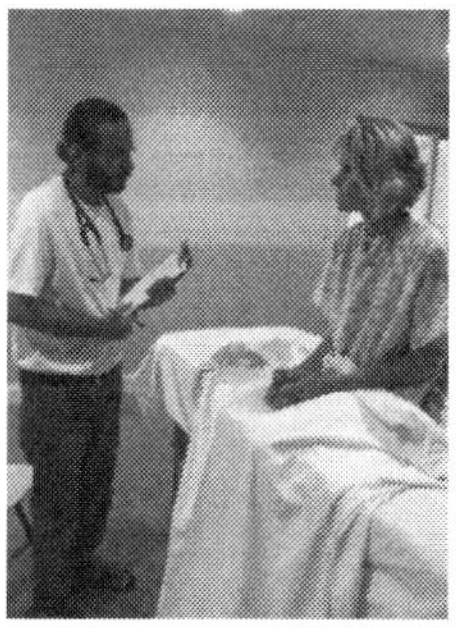
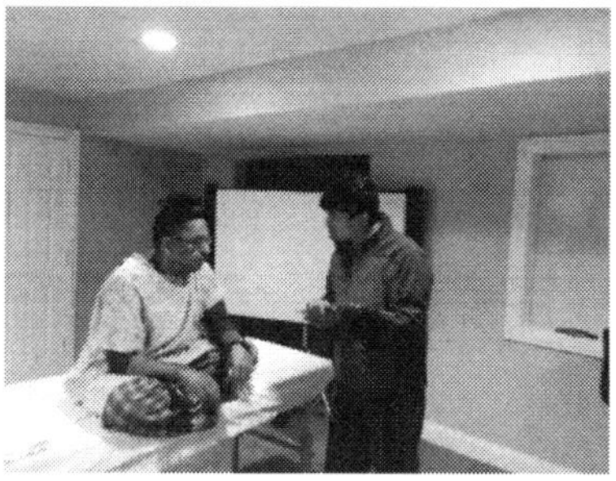
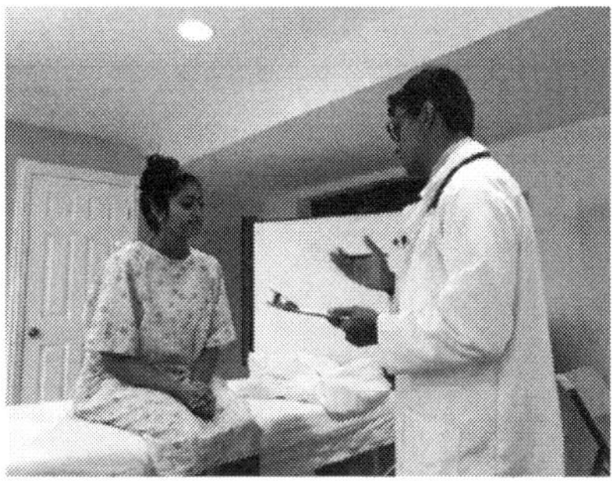
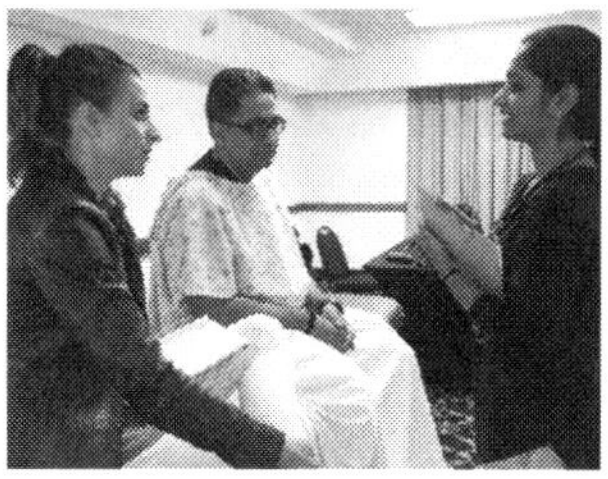
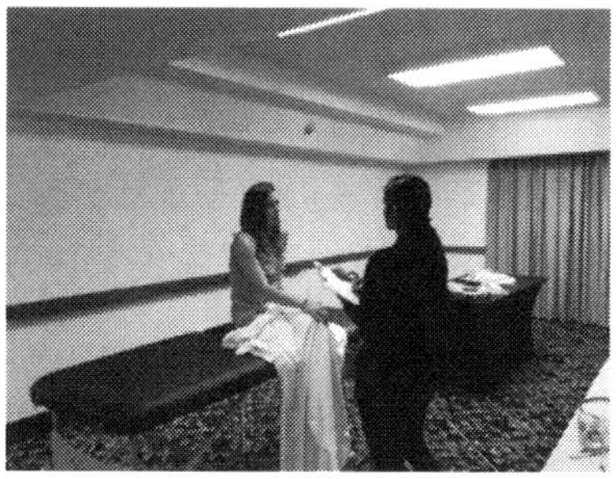

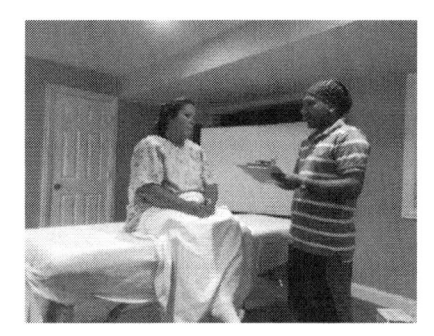

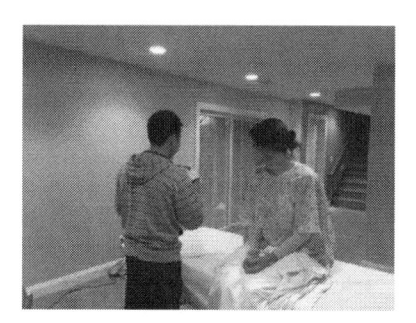

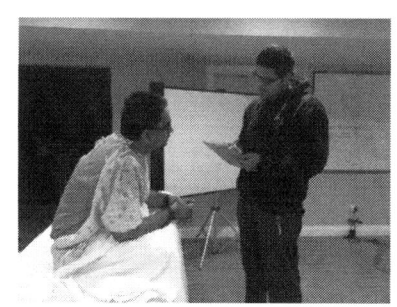

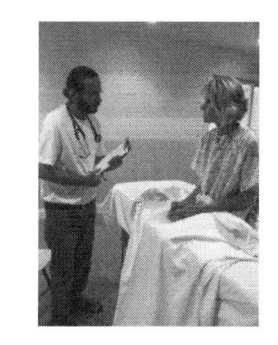

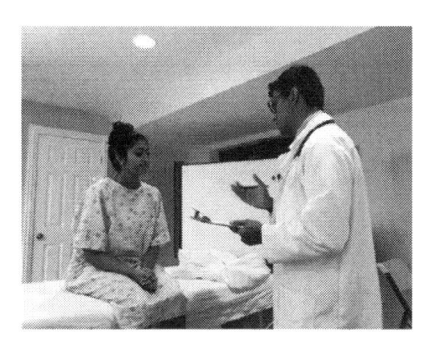

Putting yourself in your patients' shoes: Communication is about emotions

I saw an amazing video on Empathy: The Human Connection to Patient Care (https://youtu.be/cDDWvj_q-o8) published on You Tube by Cleveland Clinic. Dr. Toby Cosgrove, MD shared this in his 2012 State of the Clinic address. This video shows that patient care is connecting people with head, heart and hands. Not only this, this video proves that if you put yourself in patients' shoes, you would treat them differently.

One of my teachers—Dr. Robert Camp (Hospitalist-Spectrum Health) used to say that when in doubt about the treatment plan for your patient, always assume that you are treating your mother and things will fall in its place.

I have realized the importance of listening to my real life patients by portraying clinical scenarios for my students, and this has helped me to improve my clinical practice. I have used business theories—Theory of Constraints and Lean Principles to develop Vital Checklist Workshop. These theories are not mine; I have adapted to make my students and patients life easier.

Theory of Constraint + Lean Principles = Vital Checklist Workshop

At Vital Checklist Workshop, I use Eliyahu Goldratt's, "Theory of Constraint" (TOC) to coach medical students. Focusing on one problem at one time and overcoming bottlenecks is our central premise. Not only the medical students benefit from this, but I have enjoyed this as teaching has helped me to improve my clinical practice. After using TOC, I use lean principles to structure the thought process of the students for the Step 2 Clinical Skills exam as time is the major constraint.

Eliyahu Goldratt has defined five steps:

1. Identify the systems constraints
2. Decide how to exploit the constraints
3. Subordinate everything else to the exploitation of constraints
4. Elevate the system's constraint
5. If any constraints have been violated, repeat the process

At Vital Checklist, I try to focus on the bottlenecks of the students by diagnosing their first problem. After that, I overcome the constraints by consistent training and bring inline all the resources to master them. If the students cannot master them, I give them special attention. Step 2 Clinical Skills exam is a tricky exam, and I keep on breaking one bottleneck at one time. I will be explaining this in my upcoming books.

An easy to remember and hard to forget way to recall the steps:

Dr. Singh MD	How to remember the steps?
D	*Diagnose* the problem
R	Past *records* of your problem
S	*Step up* to get a maximum capacity
In	Bring *In-line* everything around the constraint
G	*Get* an upgraded investments for this constraints
H	Stop *Hibernation* and challenge the status quo
MD	*Measure data* again and again until improvement starts

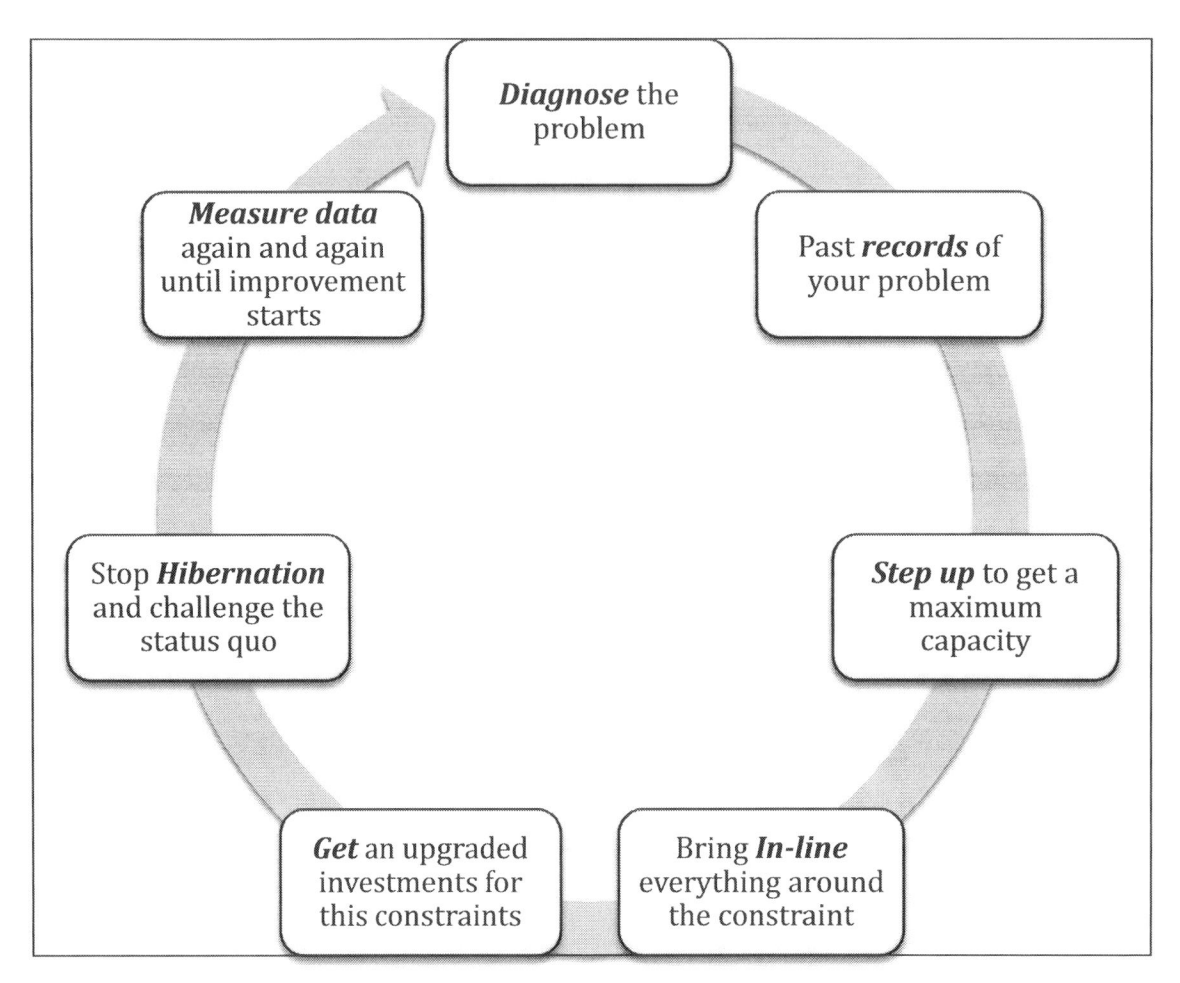

Theory of Constraint was elaborated, explained and designed by Eliyahu Goldratt in his book—The Goal.

*Disclaimer: I have **not** developed this theory. I have made a checklist for an easy memory— DrSinghMD*

Health Care Strategy: Connecting VitalChecklist.com and iCrush.org

Nowadays, writing a book is an easy task. However, changing a healthcare culture is very difficult. Bringing a brand new healthcare strategy to fruition requires proper plan of action, value chain analysis and assimilation of many business concepts into a simple and an easy to remember idea. This is what I have done by combining Vital Checklist for health caregivers and iCrush for patients. For this I have used Michael Porter's five forces. I am extremely indebted to Joan Magretta's book— Understanding Michael Porter and 80/20 Sales and Marketing by Perry Marshall from whom I have adopted these concepts. [i]

Why VitalChecklist.com and iCrush.org?

This is the first question—Rajnikant Gupta, a friend of mine asked me when I visited him in San Diego. He asked and advised me to divide into apps, products, platforms and services.
It was after a good discussion with him, I developed <u>WhatsApp Model</u> and wanted each element to interact with each other. More the interaction with each other more advantageous it becomes for the business. Nowadays, businesses are based on dynamic models and every element i.e. services, apps, products, platform must interact to make it more profitable.

WhatsApp		Medical Students	Health Caregivers	Patients
What	Is the Goal	Pass in Step 2CS in the first attempt	Improved HCAHPS and CGCAHPS score	Patient Satisfaction
s	Services	Vital Checklist Workshop for Step 2 CS	Vital Checklist Workshop for Patient Experience	(iCrush) Lifestyle Institute
A	Apps	Vital Checklist Apps where the data is fed by the patients and it communicates with the electronic health records		
p	Products	R2U book	LeanPX book	(iCrush) Disease
p	Platform	VitalChecklist.com	VitalChecklist.com	iCrush.org
R2U stands for Road to USMLE and LeanPX stands for Road to Patient Experience				
WhatsApp is registered trademark of WhatsApp INC and owned by Facebook.				
2016 © Harpreet Singh MD, FACP	Vital Checklist	(iCrush)				

Table: WhatsAPP—An Easy To Remember and Hard To Forget Vital Checklist for how services, apps, products and platform influence business strategy. In the case of Vital Checklist and (iCrush) standpoint, we have shown how they interact with each other.

Vital Checklist is a D.B.A. of 99Percentile LLC, which started as the USMLE training workshop for Step 2 Clinical Skills. After I received many thank-you cards and testimonials from the patients, Vital Checklist soon evolved into patient experience company. Now I was training PAs and Nurse Practitioners along with medical students. We pivoted from the name 99Percentile to Vital Checklist. We wanted to keep Lean Checklist, but the domain name was not available. Then on further discussion, we kept Vital Checklist, as it was similar to Vital Signs. We launched patient education videos, however, patients got confused when they clicked VitalChecklist.com.

Should I have a separate website or just a separate section was my question to Dr.Google and I came across an article written by Andy Crestodina of **www.orbitmedia.com**.

My patients were getting confused, but I did not want to create a separate platform because this will decrease search engine optimization. However, reading Andy Crestodina article, it made complete sense to have an independent platform for patients. As per him, when you are in dilemma of separate section or website you always ask yourself these two questions:

- ➢ Question1: Would the new site have a different audience?
- ➢ Question2: Would the new site have different goals?

- ➢ Answer 1: Patients, Businesses, and Lay People
- ➢ Answer 2: Health, Wellness and Disease Prevention.

Then I read a book—Understanding Michael Porter by Joan Magretta, and this consolidated even further the importance of having the separate platform for the patients. I have devised to-do list to remember Michael Porter's forces and the tests to be conducted in any business strategy.

		Warning Signs for Business Strategy
W	1)	**W**hatsApp Model (as explained above)
A	2)	**A**lternates (Threats of Substitute)
R	3)	**R**enegotiate (Bargain with suppliers)
(R)	4)	**R**enegotiate (Bargain with buyers)
N	5)	**N**ew Market –Globalization (Threat of New Market)
I	6)	**I**ndustry Competition
N	7)	**N**ew entrants (Threats of New Entrants)
G	8)	**G**overnment Regulations
S		**S**uperior and Unique Value chain which can be tailored
I		**I**nteractive (fit)
G		**G**ive and Take (Trade-off)
N		**N**ever cease to grow (continuity)
S		**S**ocial media strategy based on 80/20 principles

I have not invented the Porter's Five Forces. I read Joan Magretta's Book—Understanding Michael Porter and thought to use for my ventures. I read online critique for Porter's forces and have tried to assimilate the missing links in this Vital Checklist. Again, please note that this is not my work. God has given me the knack of making mnemonics/checklist and being a pawn of Lord almighty, I want to help people and businesses

—Dr.Harpreet Singh MD, FACP

© 2016 | Harpreet Singh MD, FACP | Vital Checklist | (iCrush)

Warning Signs—An Easy-to-Remember and Difficult-to-Forget method to remember Michael Porter's Forces.

I have explained in detail this concept in my upcoming book on Business Strategy—Warning Signs. Explaining this in this book is beyond the scope.

iCrush.org is a movement where I want to provide a platform for the patients to understand the disease process in variety of ways with various touchpoints—(iCrush)5k, (iCrush) T-Shirts, (iCrush) Patient Education Videos in different languages, (iCrush) Disease Book with Vital Checklist in different languages, Communication Box, Communication Cards, By The Way, Doctor! Flash card, Scan and Spot Weight Loss Workbook, Scan and Spot Table Mat, and most importantly (iCrush) Lifestyle Institute's health, wellness and disease prevention Workshops for lay-people, businesses and communities.

Every patient is different and learns differently. Some patients learn by reading and writing, some are visual learners, some can just hear and assimilate what has been told to them and a few are kinesthetic learners. As per John Medina of Brain Rules, more handles you provide for learning, better is the learning process. Dr. Google and Dr. Bing are already making smart patients but our main objective is making "smart patients smarter." I cannot do this alone and need help of the entire community and especially the medical students to help me with translating videos in different languages. Let's join hands and "flip the healthcare". I am indebted to Khan Academy who has taught me how to do the "FLIP."

Excerpt from Brain Rules by John Medina

"We know that information is remembered best when it is elaborate, meaningful, and contextual. The quality of the encoding stage—those earliest moments of learning—is one of the single greatest predictors of later learning success. What can we do to take advantage of that in the real world?

First, we can take a lesson from a shoe store I used to visit as a little boy. This shoe store had a door with three handles at different heights: one near the very top, one near the very bottom, and one in the middle. The logic was simple: The more handles on the door, the more access points were available for entrance, regardless of the strength or age of customer. It was a relief for a 5-year-old—a door I could actually reach! I was so intrigued with the door that I used to dream about it. In my dreams, however, there were hundreds of handles, all capable of opening the door to this shoe store.

"Quality of encoding" really means the number of door handles one can put on the entrance to a piece of information. The more handles one creates at the moment of learning "is to be accessed at a later date. The handles we can add revolve around content, timing, and environment."

Taken with permission from John Medina

John Medina explains with an example of shoe store and number of handles. More the number of handles, better the quality of encoding. This quality of encoding depends on timing, content and environment. We are not saying to replace the patient education material printed by the electronic health record.

What we are saying is adding more handles for better memory.

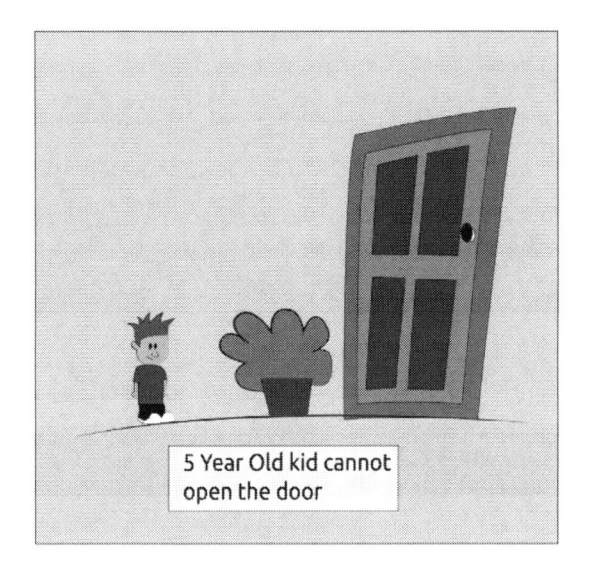

One handle and 5 year kid cannot reached

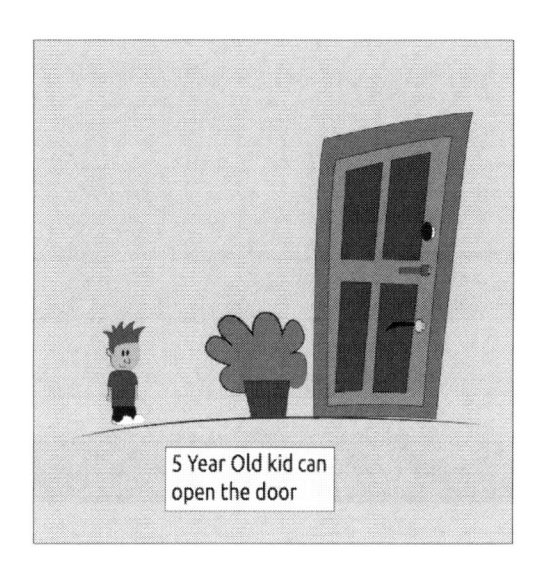

5 year old kid can open door as now handles are placed at his level

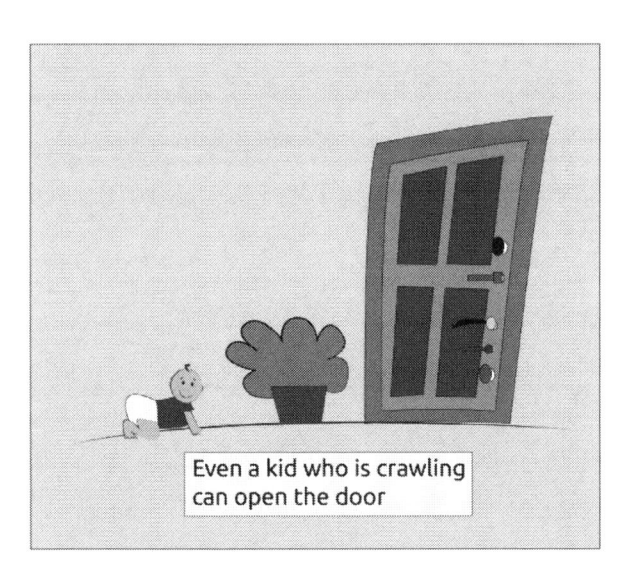

Even the kid who is crawling can open the door

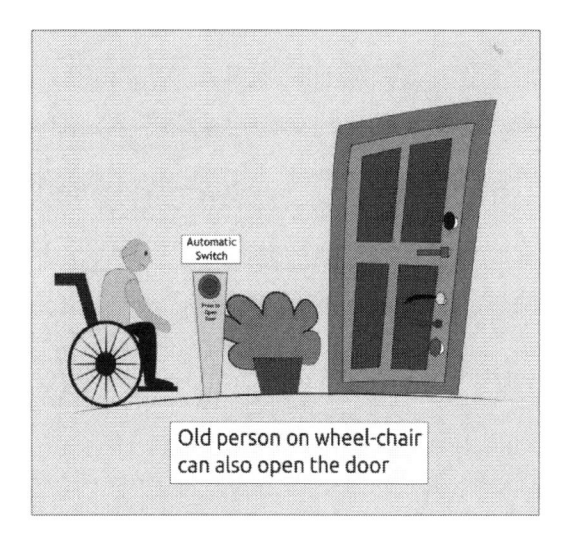

More options to open the door.

Figure: Handles and Learning: Adapted from John Medina Book

(iCrush) Mission, Vision Goals and Objectives

Mission:

"Early to diagnose, early to treat makes patients healthy, wealthy and wise."

Vision:

"Healthcare education at the fingertips."

Goal:

"Flip the Healthcare."

Objectives:

"Smart Patients Smarter."

Let's save healthcare dollars and improve patient experience together.

Section N
Testimonials

Section N - Testimonials

Student Experience: Praise of Vital Checklist Workshop for STEP 2 CS

I highly recommend Dr.Singh's course Vital Checklist to all my friends who are looking for help with the preparation for CS. His Clinical Skills Workshop simulated case is a very close to the actual exam. I had looked other materials that are out there for CS but after taking Dr. Singh's workshop i realized that the way he teaches is actually what is needed to pass the real exam with the standardized Patients. It is money well spent. I am very grateful to Dr. Singh for helping me. His passion for teaching can be seen when you take his workshop, also his excitement as you progress through the workshop and as your skills improve. At the end of the workshop you leave with strong self-confidence and knowledge in your ability to undertake this exam. He is always there for his students even after the course is over.

Dr. Syed

I met Dr.Singh during my step 2CS training. He is a wonderful teacher and doctor. He is very selfless and Always ready to help others. His patients love him,his students love him,in short everybody loves this wonderful man. He has a beautiful family and I am so glad I met them. I will definitely recommend him as a doctor and a teacher. He always spend maximum time with his patients so that they know what's going on with them. I love his approach of treating patients and we need more doctors like him :)

Navneet Toor

Dr. Singh's webinar for Step 2 CS was really helpful Interesting teaching style. Looking forward to many more sessions in future!

Prerna Bansal

I was fortunate to learn the art of clinical case taking from Dr Singh. The tips and tricks he offers are of immense help and are not provided in any book or Internet Blog.

Aman Chauhan MD

It was all your effort and motivation that we could do that good in our CS exam. You helped discover the confidence which I never thought existed in me in regards to interact with an American patient.

~Gaganpreet Khangura MD

This is a course that is much more than just the Step 2 CS exam. Dr.Singh takes a personal interest in every student and caters things to their needs and weaknesses. The way he teaches about H&Ps, counseling, patient interaction and the nuances that are required to excel in the American Medical System - it will stick with you for your entire medical career. He simplifies everything to the absolute basic with attention to every little detail. He has come up with innovative ways and such an easy algorithm to follow that there's no way you can mess this up.

Ana Maheshwari MD

Your way of teaching communication skills, including closure and counseling, were awesome. I remember the first day, when I took my first case in 25 minutes. On the last day of workshop at Vital Checklist, I took only 13 minutes. Your time management technique helped me to gain extra confidence and stay calm and collected"."His very innovative acronyms and systematic approach made history taking a lot simpler. His style of teaching was adaptive to each of us and addressed our own personal weaknesses. The training was intensive and covered almost every possible case under each system. What seemed like a daunting task in the beginning (Thorough history + examination and counseling in all of 15 minutes!), became second nature to us.

Kavitha Srinivasan MD

"Your training is going to help me in my residency and will make me a better physician. Dr. Singh, You are an awesome teacher. Your SP's are great and helped to make me perfect. The lesson I received from your workshop is one of the best lessons in my life. I wish success of your team in every step. God Bless you and your team".

Bilori Aasht

"The training Vital Checklist gave me was excellent and I received very extensive practice on cases. It boosted my confidence and now I feel more prepared, not only for CS but also for clinical electives. The best part was learning all of my mistakes after each case, so that there is no chance I'll make the same errors at the USMLE step 2 CS main exams. It's a "must take" course for all who desire to pass their step 2 CS on their first attempt".

Shweta Kochar MD

"Thanks to the Vital Checklist team, as I was able to pass my exam in the first attempt. As an International Medical Graduate (IMG), I had several fears about Clinical Skills. Your coaching is 100% perfect. It helped me a lot with my time management as well as building my confidence to deal with S.Ps and their questions. He taught me exactly what to stress during patient encounters. Your S.P's exactly matched those I saw in the exam. I would also like to add that your personal interest and effort toward my success was outstanding. I have no doubt that what you taught me will help me in residency. I wish you all the best."

Amandeep Brar MD

"I am very fortunate to have the right person guiding me with the preparation of personal statement".

Meera Shastry MD

"With immense pleasure and gratitude, I wish to inform you that I have passed the CS examination. I owe a lot to the valuable guidance, information and skills taught by you. The self-confidence and courage you instilled in me shuttled me light years ahead of where I was before coming under influence. Your friendly approach, amazing sense of humor and above all genuine concern for me has filled my heart with endless respect and thoughtfulness for you. I highly recommend your guidance to everyone who wishes to pass his or her CS examination in the first attempt, without wasting much time, effort or money".

Deepak Verma MD

"In just 3 days' time you taught us everything from history taking, examination and a mind blowing way of counseling. The way you teach is not just good, it's truly an honor to have been taught by you. Your coaching goes way beyond just passing the CS exam; it will stay with me for the rest of my professional life".

~Taran Jolly MD

"Every tip you gave me was of utmost benefit on the day of the exam. Your acronyms were amazing. It gave a continuous flow for my thought process during the exam".

~Kishan Nallapula MD

"Given the huge amount of effort, time and expense involved in taking the Step 2 CS and more importantly the grave prognosis on USMLE prospects and terrible mental stress that a CS failure can impose, there is little doubt that a proper guidance is a requisite to sail through the exam safely. Vital Checklist is a real boon for IMGs appearing for the CS".

~Dr.Karthik MD

Patient Experience: Praise from Real Life Patients

Dr.Harpreet Singh has received many testimonials during his residency, then as a hospitalist and then as an internist. Some of the names are crossed out as we were not able to secure permission from them. You can find these cards, thank you notes, and appreciation letters on www.vitalchecklist.com/testimonials-patient-experience-letters

Dr. Singh,

I don't know how to describe my gratefulness or express my appreciation for the care you gave my wife in the emergency room the day of her stroke.

I thought after her 13-year battle with cancer, chemo, multiple surgeries and radiation we were prepared for anything. I was wrong. I thank God that you were the doctor in Emergency on December 26, 2010.

You gave exceptional and immediate care to insure my wife's survival. You kept my family and me up to speed on her prognosis and what was being done for her during the most frightening and difficult time of our lives. You did this with gentleness, kindness and compassion that I will always be grateful for.

*Even after being told by the head neurologist that we should not expect much in the way of **Xxxx** speaking again you continued to say she was young and capable of recovery beyond that we could imagine. Your care and communication went way above and beyond what was required.*

Your help and follow up continued with us long after she was out of your care and living in a rehab facility.

*You are a wonderfully talented doctor, but more importantly a wise, kind compassionate and confident caregiver. I feel you did everything you could for not just my wife but for our whole family as well. My wife and I will be always grateful and have a special place in our hearts for you. Almost one year later **Xxxx** is home- living, speaking, driving and being the wonderful Mom and wife she always was.*

I thank God and you every day for this second chance. I am forever in your debt.
Sincerely,
Xxxx

Dearest Dr.Singh,

God Bless you; I will never forget you as you took time to hold my hand and comfort me which I needed so bad that day which I needed so bad that day. I was so scared and wouldn't make it through.

If I am ever re-admitted that you will be my doctor. You are truly a god send. I pray for you daily.
Xxxx

NURSE Recommendation

I would like to acknowledge the time Dr.Singh has taken to speak with the patients and their families on our unit this week. Not only has he called or sat down with each family member that asked, but also he called the family of each patient he saw without anyone asking him to. This makes such a difference for families, and the RN's caring for them. Thank you Dr.Singh for the time and the compassion you gave.
Jennifer Xxxx

NURSE Recommendation

Both Dr.Singh and Lisa spent all morning in the unit for not one but 2 of our patients that were in crisis. They were not even assigned to these patients but came up to help anyway. They did an excellent job treating the patients and were wonderful with speaking with their families. We could not have asked for more and cannot thank you both enough.
Natalie Xxxx

Dear **Xxxx**,

The attending physicians primarily Dr. Xxxx and Dr. Singh were thorough in their care, their explanations and unending in the compassion displayed. Dr. Harpreet Singh's support went far beyond her doctor. He rapidly became a friend and confidant. When the diagnosis of cancer occurred, he personally called my brothers in California and Hawaii, leaving his personal cell phone number to make sure they had all their questions answered. We recognize that the surgical course my mother followed was unusual for someone 92-year old but Dr.Singh assured all she was strong enough to come through with expectations of quality time ahead.

During her convalescence in the unit she was continuously supported and encouraged by the entire staff. Since her transfer to rehab, she has grown continually supported and encouraged by the entire staff. Since her transfer to rehab, she has grown continually stronger and returned to her apartment the day of Thanksgiving. She's got a ways to go but that journey gets shorter every day.

Again, thank you and your staff from the entire **Xxxx** Family. The care and compassion of your staff are truly appreciated.

Sincerely,
Xxxx Family

Dear Dr.Singh,
Thank you for making my Christmas "merry" by healing my eye.
*May God bless you as much as you have blessed **Xxxx** through your knowledge and good care and comfort.*
Your kindness towards Xxxx, as well as to us was true blessings.
Xxxx's sisters
Xxxx
Xxxx

Dear Dr. Singh,

Thank you for being so kind to our family. We felt so confused and lost until you came to us.

We appreciate that you took the time to show and explain to our family **Xxxx**'s CT scan. We also appreciated you giving us printouts. It was comforting to have when things were quiet at home we could look over the information you gave us and try to digest it. It just felt good having something to hold on to.

We can't thank you enough for coordinating everything. People would say they would be right back but never returned. You always returned when you said which was very comforting to our family. You were so dependable and our family needed someone to rely on.

We also appreciated the fact that you coordinated things with your brother at the Hospital. Knowing you were setting everything up for **Xxxx** made us all feel better because we knew it would be done correctly and we would be kept informed.

The surgery did not go the way we were hoping for but you taking time to stop by to see **Xxxx** and our family at the Hospital meant so much to us.

Our family would never forget you and how wonderful you were to us.

We enjoyed meeting your brother and please thank him from us for getting **Xxxx** in so quickly in so quickly to see him. We all appreciated the sense of humor "yank it out" you showed us. We are still laughing about it. Nice to have something to smile about.

Thank you for being so caring.

Xxxx and Family

I am writing to thank Dr. Harpreet Singh for all his help and assistance. You are the best! From the bottom of my heart I sincerely appreciate you. I am glad you were on duty.

Xxxx

*To **Xxxx***

*I just wanted you to know that the care my friend **Xxxx**, received at Xxxx from Dr. Harpreet Singh was wonderful! The change he has made in her medication and his total devotion to her as his patient has significantly improved her health condition. **Xxxx** would like to keep Dr. Singh as her physician when she is discharged from the hospital.*

*In my many years of being a geriatric nurse, I have never met another physician like him, so I can understand why **Xxxx** has so much confidence in Dr. Singh. Xxxx is 91 yr. old and deserves the continuity of care and peace of mind that Dr. Singh attention would allow her. Please consider making an exception to Dr. Singh, s contract so that my friend **Xxxx**. can be cared for by a physician that truly cares about her as a geriatric patient, is knowledgeable about her geriatric conditions, and can put a smile on her face that says it all. Why couldn't Dr. Singh be both?*

Sincerely:

Xxxx

To Dr. Singh

*Some impart wisdom or comfort and care. Some point out the path, and some take you there. Some warm the heart with a human touch. You have all these gifts Thank you so much for your excellent care and concern for **Xxxx** and his family during his family during his stay at **Xxxx** from 10-20-10 to 11-1-10*

Xxxx

Dr. Singh,

Thank you for taking such good care of my dad when we brought him from Florida. You were so kind & gentle; you really helped him to adjust!

My dad is home still an IV antibiotics & with a drainage tube due to the pleural effusion. He does feel great, though!

Blessings,

Xxxx

Dr. Singh,

Thank you so much for all the work you are doing –both with yourself and your practice style as well as that with your present PA's/NP's. I appreciate your willingness to teach as opportunities present themselves. I hope you are able to see the benefits of the changes you have made thank you for your continued commitment.

Emily

Dr. Singh,

Thank you for your commitment to education & for all the time &energy you put into the case studies for journal club. Your willingness to do that is hugely valuable to me & HOWM as a group.

Thank you again keep smiling

Emily

Dear Dr. Singh

It is with both pride and pleasure to write you this note. You were one of my attending physician during my stay at spectrum health center also I was given a dual chamber pacemaker by Dr. Rosenblum . I truly appreciate your professional medical services and appropriate communication you and your personality has helped me to attain minimum health status.

Thank you so much.

Xxxx

Dear Harpreet Singh,MD;

Our records indicate that during the 2008 academic calendar year, you served as a clinical preceptor for the Grand Valley State University Physician Assistant Student. As an expression of our sincere gratitude for your services, we are giving you a certificate of appreciation. We look forward to continued relations with you for our students and for the future of health care. We are also looking at ways to strengthen our program and ask you to email any feedback to us at pas@gvsu.edu. If there is anything that we can do for you, please do not hesitate to contact us.

Respectfully;

Wallace D. Boeve, EdD, PA-C

Program Director

Physician Assistant Studies

College of health professions

Grand Valley State University

Thank you so much for all your care, advice and kindness! Blodgett Patients are so lucky you are there! Being there with my sick mom was so stressful for us and you made both of us feel better just by your presence … good vibes from a good guy! Take care …be good

Thank you.

Xxxx

Xxxx Patients

I am writing to Thank Dr. Harpreet Singh for all his help & assistance. You are the BEST! From the bottom of my heart I sincerely appreciate you. I'm glad you were on duty.

Xxxx

To Whom It May Concern:

I just wanted to do a special Thank you to Dr. Singh. He was very caring and right on top of my care. I had back surgery on nov.13 .2008. I needed units of blood and got really sick. Dr. Singh took the extra mile even calling while at home during the night to check on me thank God for people like him who put the patients 1st.

Thank you

Xxxx

Dr. Singh,

We are extremely grateful for your help in the matter of **Xxxx**. *It was a great relief to find someone who shared our sense of urgency and need for compassionate care of our patient. I sometimes feel that many in medical profession have lost the sense of service that supposedly would have bring them into this field in the first place.*

Thank you for caring for our patients, and thank you retaining our faith.

David L. Pastoor M.D.

I do have to say, "Dr. Singh who is on the floor of the hospital ", is one of the Best Doctor you have had in a very long time. He listens to your complaints and does what he think is best for the patient.

Dr. Singh has showed his continued concern by contacting me several times to find out how I'm doing and where my labs are going. I feel he is such a knowledgeable doctor and cares about my illness. Now days, so many doctors just walk in and out of patients life. We believe God is in charge of our lives and that he worked through Dr. Singh that day. We will forever be grateful to have had Dr. Singh walk into ours. He truly cares about his patients.

Xxxx

Dr. Singh,

"I thank my God through Jesus Christ for you …"

Your care for my husband **Xxxx**, *while he was hospitalized was "over the top ". Thank you so much for your patience with all of our questions. It helped a lot to be heard and understood. The world of "blood clots" was a "foreign land" for us and it helped tremendously to be able to really talk with you!*

As much as we wish you were an outpatient doctor, your services are invaluable to in patient care. We wish every doctor were more like you

Thank you again, Dr. Singh for everything!

Xxxx

To Whom It May Concern:

I gladly write this letter for Dr. Harpreet Singh. On a personal level, he is pleasant, congenial, honest and a good family man. I have seen him on professional level as well. I feel strongly he is thorough in his evaluation, very knowledgeable regarding medicine and feel he gives "good patient care. "He was very helpful on the professional level with education I needed about my health. He was clear in his direction of care and made my exam very comfortable. I have enjoyed getting to know him. I would not hesitate to seek care from him and would recommend him to others.

If you would like to discuss this recommendation further I would be glad to talk with you. Please feel free to contact me.

Thank you.
Sincerely,

Steven P Delaney
Court Administrator
Magistrate- District Court
Mecosta County

Dr. Singh,

It has been a pleasure getting to know you and working alongside a physician such as you. You have demonstrated a terrific sprit with such respect and compassion for patients and colleagues alike.

"It is true; life is really generous to those who pursue their personal legend." Paulo Coelho

RN Lisa *Xxxx*
RN Britney *Xxxx*

Dr. Singh,

I just wanted to thank you so much for taking me under your wing .You are a great doctor and I learned a lot. I really enjoyed the teaching time. We had together and I appreciate your time (I know its valuable) thank you for the consistent encouragement and the great advice!

Chistina

I am feel honored to be able to write a testimonial for Dr. Singh. He has given me the necessary tools to succeed in my weight loss journey. He explained things step by step and used drawings which helped me better understand. At each visit he would supply new information and assign me a new task to complete. He showed me how to keep a food journal, read labels and make better food choices when shopping. I never felt overwhelmed when given a new task to complete. Other doctors said to lose weight but never took the time to explain how and then follow through. Because of Dr. Sing I have lost almost 30#. He is kind,caring and sensitive to his patients. I thank him from the bottom of my heart. Without him it wouldn't have been possible.

Pam *Xxxx*

My first encounter with Dr. Harpreet Singh came by chance & at a very low point in my life. I wasn't able to see my practitioner at the time, so I went ahead & booked with him. It was important that I keep the ball rolling,as I knew I needed help.As a healthcare professional myself ,I found myself overwhelmed on the job.Tired and drained of the things that truly matter...Compassion, Hope, Kindness & Empathy. Soon you realize you cannot give to others what you are not giving to yourself.

The stress of my job had gotten so bad, I just bottomed out. Working long hours in a very stressful environment,with little to no support from mgmt,trying to satisfy an insatiable physician, left me very depressed and defeated. It was time for me to take care of myself.Dr Singh was the answer to many prayers. He listened to me helped me see things in other perspectives so that I could move forward and become stronger .....physically, mentally & emotionally.

He always amazes me with his thought processes. He sees outside the box on many levels, including Spiritually. He does not fit the mode of a "pill doctor."Sure, he recognizes prescription mgmt in his practice but he does so much more. He is a great teacher and is known for drawing pictures with explanations. When you leave the office you feel informed and confident in your choices. That's the feeling I want in my Heath management.

If the Business of Healthcare continues in the Direction of Business and not Healthcare, it is apparent that the stresses will continue to target people working in it. There will be more anger,more demands, less patience, less support.

Thank goodness for the people who continue to put the CARE in healthcare.We may stumble but we get up & keep going every day. To make a difference, to care for those you love,to do the right thing in this world. Dr.Singh is one of these people.If ever you should stumble ,no matter who you are or what you do, Dr.Singh will help you get back on track. He certainly made a difference for me.

Xxxx

It gives me great pleasure to be writing a reference for Dr. H. Singh. I have enjoyed knowing Dr. Singh and working with him these past years. As a Physician Recruiter, I come in contact with physicians of all specialties, shapes and sizes and I can tell you that Dr. Singh's clinical skills, and bedside manner are among the finest. In my opinion, anyone would be in good hands if Dr. Singh was handling them as a physician or in any business venture. I continue to be amazed at his great outlook on life in general and can tell you his reputation with patients is wonderful. This is thanking Dr. Singh for the pleasure of knowing him, and wishing him success in the future.

Cindi Whitney-Dilley
Whitney Recruitment, LLC

Video Testimonials for Dr.Singh
www.vitalchecklist.com/testimonials-patient-experience-videos

Patient Testimonials

Barb—Dr. Singh Has Changed My Family's Life

I met Dr. Singh for the first time, and met someone who changed my life, and the life of my family forever. I have never met a doctor who cared more, or who wanted to be more of a patient advocate for me than Dr. Singh.

I had seriously started to consider whether or not I was a hypochondriac. I had gone to numerous doctors, paid numerous bills, trying to figure out what was going on inside of my body that was making me feel ill and tired, and I didn't have a zest for life anymore. I decided to give a doctor, a new doctor, one more chance to figure out, and diagnose if this was all in my head or if this was something going on with my life, and I met Dr. Singh.

I was reborn the day that I met him. And I say that because I got my life back. I gained energy and strength. I had my zest and zeal back for life because he figured out what was going on with me. I was diagnosed with celiac disease, and then my daughter was tested and diagnosed. Our lives have dramatically changed for the better.

Dr. Singh is an amazing man, an amazing doctor. He not only thinks outside of the box, but takes the time to draw you a picture that you can understand what he's talking about. Dr. Singh, after he diagnosed me with celiac disease, let me know that it was a hereditary disease. My daughter started seeing him a month later, and was diagnosed as well with celiac disease. So instead of her having to go through the trials and tribulations that I had to go through in my 30s and 40s, my daughter is now healthy because Dr. Singh is in our life. And I have not met a doctor who has cared more, or wanted to be more of a patient advocate than Dr. Singh.

Gail—A Real Patient Talks About Diabetes

I was very impressed that, not only as I started to explain some of my complaints that I was having with health issues, with Dr. Singh, that he began asking more questions, and more questions, and at the same time, drawing pictures explaining to me the things that I was telling him, that I had never had a physician try to figure out in front of me with questions and drawing of pictures. So I became really tuned to what he was saying and how he was talking to me.

I think the biggest impression I had was the acronyms that he used to try to educate a patient as to what they were dealing with. I watched him as he used the acronym "iCrushDiabetes". I was so impressed with that. He had an explanation for every letter of that word. And every one of them I could apply to the ailments that I was going through. In receiving my answers, he would say, "we need to do this test," or "we need to do that test." Every time he got results from those tests that were done, he would call me.

Even that day of my appointment, he called me that afternoon and said, "What are you doing at six o'clock this evening?" So again he goes through the acronym of the iCrushDiabetes. That was another three hour appointment of which we were not on his schedule.

That was a concern of his. He wanted to make sure we understood, and a lot of time when you go to the doctor, you come out of there thinking, "What did he say?" And you don't know where to go, or where to turn. But he is very careful to explain to you enough that causes you to ask more questions, which causes you to understand what he is trying to tell you. After that evening, I was so impressed with what he tries to do with patients in that education process.

As a patient if you don't understand what the doctor is telling you then you're not going to take the best care of yourself. We are still in the process of going through tests. I have more tests coming up, of which will give him a better picture of what my diagnosis should be. So I don't have a diagnosis yet, but I have a better understanding of why I'm feeling the way that I am, and what is going on with my body.

Leah—Dr. Singh is a Great Detective

"When I first met Dr. Singh it was the end of June and I had been experiencing shortness of breath and weakness and fatigue. I had no explanation because I was very active and did aerobics three times a week and had no idea what was going on. So, I went in and he greeted me very warmly. I was instantly reassured that he was listening to me. I was telling him my story and he took me seriously.

And then ordered some tests, an echocardiogram. That echocardiogram showed that I was in congestive heart failure. Big news to me. I have a history of hypertension and high blood pressure, and he knew that from his questions, and that was the reason for ordering the test. So diagnosis, congestive heart failure, but Dr. Singh wasn't satisfied that it explained all my symptom. I didnt know that there was more to be explored.

But when I went back for the second appointment, he ordered some very unusual tests. A kappa lambda lectin test, I had no idea what that was, I couldn't even look that up. I look everything up, but I couldn't even find a way to look that up.

I saw him the first time June 26, by the end of July, just one month later, he had discovered I had plasma cell leukemia, as well as congestive heart failure. He had me hospitalized in Grand Rapids that day, they started chemo the next day. And three months later I was in remission. Dr. Singh saved my life, and it still brings tears to me,.I am so grateful to this man for being such a good detective, for being so thorough and for being so kind throughout the process. "

Leah S.-- Plasma Cell Leukemia--Dr. Singh Provides Hope

'They did a bone marrow biopsy and confirmed the diagnosis of plasma cell leukemia, and started chemo that day. I asked the oncologist "If we hadn't found this, if we hadn't treated this what would have happened?" He said " Your life expectancy would have been two to four months."

It's been four months. Here I am and I wouldn't have been. One of the things that has been so helpful to me with Dr. Singh, is that he believes in empowering his patients. What that means to me, I have a fairly good background in some medical knowledge as a psychotherapist for thirty years, but there are so many things I don't know that he does know. He explains them to me, he draws diagrams and uses acronyms a lot. He also takes a personal interest in me.

With my permission, he talked to my son and daughter-in-law, and my daughter about my situation, and suggested to them that they accident proof my house, because at that time I was very weak and using a walker. He took that much of an interest. He came to the house for a home visit. He was so kind to my family. They all think he is so wonderful . He came to see me in the hospital in Grand Rapids. I could watch him sort of watching everyone, coordinating the treatment, just checking that I was being taken care of. He is that thorough and he is that kind, and he is that interested in the health and well-being of his patients, of me. And that was wonderful, and very reassuring."

Jenny-- A Daughter's Story--Mom Has Plasma Cell Leukemia and Congestive Heart Failure

"I was talking to my mom on the phone, I talked to her on the phone because I live 1,000 miles away, so most of our conversation is phone conversation. She was short of breath and saying she wasn't feeling well, which isn't like her because she is very high energy, so she had some testing done.

We found out she had some heart issues, which was devastating enough because she is young and active, and high energy, and meditation, and yoga, and aerobics, and fun. A young 68. More testing, more blood work. She called me and said, "I'm going to Butterworth tonight." The next day my brother and sister -in- law called and said, "You need to come right now", and my brother said, "it's cancer."

And when you hear the word cancer your whole world stops, whether it's you or a family member. So I jumped on the next plane and made it to the hospital. She had already had a bone marrow biopsy and they confirmed the plasma cell leukemia. Our family spent the entire week together digesting, researching, talking to Dr. Singh.

It was Dr. Singh who had done the blood work and said this doesn't make sense. This woman's symptoms and diagnosis so far doesn't make sense, and he ordered the test. The other doctors said if she would have gone untreated she would have had two months, so we wouldn't have known, we wouldn't have known, she would have passed away, and we wouldn't have had the time with her that we have had.

The heart diagnosis didn't make sense, the decline didn't make sense, the quick decline and her feeling so tired and the lack of energy. Maybe ok, its just a heart problem, and that's it, and we leave it and we don't do anything else. Dr.Singh wasn't satisfied with that, and he ordered more tests, and that's how we found the cancer.

I think it's his instinct, his ability to connect with his patients as people and take in the whole picture rather than just the lab results, and the number on the paper. I think it's his ability to say it doesn't make sense because of her life style, who she is, her personality, her communication when she comes in. The lab work confirms all the heart issues, but there's something else. I call him the investigator.

This year, again when you hear the word cancer, your life stops, everyone's life stops. The daily living and all the silly things, they don't matter anymore, only the important things matter. We didn't make it for Christmas day, so this day, two days later was our Christmas, and I don't think anyone knew the difference. We spent yesterday, the whole day giving each other very memorable gifts, and laughing, and joking, and taking pictures, and me and my brother wrestling like we always have, even though we're full grown adults, sort of.

We spent the whole evening looking at pictures, and talking about memories, and making new memories, and watching the three little cousins run around and make snow forts. Those memories, it doesn't matter what was under the tree, all those memories we wouldn't have had. And when you realize that you have the time to make them, that you get the opportunity, you say this is plasma cell leukemia, there is no cure, so let's give you as much time as you can, thats what you do. You spend that time making as much of it as you can.

If we didn't have Dr. Singh investigate, if he had stopped at the heart failure, and said we're going to do the best we can, no one would have known about the cancer, and it would have given her two months. She wouldn't be here, we wouldn't have had this time. We wouldn't have these memories."

Jenny--Dr. Singh is Dr. House with a good personality

"I thought that was very fitting. He is Dr. House with a good personality. I came home the first time and I wasn't able to see Dr. Singh because it was a quick trip and we went back to the house. I had not physically met him because I was far away. He shook my hand, talked to my mother, who was not doing well at all. He asked her questions, asked me questions. Took my cell number, texted me, introduced me to the doctors. He told me what was happening, looked at her records, made sure that his patient, made sure everyone there knew that she was his patient. He was the general doctor and filled everyone in, made calls, coordinated her care. throughout the entire week was in contact with me every day.

He came in and drew pictures. Dr. Singh loves to draw pictures. Drew pictures of what systems were at work, how the medication would work, how it enters the body, how it's different from other medications, what works, why she's sensitive to some and not others. He becomes part of your family, you become part of his family. He took an interest in me being out of town, making sure I'm okay, would I meet with some of his other patient's families who had agreed to meet with other patient families?

He's a coordinator of care for everybody on every level, and thank God that we had him. Thank God we had him to make the diagnosis. When the first two rounds of chemo were so hard, and so devastating to her, he was saying its' okay, it's going to be okay, this is just the rough part, its' going to be okay. It was. After the first two rounds she started getting better. She's had eight rounds now, she's up and walking around.

We had a beautiful Christmas. She's up in the kitchen working, doing things and making food, and having her entire overwhelming family at her house. She's here, and she had Christmas with her grandchildren. Christmas with her children, and it was a very touching, loving, heartfelt Christmas. I don't think anybody is taking one minute for granted right now. If he had stopped at the heart, she wouldn't be here. If he had stopped at the heart, we wouldn't have had Christmas.s

He just doesn't stop, he just doesn't stop investigating. With every symptom, with every side effect, with every pneumonia, every reaction with a drug, every new lab work that comes back, he looks at it like it's brand new information, not just par for the course treatment. What is different for you and your body, what do you specifically need? That's what he looks at. One of the women that I met through him, one of his patients that had agreed to meet with me, help me, called him Dr. House with a good personality, and I thought that was very fitting."

Jenny--Dr. Singh's heart is for people first, medicine second

"He's an amazing person. He's a people person. His heart is for people first, medicine second because that's what he does. That's his family's heart.

So we're a thousand miles away, and I have this experience with this wonderful doctor that is taking such good care of my mother. And I have a family where I live now that is not my blood family, but they are just as important to me. They're supportive and loving and, what can we do? And I tell them this story about Dr. Singh, and I come home and this is what happened, and this is what the doctor did, and he's texting me and explaining things. People can't understand that level of caring and involvement from a doctor.

My daughter, one of my children has had tremors. She has been tested by several doctors, wonderful doctors. She's been to several neurologists, and had MRIs and scans, and there's no conclusive diagnosis. The problem seems to be that we go to one specialist, and they look at a certain result, and we go to other specialists, and its hard to coordinate all the symptoms together.

Knowing Dr. Singh now as well as I do. I decided I would want to send him my daughters information, I would love for him to look at it and see what he thinks. Right away he asked a bunch of questions, asked for every single paper from her birth on, and she's 21 now. He wants to know everything that she's been tested for. He knows I'm a thousand miles away, he says we're going to Facetime, Skype the appointments. He's already discussed a few tests, a few specialists. I'm relieved. I'm relieved to say that okay, whatever this is, it's going to be okay. I have trust now, I have faith that my daughter is in good hands. We have someone who is going to say, " We're going to figure this out, we'll do whatever it takes." So we're starting that process now because of what my mother went through and her trust in him.

I'm just thinking of one of the things he did in the hospital that first night. The first night I met him, when he came in late at night again, on his own time. He knew one of the nurses, and he introduced us as well. He was chatting with her. My mother was having one of her worst nights. He talked to the nurse, and said, " Do you know this about Leah? Do you know what her last name means?" He talked about her more as a person than just a medical number. I saw the nurse connect more with my mother, more than just look at her lab work, her results, and the numbers on the machines.

That's what he does, and now he's a part of our family, and he'll connect to my daughter that way.

I don't know when the man sleeps, I don't know if he sleeps. I have asked him, "Do you sleep?" He assures me he does. I had the privilege of meeting his wife as well. I couldn't say enough about them as people. People first, medical professional, yes, but as people first. They came in on Sunday on their own time, because they knew I was only going to be in town for so long, they went over everything, looked at the medications. They asked me how I was doing? they offered to help me in any way, knowing i was from out of town and staying in a hospital bed next to my mother. Is there anything we can do for you? Phenomenal people."

Barb--This is not cookie cutter medicine

"What makes Dr. Singh unique is that he takes the time to show you, not only just on the internet or something, but in a drawing to explain to you what is going on inside of your body. You're not a cookie cutter with him, he doesn't lump you with the masses. My symptoms don't equal a disease necessarily, that is normally diagnosed in others by other doctors. Dr.Singh takes the time to get to know who you are as a person, what your life experience has been, and he diagnosis you with that information. With that and his knowledge paired together, it's an amazing experience. "

Barb--Vital Checklist described by a real patient

"When looking for a doctor, you can't research good bedside manners in doctors. So when I ran into Dr. SIngh and I learned he had developed Vital Checklist, it speaks to him as a doctor. the fact that he wants to reach people, more than who he can just physically come in contact with. He developed this program the blew my mind, and that helps us become our own patient advocate. Dr, Singh is on the leading edge of helping us, the patients, better understand our own body's . It's not like other sites where you plug in your symptoms and it pops up a diagnosis of what you think you might have. This is deeper, deeper and more personal. This is specifically for you. It's like he takes your DNA and discovers what is going on inside your body. It's amazing.

Val's Belief-- Consulting for Diabetes and Dementia

We're going to continue with Dr. Singh because we're really happy. What I like most about Dr. Singh is his two fold background in both diabetes and dementia. This is a really tough combination to treat, and to have someone who is really knowledgeable in both directions is just really great for us. I like that when he runs into a stumbling block he recommends that we see the nerve doctor, he sets up an appointment for us, because the nerves in Tom's legs are totally shot.

Secondly, because the dementia has never been totally diagnosed, a written diagnosis, Dr. Singh isn't just interested in Tom and I, he's interested in the entire family. He wants to know that I have care and support in giving care to Tom. So he actually wrote down his cell phone number and asked my daughter, who lives out of state, to call him. They would talk about what we're doing with Tom, and his care, just so someone else in the family feels comfortable with what we are doing with Tom. I think this is extraordinary. To have his home phone number and to feel comfortable to call at any time."

Val (wife of patient)-- Husband has Diabetes and early onset Alzheimer's

"My husband is diabetic and has been for almost forty years. He also has early onset Alzeimer's We have a new problem now. He keeps falling. His balance has gone from decent to not good at all. So we came into the doctor to see about the balance issue and what might be causing it. Right away Dr. Singh had Tom stand up and hold his arms out, and did some manipulations. Tom sat down and Dr. Singh nailed the problem. He found why Tom was having balance issues. Then, what I really like about Dr. Singh that makes me feel comfortable, is that he gets out his pen and his paper, and he explains things in layman's terms, so that I can understand what is happening with Tom. So we'd only been there maybe ten minutes, and I really felt comfortable with Dr. Singh."

Kathy-- How Dr. Singh saved my big toe

"I had a cyst on my big toe. It was right above my big toenail on my big toe. I went to a doctor and had it removed, but they didn't get it all, so they had to go back in and do another surgery. But this was a process of about four or five weeks.

Long story short is my toe got infected and I couldn't get ahold of the doctor that had done the surgery. So because I had this relationship with Dr. Singh, always taking care of me, I called up and I said, "my toe looks like Rudolph." It was hurting and I was crying. It was excruciating pain, it was infected. Immediately he gave me a shot for the pain, and to try and help calm me down. He calmed me down, and right there in his office, he takes his phone out, and calls one of his friends in Grand Rapids that was a specialist. He got me in the very next day. They lanced my toe. I honestly think I would have lost my toe.

I am just so grateful for that. he's the kind of guy that, if you have an emergency, or a problem, (yes I could have gone to the emergency room but instead I called him and came right in), you don't feel like just a number. You're a patient."

Kathy--talks about Dr. Singh from a patient's perspective

"Would I refer Dr. Singh? Absolutely I would refer Dr. Singh. I have referred him because he is very different. He cares about people, he will keep looking until he finds what the answer is. I actually had an employee who had been going to a doctor for about month, and had been off work sick and they couldn't find out what was wrong with him. I told him, "you just need to see my doctor, because he'll find out what's wrong with you." He just keeps going and keeps going until he finds out what it is, and he keeps in contact with you. He reassures you that you're going to be okay, and that we're going to figure out what's going on."

Kathy-- Dr. Singh is really there to help

"I had never had a doctor like him before. I have had a lot of good doctors, but my doctors help me when I call and make an appointment, and go in. They don't follow up, or the nurse follows up, or you call and get a nurse, and then maybe you get the doctor to sign off on something. It's like Dr. Singh does everything himself. hes the one that calls me to say, "How are you feeling? How is your blood pressure this month? Hows your toe?" He is the one, he makes you feel like he cares about you. I believe he truly does care about you. It's just a whole different relationship than I've ever had with a doctor before."

Manmonhan-medically impressed with Dr. Singh's personal approach

"The first time I talked to him I knew that he is really a doctor that understands patients, and ready to discuss more rather than just having a superficial discussion. He went really in depth and explained to me so that I can better manage my own health. The best thing about him is that he has a personalized approach. He will sit with you and talk with you as a friend and as a doctor. Especially with someone like me, who goes on the internet to look up everything and then goes to see a doctor. When I went to him and presented my point of view, he was very perceptive of my points, which I haven't found in many doctors."

Gail and Jim-- a friends recommendation of Dr. Singh

"The first time I met Dr. Singh, was after a variety of conversations with a couple of people. One of the nurses in the office, I was looking for friends to find a doctor, an internist, and I attended that appointment, but stayed in the waiting room. They were in there for three hours with Dr. Singh. (Gail)

We want to say that we couldn't believe that a doctor in this day and age would sit and explain and talk to you in terms of wanting to be on the team with you to help discover what was necessary to treat my wife. (Jim)

By the time they came back out, it was very evident they were very pleased with the examination that he had provided, the information he provided. They were just in awe of what was about to take place after that visit. (Gail)

I found him to be just remarkable. We never experienced anything like that with any of our doctors, in the seventy years we've been going to the doctors. (Jim)

Took the time to explain to them what the real issues were that she was dealing with. Had an outline of where they were going to go from there. (Gail)

HIs thorough knowledge, and on top of that describing with pictures that you would draw on paper. He was very knowledgeable, wants to make sure all the tests he was recommending would start to lead us to the causes, and how we can take care of the problems that my wife was facing. (Jim)"

Jim--a real patient's experience

"And he says, "We will find the answers". After that appointment my wife started taking all the required test that he requested. I set up an appointment with him, and went back about two weeks later. He was so thorough, it was remarkable. When I didn't understand, he tried to explain to me in layman's language what I was experiencing, what he thought I was experiencing. He invited me and my wife to have dinner with him and his wife. He would talk about diabetes and what problems that could lead to. Again, another understanding of what was going on and why we needed to be concerned. Looking at all the acronyms he uses, how he identifies every symptom that we may have by the letters. My wife and I were very very impressed. Since then we have been back for appointments and test results, and movement on all of the different tests, and results, and more tests, and more results, so that he starts to zero in closer and closer, to what is a possibility of maybe not a complete cure, but a way of extending my wife's medical treatment. He advises us and whatever he has done is remarkable... He helped her not have to use a walker, less time with oxygen. We're just really thankful so far for what we have found with him, and we highly recommend him to all of our friends."

Jim--understanding labels for better nutrition

"With Dr, Singh, I found as a person is a real likable guy. Enjoyable, funny, yet real understanding. Hes interested in what we do for a living, interested in our family make up. He shares with us with his family and their makeup. Of course him coming here just nine years ago with just a little money in his pocket, hes where he is today because hes success driven, and he's so thankful for where he is today and what's in America. One of the things out of all of this that has stuck with me is, I go through the supermarket to buy different food for the home; I look at the labels. I never looked at labels before. I didn't pay any attention to what it said. It didn't make any difference what it said, if it

tasted good, I loved it, and if it didn't taste good, like spinach, I didn't eat it. Now my appreciation, and I look at everything I buy now, its the three S's. The sugars, the saturated fats, and the sodium. Those three are looking at whether it's 5%, 10% or 15%, but no more than 20. Almost everything I buy now, if it doesn't fall within those guidelines, it's left on the shelf. I have to say, I understand what he's saying, it has made a difference, I am losing weight. I am watching my wife's and I can see the difference. What we're eating daily has helped her continually lose weight. He's just a fun guy, I like him."

Nancy--a daughter of a patient shares her experience

"I first met Dr. Singh in January 2013 when I took my mother to see him after she had had some health issues. I was very impressed with his gentleness. When I explained that she was hard of hearing, he was very good at making sure she understood the questions. We followed up with Dr. SIngh, and he ordered some tests. She really liked Dr. Singh also. I highly recommend Dr. Singh as a primary physician because of his knowledge, his caring, his concern, and his ability to communicate with patients and the family."

Nancy--wife of a patient

"Dr. Singh saw my husband for a pre-op consult and I was in the room with him. Dr. Singh looked at his lab work and decided it wasnt quite right, and wanted to do more blood tests. He was drawing pictures for my husband trying to help him understand, and tell him exactly what he was concerned about. Then Dr. Singh went on the to try and understand the medications another doctor had put my husband on. We didn't know the answer. He went on the computer, read back on all the specialist notes, and finally told us that because my husband had very low blood pressure, he had to take the medicine twice a day instead of once a day, so that his blood pressure didn't fall or he didn't lose consciousness. I highly recommend as a primary care physician because of his knowledge , his caring, his concern, and his ability to communicate with patients and their family."

Nancy-- sharing her experience as a co-worker

"Dr. Singh is very unique. He has a wide range of knowledge with medical conditions, such as diabetes. Patients have noticed and commented on how knowledgeable he is. He has a very gentle manner about him. He is very kind. He is not a harsh person, he is very easy to understand. He likes to draw pictures so that patients have a good understanding of what he is trying to communicate to them about their medical condition."

Char--appreciating Dr. Singh for taking care of her father

"Dr. Singh came in, introduced himself. Right away he realized that my father was Irish because he has a trigger finger. He sat and looked through some of his records I had brought from New Mexico. He discussed everything and did a physical on my father, and discovered a lot of things off of the reports that they weren't even handling in New Mexico. We ended up staying for the first visit an hour and a half, and learned more in that time than I did in a month and half of visits in New Mexico.

I was amazed, I didn't realize that there were still doctors out there that would give you time like that, and put a schedule off just so when you left you were confident about where you were going from there. Dr. Singh is unique because hes a doctor that cares about the family and the patient. I am my father's daughter and he wants to make sure that I am fully knowledgeable about everything that is going on with my father. He goes through it step by step.

Dr. Singh is actually attacking the dementia from a lack of blood going to his brain, from problems with his heart, his medications and all the other areas. His cholesterol was out of balance, and he's attacking the cholesterol, and just trying to patch him up and come from all directions to handle the dementia.

I would recommend Dr. Singh to anyone. He's phenomenal. He cares about the patients, he care about explaining everything. He's not worried about his schedule running late. The second appointment we had to wait 45 min, and it was well worth the wait, because I knew exactly what those patients were getting. The same thing he gave me and my father. Hes amazing. I never in my entire life have ever seen a doctor put so much forth for a patient with his explanations.

My dad is very comfortable with Dr. SIngh. They joke with each other, with the Irish and everything else. My dad wanted to know what nationality he was, and so they joke about that. He puts my dad at ease when he's in the room with him. My father's not tense and he listens to Dr. Singh. When he tells my dad not to do something, my dad actually remembers not to do it. He has a very good report with Dr. Singh."

Char--as a caregiver

"He's just an all-around positive physician. The concern, the care for his patients, even the delay in his schedule. I get the feeling that he actually cares for each and every individual that enters his office. He wants to do the best that he can with each and every one of them. This is the one physician, and I'm 57 years old and have had plenty of physicians and doctors in my life, and this is one that he just stands out above all the rest. It's not like passing through an assembly line, he takes his time with each and every patient, until they're thoroughly content, walking out of there very knowledgable.

He's all about helping the patient and putting their minds at ease that there is a brighter side to the illnesses, and we're going to attack it from every different way. When you leave there you just have confidence that this is a doctor that is going to follow through and take care of it all the way.

He drew several pictures. When he read the report from New Mexico, from the cardiologist, there's actually a part of my father's heart that is working backwards, he drew me a picture what aprt is working and how, and how its diminishing the blood flow to my father's brain, which is adding to the dementia. I still have those pictures.

By showing me with the pictures I fully understood what he was saying. a lot of the time I think I kind of understood but not fully. With the picture I grasped the whole idea of what he was telling me. I know exactly what is going on with my father now. When I was in New Mexico, they didn't have the dementia meds, I felt like they had given up because he was 81 and they didn't want to battle anything to make it easier for my fathers life. That upset me.

I didn't realize how upset I was until I met Dr. Singh. He opened my eyes up to a lot of things. I learned more than I did in a month and a half in New Mexico. We met with his primary care physician down there five times, there was surgeon that removed a tumor, that recognized the dementia. There was his cardiologist that knew about the reverse effect in his heart had put it into the chart, but never took any steps to rectify the problem.

I came here and see how Dr. Singh is attacking and going with different tests and specialist, I realize these are things that benefit my father. I just thank God I was lucky enough to find him. My dad's demeanor and personality is much calmer. We laugh together and we are making happy memories together instead of all the angry ones. That means a lot to me.

I feel better because I feel I am getting him adequate care, and I found it all in one doctor, and thats Dr. Singh."

Char--learning perspective on dementia

"I went into this blindsided, because I don't know anything about dementia. I have never been around anyone with dementia, and I have kinda had to learn on my own in the daily process of staying with my dad. Dr. Singh let me know what's going to happen, what we're going to try and do to halt this. I have a little more confidence in myself to be able to get along with my father and handle the situations that come up with him because of Dr. Singh. It makes my days a lot more pleasant, it really does.

I can't speak highly enough of him, I really can't. What he gives to his patients words can't describe. You can sit there and try and say what you want about Dr. Singh and its still not as much as it should be. There are special people that come along, and I think Dr. Singh is one of those special doctors. Words cant describes it.

The pictures that I got to bring home, what was nice was that when my step sister came down, I was able to show her the pictures and explain it just life Dr. Singh did, so she understood it also. Instead of just trying to relate you know, all the doctor words and that. The pictures make it so much easier, it's like teaching kindergarten. He's not the greatest artist, but good enough that I understood."

Ed and Bev--a couple share their story about Dr. Singh

"He just seems to be so interested in what's going on and wants to get to the bottom of things. He wants to make sure that he gets answers. I I usually go into doctors visits with Ed so that i can hear what's going on, and we can both can get an idea whats taking place. Sometimes he hears differently than what i hear, and so then we can put it together and maybe get an answer. (Bev)

Dr. Singh is so thorough when he investigates what your problem is. He really takes his time and asks you the proper questions to get a good diagnosis. He is so patient with us, and takes his time with us, that we are really enjoying having him as our family doctor. (Ed)

His patients and thoroughness, because not every doctor will take the time to let you know how he feels, and to let you know what you might be facing or what he can do to help. He really has an interest in his patients. (Bev)

When the office girl asked us if we wanted to switch over, she said, "we are having such good results with him." (Ed)

The girls in the front office realize how much time he takes with his patience, of course that kind of throws them off a little bit, but they know I'm sure how good he is. (Bev)"

Ed-- why I come back to Dr. Singh

"I wasn't feeling well and I wasn't able to meet with my regular doctor.. The technician suggested I see Dr. Singh and the first visit was a terrific success. So from that point on I have been seeing him on a regular basis.

My impression was so good because of the time he took and the uninterrupted question and answer about my condition. Dr. Singh is so careful to diagnose the problem and ask you the question that are pertinent to the case, gives you his undivided attention. We are pleased to recommend him to anyone who needs assistance."

Dr. Sweta Kochar--how to pass step 2 CS exam on the first attempt

"I did my step 2 CS class three years ago when I came to the US. It was an excellent experience, especially Dr. Singh. he was very helpful, very informative, and he worked on a very personal base level. He worked on my shortcomings, my weakness, at the same time appreciating my strengths, and giving steps to improve them further.

I passed my step 2 CS on the first attempt. After the exam, he helped me to do a good SOAP Note for example, which helped me in my clinical electives at the University of Michigan. It also helped me throughout my residency.

Step 2 CS is is just a beginning, just a planning for the future now, because it helps you perfect your technique, the skills you will actually be using the real world, especially during a residency. Using those skills helps you to do your job, helps you have good patient satisfaction scores, have good timing. Working your cases, working with your patients, at the same time giving them happiness."

Dr. Sweta Kochar--How step 2 CS exam helps with residency

"Step 2 CS not only helps you clinically, but also Dr. Singh has been very helpful with all my questions. I learned good patient skills, but at the same time you deal with different challenges during residency. Those weren't very hard because I had someone to help during residency. Dr. Singh has been the person, has been an excellent mentor.

Vital Checklist is not only essential for passing Step 2 CS, it is essential for being a good, humane doctor, so that you can perfect your techniques, and have a good residency.

For example, in the Step 2 CS Exam, you have to do a patient encounter in 15 minutes. In residency you feel that it is not possible to do that when you have more complicated patients, and not a perfect scenario.

Dr. Singh creates a good scenario which made me feel comfortable in a busy ER, even mid shift. WIth a bunch of admissions in your hand, you can get a good history and physical exam without missing essential points, and at the same time having good time management. You can get a good history and physical exam in 15 minutes."

Dr. Sweta Kochar--Step 2 CS Exam helps with interviews

"After my course in Vital Checklist, Dr. Singh has always been in touch, and always been available for my concerns and questions, and guiding me through the interview process.

The interview process, he helped me with the matching list, he helped me know what to look for in a program. That has helped me a lot because the program I am at right now has an excellent patient encounter exposure. The people there are excellent, and the work environment is so good that I don't feel stress from working there.

After going through the interview process and getting matched with my residency program he has still been in touch. for example, I'm in my third year of residency currently, so I called him and asked him how should I start? And he says, "Send me your CV and I will send it to the CEOs of the main, big, hospitals that are really good," in the area I was looking at. Then they called me. They were very happy to have a connection with someone who can talk about me. He reviewed my CV so that I cross my T's, dot my I's. It makes a good meeting in an organized manner.

He has been very accessible, very approachable, like my own brother. He has been very helpful."

Dr. Sweta Kochar--Step 2 CS training provides skills for patient care

"Another important thing I learned from Vital Checklist and Dr. Singh is how important it is to explain to patients in their own ways and their own language. I am always getting comments and appreciation on that particular skill. He helped me be able to use diagrams and mnemonics. Especially, for example, Heart Failure patients, who are frequent fliers with readmission problems, and hospitals aren't emphasizing so much on.

After my cardiology rotations, my attendant put in my evaluation that I have been very thorough in getting my patient's morning weights every day, because I would push in a cal, bring in the weighing machine, and tell them how to weigh so that everyday make sure they learn, and make sure they get the habit, and can follow it at home.

Making drawings and pictures. I use the boards in the room to explain to the patients what is going on. A couple of the patients said that I was the first one to explain to them what is going on. All these qualities i got from Dr. Singh, and I thank him for that."

Amit Javed--Step 2 CS Coaching

"I'm Amit Javed. I am an international medical graduate from New Delhi India. I have been preparing for the USME exams to pursue a residency in America. There are a lot of challenges that an international graduate faces.

The most important of all is the anxiety about an exam for which you've never been trained. It's coming to a country just only for a day. You are totally unaware of the culture, the customs, the problems these people have. You are coming into unknown territory to take an exam.

Most of us have a lot of anxiety about this exam. A lot of the anxiety comes from not knowing how the exam is going to be. Will you be able to understand your American patients, their accent, their concerns, their issues, because we are trained in a different environment.

So when we are looking for a training course, we are looking for a course that understands our concerns, that understands our culture.

Dr. Singh's Vital Checklist is a unique program that is aimed to help international graduates like myself. The program is designed in such a way that it gives you an insight into American culture, their problems, issues, and concerns. Dr. Singh teaches three to five students at a time, and the biggest advantage is you get one- to-one teaching from him. He's an excellent teacher and amazing and very challenging.

Mrs. Singh is an amazing SP, I would say she is even better than Dr. Harpreet Singh. If you can face Dr. Singh and Mrs. Singh then I would say you could face even the most challenging SPs on your examination.

Dr. Singh not only trains you for this examination, but trains you for life as a resident. I strongly recommend Vital Checklist for any international graduate who wants to come to the US for training program or residency. The most vital thing is being here, I felt at home away from home."

Cases: Table of Content

A. Central Nervous System

1. Headaches - Unilateral headache
2. Headaches - Bilateral headache
3. Muscle weakness
4. Gait abnormality
5. Dizziness
6. Loss of Consciousness
7. Numbness or tingling
8. Tremors
9. Seizures
10. Loss of vision
11. Memory loss
12. Confusion
13. Hearing Loss

B. Cardiovascular System

14. Chest Pain/ Pressure
15. Palpitation
16. Shortness of Breath
17. Light-headedness
18. Hypertension Medication Refills

C. Respiratory System

19. Cough
20. Shortness of breath
21. Chest pain
22. Phlegm
23. Sore throat
24. Snoring

D. Gastrointestinal System

25. Abdominal Pain - Right Upper Quadrant
26. Abdominal Pain - Right Lower Quadrant (Female)
27. Abdominal Pain - Epigastric
28. Abdominal Pain- Left lower quadrant
29. Dysphagia
30. Weight loss
31. Vomiting
32. Diarrhea
33. Jaundice
34. Bloody Vomiting
35. Bloody stools

36. Fatigue with Pallor

E. Endocrine System

37. Polyuria
38. Diabetic medication refills
39. Fatigue
40. Weight Gain
41. Neck mass

F. Musculoskeletal System

42. Knee pain
43. Ankle pain
44. Elbow pain
45. Shoulder pain
46. Back Pain
47. Trauma patient
48. Fatigue

G. Urology and Reproductive system

49. Bloody urine
50. Burning urination
51. Incontinence
52. Lower Abdominal Pain
53. Pregnancy
54. Unable to conceive
55. Erectile Dysfunction
56. Amenorrhea
57. Vaginal Bleeding
58. Pain during sex
H. Psychiatry
59. Depressed mood
60. Hallucination
61. Anxiety
62. ADHD
63. Insomnia
64. Abuse- Young
65. Abuse- Old

I- Pediatric case

66. Dehydration

67. Seizure
68. Bedwetting
69. Wheezing/ Difficulty breathing
70. Fever
71. Behavioral Problems

J- Others

72. Pre- employment Checkup
73. Pre- surgical clearance
74. Telephone case
75. Fever

Section O
Authors

Section O – Authors

Associate Authors

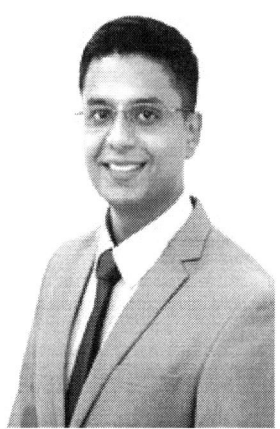

Dr.Himanshu Deshwal
PGY-1

Dr. Himanshu Deshwal is a currently resident physician in Internal Medicine at Cleveland Clinic Foundation Program, Ohio. A graduate of Armed Forces Medical College, Pune. Dr. Deshwal has been an enthusiastic young doctor who strongly believes in patient experience and empathy. He has a keen interest in the academic field of medicine and is always on the lookout to improve clinical practice, knowledge, and communication with the patients. He has helped medical students and colleagues to develop communication and clinical skills is beyond commendation and has played a vital role in "Road to USMLE Step 2CS". He has a unique ability to draw pictures and metaphors to make patient education easier and actively took part in community seminars. He has illustrated over 200 illustrations for Vital Checklist™, (iCrush)?™ and Arts Plus Medicine™. He has co-authored many books with Dr.Singh and has to lead many teams. He loves taking part in competitive sports and athletics, and now he wants to help his patients in improving their health and wellness.

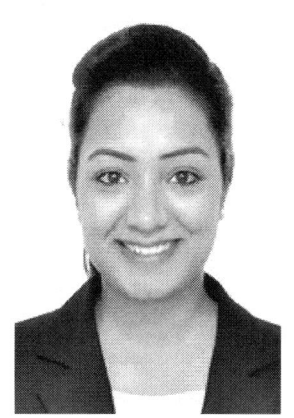

Dr. Avantika Singh
PGY-1

Dr. Avantika Singh is currently a resident physician in Pediatrics at the Children's Hospital of Wisconsin, Medical College of Wisconsin, Milwaukee. She is an alumna of Vardhman Mahavir Medical College and Safdarjung Hospital, New Delhi, India. After completing medical school, she pursued a Post-Doctoral Clinical Research Fellowship at Harvard Medical School in neonatal neurology, where she worked at Boston Children's Hospital, Brigham and Women's Hospital, Mass General Hospital and Tufts Medical Center. She is passionate about innovation in teaching and has held several leadership positions throughout her career. She loves fusion cooking and graphic designing in her spare time.

Dr. Ankur Sinha is currently a resident physician in Internal Medicine at Maimonides Medical Center, Albert Einstein College of Medicine, New York. He is an alumni of Armed Forces Medical College, India and trained at the Royal Liverpool Children's Hospital, Liverpool, UK. He is passionate about scholastic as well as clinical medicine and actively takes part in teaching and research activities. Further information about Dr. Sinha can be accessed at www.drsinhamd.com

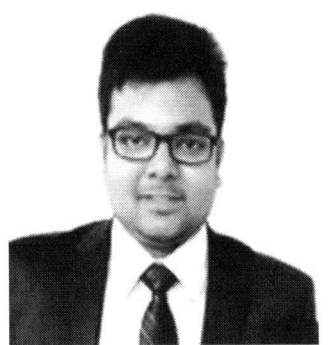

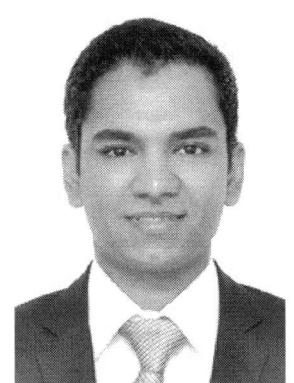

Dr.Ankur Sinha
PGY-2

Dr. Krishna Adit Agarwal is currently a resident physician in Massachusetts. He is an alumni of Vardhman Mahavir Medical College & Safdarjung Hospital, India and has trained at Harvard Medical School. He has been an innovator, leader, and mentor for many. Besides pioneering MEDSICON™ and I-MediSTAR™, he is also the author of leading books, 'Road to USMLE™' and 'Review of Surgery for Students'. Dr. Agarwal takes immense interest in guiding medical students in their chosen career paths and in taking new student-led projects to fruition. You can get in touch with him at www.DrAgarwalMD.com

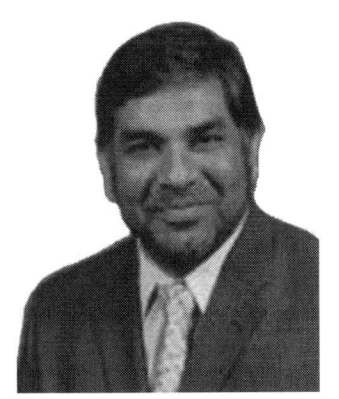

Dr. Krishna Agarwal
PGY-1

Dr. John R. Lobo is a Urologist in an independent practice in Grand Rapids, MI. He completed his undergraduate education at Brooklyn College, Brooklyn NY, with a B.S. in Chemistry. He attended the State University of New York Downstate Medical Center where he received his M.D. in 1999. He completed an Internship in General Surgery and Residency in Urology at Mayo Clinic in Rochester, MN in 2005. His practice interests include most aspects of general urology, including urologic cancers, voiding dysfunction, and urinary stone disease. Dr. Lobo has contributed to the Urology Section.

Dr. John Lobo
Consultant Urologist

About Harpreet Singh MD, FACP

Chief Medical Author

Dr. Harpreet Singh is a renowned medical doctor, co-host of Talk Medicine radio show on WBRN, medical author, speaker, founder of Vital Checklist and iCrush.org. He started his American Dream on September 23, 2003, with 54 dollars and an M.B.B.S degree from KMC, Manipal, India. After completing his residency from Spectrum Health and Mercy Health in Grand Rapids, he worked as a hospitalist with HOWM and IPCM. He worked as a medical director and hospitalist with ECI Healthcare, and Hospital Physician Partners. He now practices as an internist in Grand Rapids and Big Rapids area where he has helped thousands of patients. His patients call him Dr. House with a good personality, investigator, detective, and a doctor with excellent bedside manner. One of his peers has referred to him as the William Osler of 21st century. Seeing his love for patient care and patient experience, he was appointed as Chief Experience Officer of Michigan Primary Care Partners. When he is not seeing patients, he is teaching communication and clinical skills to medical students, physician assistants and nurse practitioners via his live workshops. He trains medical students via Clinical and Communication skills workshops and webinars.

Dr. Singh has started iCrush.org where he posts his patient education videos, and his mission is to flip healthcare. He wants to build (iCrush) as a movement, a lifestyle Institute, health, and wellness program where a layperson gets benefits. He organized his first (iCrush)5k event in Big Rapids to educate people about diabetes. The second (iCrush)5k was for multiple sclerosis awareness, and this benefitted his young patient who suffers from MS. Under this umbrella, he conducts workplace healing, health, wellness, and disease prevention workshops to reduce medical costs, absenteeism, presenteeism, decreases musculoskeletal injuries thus improving return on investment (R.O.I) and return on emotions (R.O.E.). Many attendees have praised him for his Scan and Spot Weight Loss Seminar.

Dr. Singh explains patients' their disease process with the help of pictures and therefore he is called an "Artist Doctor." We already know the importance of art in medicine. However, he wants to take arts to the next level by starting online portal--www.artsplusmedicine.com.

Dr. Singh is a voracious reader and loves reading medical books and business books. He loves developing the mnemonics, checklists, and art for easy understandability and memory. His loves playing racquetball and is addicted to hot yoga. For relaxation, he meditates and prays. Presently, he is teaching chemistry to his fifth grader and learning Spanish from his kindergartner who just started Spanish immersion school.

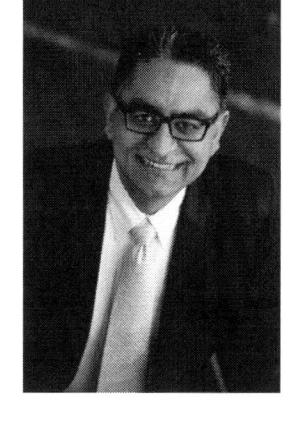

Books and Touchpoints by Dr. Harpreet Singh Coming soon in 2017 and 2018

Road to Patient Experience
How to lose a patient and win a friend?
How to be a B.A.D patient? B.A.D. means By Asking Doctors more questions
(iCrush) Ebola
(iCrush) Diabetes
(iCrush) Multiple Sclerosis
(iCrush) Tobacco and Smoking
Scan and Spot Nutrition Facts Workbook
Lucky Touch: Connecting empathy with patient experience
Vital Checklist Communication Workbook for patients
Vital Checklist Communication Apps
Scan and Spot Nutrition Facts Tablemat
iHandoffs for Nurse Communication
Communication Box
(iCrush) T-shirts
By the way, doctor! Flash Card